Skin and Soft Tissue Infections

Editor

HENRY F. CHAMBERS

INFECTIOUS DISEASE CLINICS OF NORTH AMERICA

www.id.theclinics.com

Consulting Editor
HELEN W. BOUCHER

March 2021 • Volume 35 • Number 1

ELSEVIER

1600 John F. Kennedy Boulevard • Suite 1800 • Philadelphia, Pennsylvania, 19103-2899.

http://www.theclinics.com

INFECTIOUS DISEASE CLINICS OF NORTH AMERICA Volume 35, Number 1
March 2021 ISSN 0891–5520, ISBN-13: 978-0-323-79138-0

Editor: Kerry Holland
Developmental Editor: Donald Mumford

Infectious Disease Clinics of North America (ISSN 0891–5520) is published in March, June, September, and December by Elsevier Inc., 360 Park Avenue South, New York, NY 10010-1710. Periodicals postage paid at New York, NY and additional mailing offices. Subscription prices are $347.00 per year for US individuals, $922.00 per year for US institutions, $100.00 per year for US students, $396.00 per year for Canadian individuals, $973.00 per year for Canadian institutions, $432.00 per year for international individuals, $973.00 per year for international institutions, $100.00 per year for Canadian students, and $200.00 per year for international students. To receive student rate, orders must be accompanied by name of affiliated institution, date of term, and the *signature* of program/residency coordinator on institution letterhead. Orders will be billed at individual rate until proof of status is received. Foreign air speed delivery is included in all *Clinics* subscription prices. All prices are subject to change without notice. **POSTMASTER:** Send address changes to *Infectious Disease Clinics of North America,* Elsevier Health Sciences Division, Subcription Customer Service, 3251 Riverport Lane, Maryland Heights, MO 63043. **Customer Service: 1-800-654-2452 (US). From outside of the US and Canada, call 1-314-447-8871. Fax: 1-314-447-8029. E-mail: JournalsCustomerService-usa@elsevier.com (print support) or JournalsOnlineSupport-usa@elsevier.com (online support).**

Infectious Disease Clinics of North America is also published in Spanish by Editorial Inter-Médica, Junin 917, 1er A 1113, Buenos Aires, Argentina.

Reprints. For copies of 100 or more, of articles in this publication, please contact the Commercial Reprints Department, Elsevier Inc., 360 Park Avenue South, New York, New York 10010-1710. Tel. 212-633-3874, Fax: 212-633-3820, E-mail: reprints@elsevier.com.

Infectious Disease Clinics of North America is covered in *MEDLINE/PubMed (Index Medicus), Current Contents/ Clinical Medicine, Science Citation Alert, SCISEARCH,* and *Research Alert.*

Contributors

CONSULTING EDITOR

HELEN W. BOUCHER, MD, FIDSA, FACP
Director, Infectious Diseases Fellowship Program, Division of Geographic Medicine and Infectious Diseases, Tufts Medical Center, Associate Professor of Medicine, Tufts University School of Medicine, Boston, Massachusetts, USA

EDITOR

HENRY F. CHAMBERS, MD
Professor of Medicine, Emeritus, Division of HIV, Infectious Diseases and Global Medicine, Department of Medicine, Zuckerberg San Francisco General Hospital and Trauma Center, University of California, San Francisco, San Francisco, California, USA

AUTHORS

RITESH AGNIHOTHRI, MD
Complex Medical Dermatology Fellow, Department of Dermatology, University of California, San Francisco, San Francisco, California, USA

AMY E. BRYANT, PhD
Research Professor, Department of Biomedical and Pharmaceutical Sciences, College of Pharmacy, Idaho State University, Meridian, Idaho, USA

RACHEL J. BYSTRITSKY, MD
Assistant Professor, Department of Medicine, Infectious Diseases, University of California, San Francisco, San Francisco, California, USA

HENRY F. CHAMBERS, MD
Professor of Medicine, Emeritus, Division of HIV, Infectious Diseases and Global Medicine, Department of Medicine, Zuckerberg San Francisco General Hospital and Trauma Center, University of California, San Francisco, San Francisco, California, USA

SARA E. COSGROVE, MD, MS
Professor of Medicine, Division of Infectious Diseases, Department of Medicine, Johns Hopkins School of Medicine, Baltimore, Maryland, USA

CARLA CRUZ-DIAZ, MD
Complex Medical Dermatology Fellow, Department of Dermatology, University of California, San Francisco, San Francisco, California, USA

MICHAEL Z. DAVID, MD, PhD
Assistant Professor, Division of Infectious Diseases, Department of Medicine, University of Pennsylvania, Department of Epidemiology, Biostatistics and Informatics, University of Pennsylvania, Philadelphia, Pennsylvania, USA

LISA E. DAVIDSON, MD
Associate Professor, Division of Infectious Diseases, Department of Internal Medicine, Atrium Health, Charlotte, North Carolina, USA

STEPHANIE A. FRITZ, MD, MSCI
Associate Professor, Department of Pediatrics, Washington University School of Medicine, St Louis, Missouri, USA

BRIANA M. GARCIA, BS
Medical Student, University of California, San Francisco School of Medicine, San Francisco, California, USA

ELLIE JC. GOLDSTEIN, MD
Clinical Professor of Medicine, David Geffen School of Medicine at UCLA, Los Angeles, California, USA; R M Alden Research Laboratory, Santa Monica, California, USA

SARAH E. GREENE, MD, PhD
Postdoctoral Fellow, Department of Pediatrics, Washington University School of Medicine, St Louis, Missouri, USA

TIMOTHY J. HATLEN, MD
Divisions of Infectious Diseases and HIV, Harbor-UCLA Medical Center, Lundquist Institute for Biomedical Innovation at Harbor-UCLA Medical Center, Torrance, California, USA; David Geffen School of Medicine at UCLA, Los Angeles, California, USA

JEAN-FRANCOIS JABBOUR, MD, MSc
Division of Infectious Diseases, Department of Internal Medicine, American University of Beirut Medical Center, Beirut, Lebanon

SOUHA S. KANJ, MD, FACP, FIDSA, FRCP, FESCMID, FECMM
Division of Infectious Diseases, Department of Internal Medicine, American University of Beirut Medical Center, Beirut, Lebanon

LISA L. MARAGAKIS, MD, MPH
Associate Professor of Medicine, Division of Infectious Diseases, Department of Medicine, Johns Hopkins School of Medicine, Baltimore, Maryland, USA

LOREN G. MILLER, MD, MPH
Division of Infectious Diseases, Harbor-UCLA Medical Center, Lundquist Institute for Biomedical Innovation at Harbor-UCLA Medical Center, Torrance, California, USA; David Geffen School of Medicine at UCLA, Los Angeles, California, USA

CHRISTOPHER POLK, MD
Assistant Professor, Division of Infectious Diseases, Department of Internal Medicine, Atrium Health, Charlotte, North Carolina, USA

DANYA ROSHDY, PharmD
Clinical Pharmacy Specialist in Infectious Diseases, Antimicrobial Support Network, Division of Pharmacy, Atrium Health, Charlotte, North Carolina, USA

MINDY M. SAMPSON, DO
Hospital Epidemiologist, Division of Infectious Diseases, Department of Internal Medicine, Atrium Health, Charlotte, North Carolina, USA

SHIVAN SHAH, MD
Fellow, Department of Infectious Diseases, The University of Texas MD Anderson Cancer Center, Houston, Texas, USA

SIMA L. SHARARA, MD
Research Fellow, Division of Infectious Diseases, Department of Medicine, Johns Hopkins School of Medicine, Baltimore, Maryland, USA

SAMUEL SHELBURNE, MD, PhD
Professor, Department of Infectious Diseases, The University of Texas MD Anderson Cancer Center, Houston, Texas, USA

KANADE SHINKAI, MD, PhD
Professor, Department of Dermatology, University of California, San Francisco, San Francisco, California, USA

DENNIS L. STEVENS, PhD, MD
Director, Infectious Diseases Center of Biomedical Research Excellence, Veterans Affairs Medical Center, Boise, Idaho, USA

RICHARD R. WATKINS, MD, MS
Division of Infectious Diseases, Cleveland Clinic Akron General, Akron, Ohio, USA; Associate Professor of Internal Medicine, Department of Medicine, Northeast Ohio Medical University, Rootstown, Ohio, USA

Contents

> The diagnosis of a skin and soft tissue infection (SSTI) requires careful attention to a patient's history, physical examination, and diagnostic test results. We review for many bacterial, viral, fungal, and parasitic pathogens that cause SSTIs the clues for reaching a diagnosis, including reported past medical history, hobbies and behaviors, travel, insect bites, exposure to other people and to animals, environmental exposures to water, soil, or sand, as well as the anatomic site of skin lesions, their morphology on examination, and their evolution over time. Laboratory and radiographic tests are discussed that may be used to confirm a specific diagnosis.

> Cellulitis is a common infection of the skin and subcutaneous tissue caused predominantly by gram-positive organisms. Risk factors include prior episodes of cellulitis, cutaneous lesions, tinea pedis, and chronic edema. Cellulitis is a clinical diagnosis and presents with localized skin erythema, edema, warmth, and tenderness. Uncomplicated cellulitis can be managed in the outpatient setting with oral antibiotics. Imaging often is not required but can be helpful. Recurrent cellulitis is common and predisposing conditions should be assessed for and treated at the time of initial diagnosis. For patients with frequent recurrences despite management of underlying conditions, antimicrobial prophylaxis can be effective.

> Cellulitis is a common clinical diagnosis in the outpatient and inpatient setting; studies have demonstrated a surprisingly high misdiagnosis rate: nearly one-third of cases are other conditions (ie, pseudocellulitis). This high rate of misdiagnosis is thought to contribute to nearly $515 million in avoidable health care spending in the United States each year; leading to the delayed or missed diagnosis of pseudocellulitis and to delays in appropriate treatment. There is a broad differential diagnosis for pseudocellulitis, which includes inflammatory and noninflammatory conditions of the skin. Accurate diagnosis of the specific condition causing pseudocellulitis is crucial to management, which varies greatly.

Staphylococcus aureus is the most common bacteria causing purulent skin and soft tissue infections. Many disease-causing S aureus strains are methicillin resistant; thus, empiric therapy should be given to cover methicillin-resistant S aureus. Bacterial wound cultures are important for characterizing local susceptibility patterns. Definitive antibiotic therapy is warranted, although there are no compelling data demonstrating superiority of any one antibiotic over another. Antibiotic choice is predicated by the infection severity, local susceptibility patterns, and drug-related safety, tolerability, and cost. Response to therapy is expected within the first days; 5 to 7 days of therapy is typically adequate to achieve cure.

Staphylococcus aureus infections are associated with increased morbidity, mortality, hospital stay, and health care costs. S aureus colonization has been shown to increase risk for invasive and noninvasive infections. Decolonization of S aureus has been evaluated in multiple patient settings as a possible strategy to decrease the risk of S aureus transmission and infection. In this article, we review the recent literature on S aureus decolonization in surgical patients, patients with recurrent skin and soft tissue infections, critically ill patients, hospitalized non–critically ill patients, dialysis patients, and nursing home residents to inform clinical practice.

Necrotizing soft tissue infections occur after traumatic injuries, minor skin lesions, nonpenetrating injuries, natural childbirth, and in postsurgical and immunocompromised patients. Infections can be severe, rapidly progressive, and life threatening. Survivors often endure multiple surgeries and prolonged hospitalization and rehabilitation. Despite subtle nuances that may distinguish one entity from another, clinical approaches to diagnosis and treatment are highly similar. This review describes the clinical and laboratory features of necrotizing soft tissue infections and addresses recommended diagnostic and treatment modalities. It discusses the impact of delays in surgical debridement, antibiotic use, and resuscitation on mortality, and summarizes key pathogenic mechanisms.

Skin and soft tissue infections (SSTIs) frequently are encountered in clinical practice, and gram-negative bacilli (GNB) constitute an underrated portion of their etiology. The rate of GNB-causing SSTIs is increasing, especially with the rise in antimicrobial resistance. Although the diagnosis of SSTIs mostly is clinical, rapid diagnostic modalities can shorten the time to initiating proper therapy and improving outcomes. Novel antibiotics are active against GNB SSTIs and can be of great value in the management. This review provides an overview of the role of GNB in SSTIs and summarizes their epidemiology, risk factors, outcome, and clinical management.

Persons who inject drugs are at high risk for skin and soft tissue infections. Infections range from simple abscesses and uncomplicated cellulitis to life-threatening and limb-threatening infections. These infections are predominantly caused by gram-positive organisms with Staphylococcus aureus, Streptococcus pyogenes, and other streptococcal species being most common. Although antimicrobial therapy has an important role in treatment of these infections, surgical incision, drainage, and debridement of devitalized tissue are primary. Strategies that decrease the frequency of injection drug use, needle sharing, use of contaminated equipment, and other risk behaviors may be effective in preventing these infections in persons who inject drugs.

Skin and soft tissue infections are common in diabetics. Diabetic foot infection usually results from disruption of the skin barrier, trauma, pressure, or ischemic wounds. These wounds may become secondarily infected or lead to development of adjacent soft tissue or deeper bone infection. Clinical assessment and diagnosis of these conditions using a multidisciplinary management approach, including careful attention to antibiotic selection, lead to the best outcomes in patient care.

Skin and soft tissue infections among the non–human immunodeficiency virus infected immunosuppressed population are a serious and growing concern. Many pathogens can cause cutaneous infections in these patients owing to the highly varied and profound immune deficits. Although patients can be infected by typical organisms, the diversity and antimicrobial-resistant nature of the organisms causing these infections result in significant morbidity and mortality. The diagnostic approach to these infections in immunocompromised hosts can differ dramatically depending on the potential causative organisms. An understanding of new immunosuppressive treatments and evolving antimicrobial resistance patterns are required to optimally manage these difficult cases.

Animal and human bite injuries are a public health burden. Dog bites outnumber cat bites, but cat bites pose the greatest risk for infection.

Skin and soft tissue infections are the most frequent infectious manifestations resulting from bite injury, although invasive infection may occur through direct inoculation or dissemination through the bloodstream. Although contemporary, well-designed trials are needed to inform clinical practice, preemptive antibiotic therapy after a bite injury is warranted for injuries posing high risk for infection and for patients at risk of developing severe infection; antibiotics should target aerobic and anaerobic microbes that comprise the oral and skin flora.

INFECTIOUS DISEASE CLINICS OF NORTH AMERICA

Preface

Skin and Soft Tissue Infections

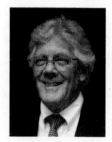

Henry F. Chambers, MD
Editor

Everyone will personally experience a skin and soft tissue infection at one time or another. Some are trivial; most are simple to manage and more of a nuisance than a health threat. Others are devastating, life and limb threatening. This issue of *Infectious Disease Clinics of North America* is devoted to the diagnosis and management of those skin and soft tissue infections that are most commonly encountered in clinical practice as well as those that present the greatest risks to health if not quickly identified and appropriately treated. The emphasis is largely on bacterial infections, although the article on how to approach the patient with a skin and soft tissue infection provides a comprehensive review of the astonishing number of potential pathogens, including fungal, parasitic, and viral causes. The article on mimics of skin and soft tissue infections is an important reminder that, as with all medical conditions, there is a differential diagnosis, and one should not overlook other diseases affecting the skin. Recurrence of infection is a problem particularly with those caused by *Staphylococcus aureus*; the article on decolonization is a comprehensive, up-to-date review of strategies and approaches for prevention and those who are most likely to benefit. The remaining articles focus on bacterial pathogens, the variety of skin and soft tissue infections they cause, the settings in which these occur, and their diagnosis and management. The

Infect Dis Clin N Am 35 (2021) xiii–xiv
https://doi.org/10.1016/j.idc.2020.12.001
0891-5520/21/© 2020 Published by Elsevier Inc.

objective of this issue is to provide a handy resource with the most current information for clinicians who are treating patients.

Henry F. Chambers, MD
Department of Medicine
University of California, San Francisco
Room 3400
Building 30 San Francisco General Hospital
1001 Potrero Avenue
San Francisco, CA 94110, USA

E-mail address:
Henry.Chambers@ucsf.edu

Approach to the Patient with a Skin and Soft Tissue Infection

Richard R. Watkins, MD, MS[a,b], Michael Z. David, MD, PhD[c,d],*

KEYWORDS

- Skin and soft tissue infection • Diagnosis • Environmental exposures
- Differential diagnosis • Laboratory testing

KEY POINTS

- The approach to a patient with a putative skin and soft tissue infection (SSTI) requires careful attention to history, physical examination, and laboratory studies to develop a narrow differential diagnosis.
- Past exposures to insects, arthropods, domesticated or wild animals, fish, salt or fresh water, beaches, soil, or spas may provide clues to the etiology of an SSTI.
- Travel itineraries often help to narrow a differential diagnosis for an SSTI.
- Behaviors such as drug use, sexual activity, hunting, fishing, hiking, swimming, gardening, or obtaining a tattoo place individuals at risk for encountering specific pathogens that cause SSTIs.
- The anatomic location of skin lesions on the body and their evolution over time may guide the choice of laboratory or radiographic tests to confirm a diagnosis of an SSTI.

INTRODUCTION

Acute skin and soft tissue infections (SSTIs) are commonly encountered in clinical practice, yet they can be challenging to diagnose and manage. SSTIs range from mild cases of cellulitis to potentially life-threatening conditions, such as necrotizing fasciitis and shock from staphylococcal scalded-skin syndrome. Infections of the skin and soft tissues may be caused by bacteria, fungi, viruses, and parasites. They may lead to significant complications, including osteomyelitis, bacteremia, endocarditis, and death. In patients younger than 65, the incidence of SSTIs between 2005 and

[a] Division of Infectious Diseases, Cleveland Clinic Akron General, 224 West Exchange Street, Akron, OH 44302, USA; [b] Department of Medicine, Northeast Ohio Medical University, Rootstown, OH, USA; [c] Division of Infectious Diseases, Department of Medicine, University of Pennsylvania, Blockley Hall 707, Philadelphia, PA 19104, USA; [d] Department of Epidemiology, Biostatistics and Informatics, University of Pennsylvania, Philadelphia, PA, USA
* Corresponding author. Division of Infectious Diseases, Department of Medicine, University of Pennsylvania, Blockley Hall 707, Philadelphia, PA 19104.
E-mail address: michdav@pennmedicine.upenn.edu
Twitter: @MichaelDavid80 (M.Z.D.)

Infect Dis Clin N Am 35 (2021) 1–48
https://doi.org/10.1016/j.idc.2020.10.011
0891-5520/21/© 2020 Elsevier Inc. All rights reserved.

2010 was approximately 4.8 per 100 person years in the United States.[1] The incidence increased dramatically in the early 2000s, largely due to the spread of community-associated methicillin-resistant *Staphylococcus aureus* (CA-MRSA) strains.[2] In a study of 12 urban emergency departments (EDs) in the United States, MRSA was the most common cause of purulent SSTIs in 2004 and 2008.[3] Recent data suggest that SSTIs in general and MRSA specifically may be on the decline, although the precise cause is yet to be determined.[4] Although risk factors for acute bacterial SSTIs such as skin abscesses and cellulitis include obesity, diabetes mellitus, injection drug use, MRSA nasal colonization, smoking, previous bacterial SSTIs, and edema, risk factors for other SSTIs are sometimes pathogen-specific. A discussion of environmental, behavioral, and host risk factors, including those related to immunocompromised persons, follows in this review. We present this information to guide the approach to developing and narrowing a differential diagnosis in a patient with a suspected SSTI.

The skin is colonized by a diverse range of microorganisms including bacteria, viruses, and fungi (**Fig. 1**). In general, the skin flora exists in a commensal relationship with its human host. But when a disruption in this balance occurs, the result can be a skin disorder or infection. For example, cellulitis arises when microbes breach the cutaneous surface, frequently in patients with fragile skin or diminished local host defenses, previous cutaneous trauma or surgery, previous episodes of cellulitis, and edema.[5] Breaks in the skin can be small and are often clinically unapparent. The severity of illness from an SSTI generally correlates with the depth of skin structure involvement. The Infectious Diseases Society of America characterizes 3 types of SSTIs: uncomplicated infections involving the superficial structures only; complicated infections involving deeper structures that commonly arise from wounds; and infections with tissue necrosis, such as necrotizing fasciitis and myonecrosis.[6] Microbial invasion of the skin induces a localized host inflammatory response that often manifests with pain, erythema, edema, tenderness with palpation, and warmth. Lesions may develop that are papular, nodular, ulcerative, or blistering. Local purulent or other drainage as well as systemic symptoms of fever, chills, and malaise also can be present.

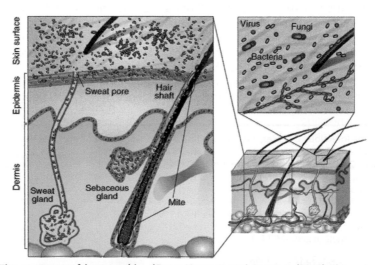

Fig. 1. The anatomy of human skin. (*From* Kong H and Segre J. (2012) Skin microbiome: looking back to move forward. J Invest Dermatol. 132:988-939; with permission.)

The first step in diagnosing an SSTI is clinical suspicion. A careful history that includes information about the patient's immune status, comorbid conditions, geographic place of residence, travel history, recent trauma or surgery, previous antimicrobial therapy, recent hospitalizations, lifestyle, hobbies, sexual activity, previous incarceration, household or other close contacts with an SSTI, and animal exposure or bites is essential when developing the differential diagnosis, as is an appropriate index of suspicion for specific etiologic agents.[6] A thorough physical examination and information about the morphologic characteristics, anatomic distribution, and evolution over time of skin lesions are essential. Radiographic studies including plain radiographs, ultrasound, computed tomography (CT), and MRI can help determine the diagnosis and the extent of the infection.

The most common pathogens associated with SSTIs have been β-hemolytic streptococcus (groups A, B, C, G, and F) and S aureus, but more recently gram-negative bacilli (GNB) have been increasingly reported, especially in polymicrobial infections.[7] Culture data are usually not obtained for cellulitis, and superficial swabs of wounds are not recommended due to the risk of culturing commensal bacteria and their inaccuracy in identifying the true etiologic pathogen.[8] Necrotizing SSTIs are often polymicrobial and can include aerobic gram-positive cocci such as S aureus, GNB such as Escherichia coli, and anaerobes including Clostridium spp and Bacteroides fragilis. Infected pressure ulcers are also frequently polymicrobial and share a similar pathogen profile as necrotizing infections. The usual pathogens in animal bites are the oral flora of the biting animal, along with human skin flora. Surgical infections are predominantly due to group A streptococcus and S aureus, although GNB such as Pseudomonas aeruginosa are also common. It is important to recognize that nonpurulent SSTIs (eg, cellulitis and erysipelas) are most likely caused by streptococci, whereas purulent SSTIs (eg, folliculitis, furuncles, carbuncles, and abscesses) are usually caused by S aureus.[9] Especially since the 1980s, multidrug-resistant bacterial organisms, such as MRSA, vancomycin-resistant Enterococcus, and GNB carrying extended spectrum β-lactamases (ESBLs), have become increasingly common causes of SSTIs both in the health care setting and in the community. Therefore, empiric therapy for patients with an SSTI must be chosen with attention to recent local patterns of resistance among likely pathogens.

Viral skin infections often present with a rash (exanthem) and involvement of the mucosal membranes. They include viral childhood exanthems (measles, rubella, erythema infectiosum, and roseola), herpes simplex virus (HSV), varicella zoster virus (VZV), Kaposi sarcoma virus, and viral zoonotic infections (eg, orf, monkeypox virus, and Ebola virus).[10] Severe acute respiratory syndrome coronavirus 2 infection causing Coronavirus Disease 2019 can result in dermatologic manifestations with various clinical presentations.[11]

Fungal skin infections are common and may occur after traumatic inoculation or hematogenous seeding, the latter being more common in immunocompromised patients. Protective immunity in the skin against Candida spp is mediated by interleukin-17–producing T cells, and, although superficial Candida SSTIs are common in immunocompetent hosts, T-cell deficiency can lead to chronic mucocutaneous candidiasis.[12]

CLINICAL PRESENTATION OF COMMON SKIN AND SOFT TISSUE INFECTION PATHOGENS AND SYNDROMES

SSTIs can present with a myriad of signs and symptoms that are mainly determined by the infecting organism (**Table 1**). The superficial infections (ie, impetigo, folliculitis, and

Table 1
Clinical presentation of SSTIs and common pathogens[5,6,9,13]

Skin Lesion or Condition	Typical Presentation	Frequent Pathogens	Comments
Ulcers	Foot ulcers associated with diabetic patients; sacral pressure ulcers in debilitated patients; cutaneous anthrax causes enlarging ulcer with black eschar	Often polymicrobial including *Streptococcus* spp, *Staphylococcus* spp, GNB, and anaerobes; *Bacillus anthracis*; *Francisella tularensis*; *Mycobacterium ulcerans* in tropical regions	If chronic (ie, ≥4–6 wk), consider underlying osteomyelitis
Nodules	Raised, firm lesions, sometimes erythematous	*Mycobacterium marinum*, *Mycobacterium leprae*, *Nocardia* spp, *Sporothrix schenckii*, *Leishmania* spp, and disseminated *Cryptococcus neoformans*, *Blastomyces dermatitidis*, *Histoplasma capsulatum*, and *Coccidioides immitis*	Hidradenitis suppurativa is a noninfectious condition associated with sweat glands, often in the axilla and groin, and may have a nodular appearance before developing intermittently draining sinus tracts
Papules	Erythematous lesions that often develop at primary site of inoculation	Cat-scratch disease and bacillary angiomatosis (*Bartonella henselae*); parasites (schistosomiasis, cutaneous larva migrans)	
Pustules	Small, pus-filled lesions associated with acne and folliculitis	*Cutibacterium acnes* (formerly *Propionibacterium acnes*)	
Vesicles	Bubblelike sac caused by fluid trapped under the epidermis	Viruses including VZV, HSV, and monkeypox	Fluid culture or DFA test of fluid from a freshly unroofed lesion may be useful for diagnosis
Folliculitis	Pimplelike lesion caused by infection and inflammation of hair follicle(s)	*Staphylococcus aureus*, *Pseudomonas aeruginosa* (hot tub folliculitis), schistosomes (swimmer's itch)	Hot tub folliculitis is caused by insufficient chlorination
Cellulitis	Localized warmth, erythema, tenderness, and edema; drainage may occur	*S aureus*, group A, C, or G streptococcus, *P aeruginosa*, other GNB	Treatment is usually empiric; *S aureus* characterized by spread from a central lesion (eg, abscess or foreign body)

	Description	Organisms	Comments
Abscess	Swollen, warm, erythematous, and tender lesion filled with purulent fluid	*S aureus* (CA-MRSA, MSSA), *Staphylococcus lugdunensis*, *Streptococcus anginosus* group	Incision and debridement are often necessary
Draining cutaneous fistula	Painful bump or boil on abdomen, communication between bowel and skin	Bowel flora, *Actinomyces israelii*, *Nocardia* spp	Most develop after intra-abdominal surgery or abdominal trauma resulting in inoculation; may or may not cause a local SSTI
Cutaneous draining sinus	Draining skin defect with subcutaneous infection, often chronic and may or may not have surrounding erythema	*Actinomyces* spp, *Nocardia* spp, *Mycobacterium tuberculosis*, nontuberculous mycobacteria	Hidradenitis suppurativa can have a similar appearance
Bullae	Blister lesions filled with clear fluid	*S aureus* (SSSS), gas gangrene (*Clostridium* spp), *Vibrio vulnificus*, *Shewanella* spp, agents of necrotizing fasciitis (see last row of this table)	Patients with cirrhosis are particularly susceptible to severe halophilic *Vibrio* spp infection
Crusted/Impetigo	Thick, crusty, superficial, yellow ("honey crusted") lesions	*S aureus* and *Streptococcus pyogenes*	Streptococcal lesions more common in children aged 2–5 y
Erysipelas	Painful, erythematous, rapidly spreading rash with sharply demarcated borders; typically on the face; can also affect extremities	*S pyogenes*	Only affects the superficial dermis whereas cellulitis affects deeper layers of skin
Necrotizing fasciitis	Often begins at site of minor trauma; characterized by fever, pain, and edema, followed by development of fluid-filled bullae; infection tracks along fascial planes deep to the subcutaneous fat	Group A streptococcus, mixed aerobic/anaerobic bacteria, *Clostridium perfringens*, *S aureus* (including MRSA and MSSA)	Predisposing factors include DM, PVD, recent surgery; called Fournier gangrene when it affects groin or genitals

Abbreviations: CA-MRSA, community-associated methicillin-resistant *Staphylococcus aureus*; DFA, direct fluorescent antibody; DM, diabetes mellitus; GNB, gram-negative bacilli; HSV, herpes simplex virus; MRSA, methicillin-resistant *S aureus*; MSSA, methicillin-susceptible *S aureus*; PVD, peripheral vascular disease; SSSS, staphylococcal scalded-skin syndrome; SSTI, skin and soft tissue infection; VZV, varicella zoster virus.

erysipelas) are mainly caused by *S aureus* or streptococci. Most cases of impetigo occur in children, and there is a predilection for the summer months (**Fig. 2**). Minor trauma such as from an insect bite or abrasion is a risk factor for developing impetigo, as is nasal colonization with *S aureus*.[14] Nonbullous impetigo begins as a single erythematous maculopapular lesion that develops into a vesicle, which ruptures and forms a honey-colored crust. Bullous impetigo occurs in neonates and develops on the trunk, extremities, or buttocks. It is a localized form of staphylococcal scalded-skin syndrome caused by toxin-producing strains of *S aureus*. Folliculitis is a superficial infection of hair follicles with perifollicular papules or pustules on an erythematous base. The most common etiologies are *S aureus* or *Streptococcus* spp. Folliculitis can also be due to *P aeruginosa* or fungi, including *Malassezia* spp and *Candida* spp.

Erysipelas usually involves the lower extremities or the face. It is characterized by a painful, erythematous, edematous area of the skin that is sharply demarcated from normal adjacent skin (**Fig. 3**). Lymphedema is a risk factor, and erysipelas tends to recur in areas of previous infection. The most common pathogen is group A streptococcus. Fever and leukocytosis are often present, although the patient usually does not develop signs of sepsis. Severe disease is uncommon and can be complicated by the formation of bullae, and the infection may extend to deeper tissues.

Cellulitis, one of the most common SSTIs seen in clinical practice, is an acute, progressive infection of the skin and subcutaneous tissues characterized by erythema, pain, edema, and warmth (**Fig. 4**). Previous trauma is a risk factor. Hematogenous spread of bacteria to the skin resulting in cellulitis can also occur. Cellulitis does not have sharply demarcated borders like erysipelas, and can spread in a patchlike fashion. Fever, chills, and malaise are present in many cases. Cellulitis is frequently misdiagnosed, resulting in unnecessary antibiotic use and considerable health care expense. In one study, 30.5% of patients who presented to an ED and were admitted for presumed cellulitis were misdiagnosed.[15] Some mimics of cellulitis include venous stasis dermatitis, lipodermatosclerosis, irritant dermatitis, erythema nodosum, acute gout, and other primary inflammatory skin conditions.[16] Some of the mimics typically have a more chronic clinical course.[17]

A skin abscess is a walled-off collection of pus in the dermis and deeper layers of the skin. A furuncle is an infection of the hair follicle with extension into adjacent tissues that leads to abscess formation, whereas a carbuncle is a group of furuncles that drain through a central opening. These 3 conditions are referred to as purulent SSTIs and are most commonly caused by *S aureus*. Patients with recurrent purulent SSTIs may be chronically colonized with *S aureus*, particularly MRSA, and should be screened with a culture of the nares,[18] and perhaps additional body sites because exclusive extranasal MRSA colonization occurs in approximately 30% of carriers.[19] Furthermore, patients with purulent SSTIs who report a "spider bite" but did not actually see a spider have a high likelihood of being infected with MRSA.[20] Pyomyositis is a purulent SSTI of skeletal muscle, often in the larger muscles of the thigh and pelvis, that frequently manifests with systemic signs of infection (eg, fever, chills, malaise, and leukocytosis) and cramping pain localized to a muscle group. *S aureus* is the most common etiology.[21]

Necrotizing fasciitis (NF) is a fulminant, life-threating infection of fascia and subcutaneous tissue with rapidly spreading necrosis of the soft tissues. Fournier's gangrene is a subtype of NF that involves the perineal and genital regions. NF often develops from a break in the skin, such as trauma or surgery. Risk factors for NF include diabetes, smoking, alcohol abuse, vascular insufficiency, and injection drug use. NF should be suspected if signs of systemic toxicity (eg, fever, chills, hypo-tension, or acute kidney injury), tenderness out of proportion to examination and/or beyond the

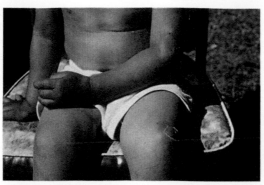

Fig. 2. Impetigo on a child's left arm and leg. (*From* the Public Health Image Library, CDC. ID #5155 PHIL CDC. https://phil.cdc.gov/Details.aspx?pid=5155.)

margins of erythema, bullae or cutaneous necrosis, edema, crepitus, or loss of sensation are present, or if there is rapid progression of symptoms.[22] Urgent surgical intervention with debridement of infected tissue is crucial to improve prognosis and survival. Indeed, a lack of surgical intervention is associated with high mortality.[23]

Common viral infections of the skin, herpes simplex virus-1 (HSV-1) and HSV-2, cause vesicles or pustules on an erythematous base that evolve over days into crusty, often very tender ulcerations, most commonly in the perioral or genital regions (**Fig. 5**). HSV infection of the finger, known as herpetic whitlow, can be misdiagnosed as a bacterial infection. VZV has 2 distinct forms: a primary infection (varicella or chickenpox), and a reactivation infection called shingles or herpes zoster. Varicella presents as vesicular lesions on the face, trunk, and extremities, whereas zoster manifests as a painful, vesicular eruption that follows a dermatomal distribution (**Fig. 6**).

Fungal pathogens are a common cause of human SSTIs. Tinea infections are most commonly caused by fungi of genus *Trichophyton, Microsporum*, or *Epidermophyton*.

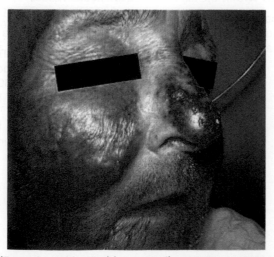

Fig. 3. Erysipelas. (*From* the Public Health Image Library, CDC. ID #2874 PHIL CDC. https://phil.cdc.gov/Details.aspx?pid=2874.)

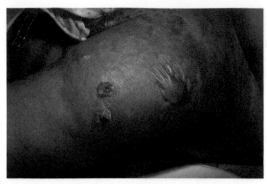

Fig. 4. Cellulitis on the left shoulder of a child after a vaccination. (*From* the Public Health Image Library, CDC. ID #4647 PHIL CDC. https://phil.cdc.gov/Details.aspx?pid=4647.)

Cutaneous manifestations are classified based on the affected body site.[24] Tinea pedis (athlete's foot) occurs on the feet and between the toes; tinea cruris (jock itch) occurs in the genital area and upper thighs; tinea capitis is an infection of hair follicles on the scalp that usually affects children but adult cases also occur; and tinea corporis, commonly called ringworm, causes a pruritic, erythematous patch with central clearing on the face, trunk, back, or extremities.[24] Candidal infections of the skin, called intertrigo, are frequently seen on obese patients and present with erythematous, pruritic plaques and beefy red erosions with satellite lesions in the groin region or in skin folds elsewhere on the body (**Fig. 7**). Sporotrichosis, caused by *Sporothrix schenckii*, typically presents in gardeners and is characterized by a small, erythematous or necrotic nodule at the site of inoculation that progresses to lymphangitic streaking (**Fig. 8**).

ANATOMIC CONSIDERATIONS IN A PATIENT WITH SUSPECTED SKIN AND SOFT TISSUE INFECTION
Location of Lesions Within the Skin and Subcutaneous Tissues

Understanding the structural anatomy of the skin and its relationships to infecting pathogens can aid the clinician in diagnosing SSTIs. The epidermis (see **Fig. 1**) provides a mechanical barrier that, when disrupted, can allow bacteria access to deeper

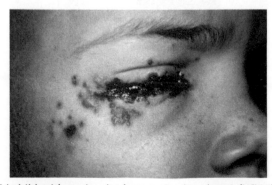

Fig. 5. A 7-year-old child with periocular herpes simplex virus-1 (HSV-1). (*From* the Public Health Image Library, CDC. ID #6492 PHIL CDC. https://phil.cdc.gov/Details.aspx?pid=6492.)

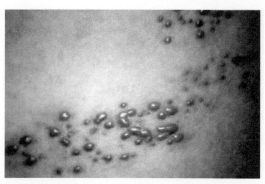

Fig. 6. Shingles along the dermatomal innervation of the T10–T11 thoracic nerves. (*From* the Public Health Image Library, CDC. ID #21505 PHIL CDC. https://phil.cdc.gov/Details. aspx?pid=21505.)

tissues and structures. For example, *Streptococcus pyogenes* infects the epidermis and can lead to obstruction of lymphatics, causing edema that is characteristic of erysipelas (**Table 2**). Intracellular infection of the epidermis through cutaneous inoculation, seen with HSV, leads to vesicle formation. The dermis contains connective tissue and embedded structures including hair follicles, glands, blood vessels, nerves, and muscles, each of which can be a local site of infection and pathogenesis. The capillary plexus can provide invading bacteria with access to the circulation and is an important site for white blood cell sequestration and chemotaxis. Metastatic spread to the plexus can result in cutaneous manifestations of a variety of infections, including disseminated fungal infections, meningococcemia, *Mycobacterium avium* complex, *Mycobacterium tuberculosis*, *Neisseria gonorrhoeae*, *Salmonella* spp, *P aeruginosa*, and *S aureus*.

Anatomic Location of Skin and Soft Tissue Infections

The anatomic location of a skin lesion, along with its initial morphology, and the evolution and progression of its morphology over time, may offer clues as to the etiology of a skin infection. Common SSTI syndromes, such as bacterial abscesses and cellulitis, may occur at any site on the skin or the mucous membranes. *S aureus* abscesses, however, are more common in areas of rubbing by clothing, such as on the lateral

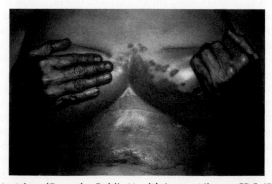

Fig. 7. Candidal intertrigo. (*From* the Public Health Image Library, CDC. ID #16702 PHIL CDC. https://phil.cdc.gov/Details.aspx?pid=16702.)

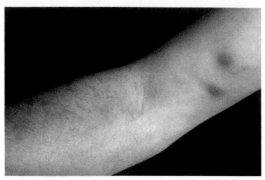

Fig. 8. Sporotrichosis, demonstrating lymphangitis spread along the arm. (*From* the Public Health Image Library, CDC. ID #16820 PHIL CDC. https://phil.cdc.gov/Details.aspx?pid=16820.)

abdomen, the buttocks, neck, or the inner thighs. Abscesses may also occur at a site of local trauma or laceration. Cellulitis may occur at anatomic sites of previous acute skin trauma, or in regions with chronic edema or chronic ulceration from any cause. Given these associations, a common site of cellulitis is in the distal lower extremities in patients with chronic edema there or in patients with tinea pedis, as these lesions of the foot offer a portal of entry for skin pathogens. However, lesions that have the morphologic characteristics of cellulitis that appear on both legs simultaneously are more likely to be of a noninfectious etiology.

Another SSTI defined by its location and local anatomy, periorbital cellulitis, also called preseptal cellulitis, is an infection of the soft tissues surrounding the eye anterior to the orbital septum. It may result from inoculation of bacteria into the skin surrounding the eye, such as from abrasions, lacerations, previous infection of the lachrymal ducts or tear sac (dacryocystitis) or eyelids (blepharitis), or insect bites. Alternatively, it can result from hematogenous spread of bacteria. Periorbital cellulitis presents with unilateral facial swelling, unilateral eyelid erythema, edema, and tenderness. Systemic features, such as fever and chills, are usually absent. Orbital cellulitis has a presentation similar to periorbital cellulitis, but patients also may have proptosis, limitation of extraocular movement, decreased visual acuity, papilledema, or chemosis. A retrospective study of children admitted to a tertiary hospital found diplopia, ophthalmoplegia, and proptosis to be features associated with orbital cellulitis.[27] A CT or MRI scan of the orbits can aid in differentiating periorbital and orbital cellulitis.

Typical anatomic locations for infectious skin lesions, associated pathogens, and characteristics of disease syndromes are listed in **Table 2**. Rarely is the anatomic location of a lesion pathognomonic for a specific pathogen. However, the location may help to narrow the differential diagnosis; for example, only a limited number of pathogens typically produce lesions on the palms and soles, including Rocky Mountain spotted fever (with a tick exposure), hand foot and mouth disease (more common in children), toxic shock syndrome (with presence of a toxin-producing strain of S aureus infection or colonization), measles (in an unvaccinated person with relevant exposure to an infected person), secondary syphilis (confirmed with appropriate serology or antigen testing), rat bite fever (with prior exposure to rats), or monkeypox (with relevant travel history and animal exposure). Certain infectious syndromes are defined by an anatomic location (eg, sycosis barbae, folliculitislike lesions in the facial region with beard growth; paronychia; or tinea capitis). Another distinctive clue to the etiology

Table 2
Selected skin and soft tissue infections and anatomic considerations in diagnosis

Frequent or Typical Anatomic Site	Disease (Other Names and Typical Pathogens)	Comments that May Guide Development of Differential Diagnosis
Scalp	Tinea capitis (Microsporum spp or Trichophyton spp)	Dermatophyte infection that may affect the scalp, eyebrows, and eyelashes; usually manifested by patches of pruritic, scaling skin[24,25]
Face	Herpes (cold sores; HSV-1 or -2)	Often painful, perioral macular lesions that develop vesicles and then ulcers; frequent recurrent lesions; spread by direct person-to-person contact[10]
	VZV	Shingles (zoster), a reactivation of VZV infection, may result in painful, vesicular, unilateral facial lesions in a dermatomal distribution; if they involve the nasociliary branch of the trigeminal nerve, sometimes suggested by Hutchinson sign (ie, the presence of VZV lesions on the tip of the nose), there is a risk of developing ophthalmic herpes zoster
		See **Table 3**
	Ameba (Balamuthia mandrillaris) Protothecosis (Prototheca spp)	Caused by a species of algae after freshwater swimming or other exposure; typically presents as painful vesicular or bullous lesions with purulent drainage; also reported as erythematous plaques, verrucous lesions, or pustular or nodular lesions; often following minor skin trauma[26]
	Erysipelas (St. Anthony fire)	See **Table 1**; although it occurs on the face, the most common site is the lower extremities
	Orbital or periorbital cellulitis (often Staphylococcus aureus)	Cellulitis (periorbital) that may also affect the deeper structures of the orbit (orbital); may occur after minor skin trauma or complicating blepharitis or dacryocystitis; orbital and periorbital cellulitis are often distinguished clinically, but imaging studies may be necessary[27] (see text)

(continued on next page)

Table 2
(continued)

Frequent or Typical Anatomic Site	Disease (Other Names and Typical Pathogens)	Comments that May Guide Development of Differential Diagnosis
Extremities		
Upper extremities	Tularemia inoculation lesion (*Francisella tularensis*)	See **Table 3**
	Fish tank granuloma (*Mycobacterium marinum*)	Often on the cooler, distal regions of the hands or upper extremity, frequently overlying bony prominences[28]; see **Table 3**
	Prototothecosis	See preceding comments
Lower extremities	Ecthyma (Group A streptococcus); Ecthyma gangrenosum (*Pseudomonas aeruginosa*)	Often follows minor skin injury such as an insect bite or scratch; appears as "punched out lesions"; more extensive, disseminated lesions should raise concern for ecthyma gangrenosum, especially in the immunocompromised (see text)
	Cellulitis (*Streptococcus* spp, *S aureus*, *Pseudomonas* spp)	Although cellulitis may occur at any site on the body, on the lower extremities it is a frequent complication of a laceration or minor skin injury, or chronic edema of any etiology (eg, lymphedema, venous insufficiency); chronic ulcers; or tinea pedis; usually unilateral[9]
	Erysipelas	See **Table 1** and preceding comments
	Prototothecosis	See preceding comments

Hands	Scabies (*Sarcoptes scabei var. hominis*)	Often in intertriginous areas, including webs between digits; pruritic burrow tracks that develop into papules; fever typically absent; also common in the axillae, elbows, and at the beltline; crusted (or Norwegian) scabies is a more severe form, usually in immunocompromised hosts, with crusting and deep skin fissures[29]
	Human bite (human oral flora)	May result from a bite or from a clenched fist injury after punching an opponent in the mouth; see **Table 3**
	Herpetic whitlow (HSV-1 or -2)	May result from nail biting and autoinoculation of HSV into the cuticles from the perioral region in a person with oral HSV[10]
	Cutaneous listeriosis (*Listeria monocytogenes*)	In veterinarians and farm workers exposed to live calf births; results from direct inoculation of the pathogen[30]
	Paronychia (often *S aureus*)	Painful erythema, fluctuance, and edema sometimes with an abscess of the cuticle or pads of the digits
	Sporotrichosis (Rose handler's disease or Rose gardener's disease; *Sporothrix schenckii*)	See **Table 3**
Feet	Diabetic foot infection	Common in DM with neuropathy after repeated foot trauma and ulcer formation; may progress to osteomyelitis; a variety of bacterial pathogens may be cultured; often requires debridement or amputation for cure, in addition to antimicrobial drug therapy
	Madura foot (Mycetoma)	See **Table 3**
	Tungiasis (*Tunga penetrans*)	See **Table 3**
	Cutaneous larva migrans (creeping eruption) (*Gnathostoma* spp, *Ancylostoma caninum*, *Ancylostoma braziliense*, and *Uncinaria stenocephala*)	See **Table 3**
	Mycobacterial furuncles (*Mycobacterium ulcerans*, *Mycobacterium chelonae*)	May develop after use of common foot baths or after nail care at a salon[28]; see **Table 3**
	Hot foot syndrome (*P aeruginosa*)	See **Table 3**
	Tinea pedis or Athlete's foot (*Trichophyton rubrum* typically)	Often affects the webs between toes and can be on the sole; causes pruritic erosions or scales and may cause blistering of the skin and predispose to bacterial superinfection, and is therefore a risk factor for bacterial cellulitis[24,25]
	Onychomycosis	Dermatophyte infection of the toenails, often resulting in thickening and discoloration of the nail

(continued on next page)

Table 2
(continued)

Frequent or Typical Anatomic Site	Disease (Other Names and Typical Pathogens)	Comments that May Guide Development of Differential Diagnosis
Palms and soles	Hand, foot, and mouth disease (Coxsackieviruses and Enterovirus 71)	Papular or vesicular lesions appearing 1–2 d after onset of fevers, malaise, sore throat, and myalgias; also have painful lesions of the mouth (herpangina); spreads via respiratory secretions, skin lesion contact, or from feces; more common in children[31]
	Secondary syphilis (*Treponema pallidum*)	Typically rash may occur 6–8 wk (without therapy for primary infection) after infection by sexual transmission; many presentations: commonly as annular lesions with a raised border, or violaceous and plaquelike lesions[32]
	Toxic shock syndrome (*S aureus*)	Most often palmar erythema and edema in the setting of typical signs and symptoms (whole-body rash, hypotension, involvement of 3 or more organ systems, and desquamation of the skin after rash develops); toxin-mediated disease associated with tampon use, minor local infection, or mucosal surface colonization by *S aureus*[33]
	Rat bite fever (*Streptobacillus moniliformis*)	See **Table 3**
	HSV erythema multiforme	Fixed bull's eye lesion that may appear <10 d after reactivation of HSV on the face or genitals[10]
	Measles (measles virus)	7–14 d after exposure to an infected person, high fever and cough are noted, followed 3–5 d later by an erythematous, maculopapular rash that begins on the face and spreads to the entire body in inadequately vaccinated or unvaccinated and previously uninfected hosts; mouth can show white "Koplik spots" early in course of disease; measles is among the most contagious of known pathogens
	Monkeypox	Most common in Congo; results usually from direct exposure to or bites of animals; fever, chills, headaches, lymphadenopathy, and backaches are common; lesions progress from macules to papules to vesicles to pustules and then scabs; they resolve in 2–4 wk[34]

Tinea pedis	See preceding comments
Disseminated meningococcemia (*Neisseria meningitidis*)	Pathogen spread via respiratory route and can colonize the throat; spreads in congregate living sites; cause of meningitis; can disseminate to the blood with life-threatening syndrome of fevers, chills, myalgias, abdominal pain, hypotension, and a dark, purple rash; palms and soles often show a petechial and/or purpuric rash; occurs worldwide although most common in the "Meningitis Belt" of sub-Saharan Africa[35]
Human monocytic ehrlichiosis (*Ehrlichia chaffeensis*)	Tick-borne bacterial illness with symptoms of fever, chills, headache, myalgias, nausea, vomiting, diarrhea, and rash appearing approximately 1–2 wk after *Amblyomma americanum* tick bite; the rash spares the face but may affect palms and soles, is nonpruritic, maculopapular or petechial, and it occurs in 60% of children and 30% of adults infected; white-tailed deer are the primary reservoir; occurs in the United States in the southern, south-central, and mid-Atlantic states[36]
Chikungunya virus	Mosquito-borne viral illness leading to severe, bilateral symmetric arthralgias and fever 3–7 d after infection; maculopapular rash may affect palms and soles; found in Asia, central and southern Africa, and the Americas[37]
Breast	
Mastitis or breast abscess (often *S aureus*)	May be associated with lactation; very tender; abscesses may require incision and drainage

(continued on next page)

Table 2
(continued)

Frequent or Typical Anatomic Site	Disease (Other Names and Typical Pathogens)	Comments that May Guide Development of Differential Diagnosis
Genitalia/Groin	Chancre of primary syphilis (*T pallidum*)	Sexually transmitted disease; a painless, indurated ulcer with raised borders appearing 9–90 d after infection, often on the glans, prepuce, or coronal sulcus in men and on the labia or the perineum in women or near the rectum; may be a linear chancre without ulcer; rarely is a painful ulcer; resolves within several days with therapy and in 3–6 wk if not treated[32]
	Intertrigo (*Candida* spp)	Maculopapular lesions typically of the groin and other skin folds that become intensely red with satellite lesions, sometimes pruritic (see text)
	Tinea cruris (jock itch) (*T rubrum or Trichophyton mentagrophytes*)	Pruritic lesion in the groin that may extend from the crural fold to the inner thigh; may be bilateral and may involve the scrotum or labia; skin irritated, sometimes erythematous or scaling; may have a burning sensation; superinfections may occur[24,25]
	Pubic lice ("crab lice") (*Pthirus pubis*)	May be sexually transmitted; lice are ectoparasites that attach to pubic hair[29]
	Scabies (*Sarcoptes scabei var. hominis*)	See preceding comments
	HSV	Painful vesicular lesions that develop into shallow ulcers; sexually transmitted; recurrent episodes are lifelong[10]
	Genital warts (HPV)	See **Table 3**
	Fournier gangrene (usually polymicrobial aerobic and anaerobic bacterial infection)	Rapidly progressive necrotizing fasciitis affecting the perineum and/or genitalia; skin color is often gray; it may occur after local trauma or with no predisposing condition; DM is a risk factor; a surgical emergency requiring rapid debridement[38]
Buttocks/Hips	Hot tub folliculitis (*P aeruginosa*) (Bikini bottom)	Folliculitis that often occurs at sites where bathing suits contact the body; "bikini bottom" is the term for firm, deep nodules in the inferior gluteal crease; may also affect the external auditory canal; in whirlpools, often lesions are limited to the submerged areas below the chest; usually spares the face and scalp[26]; see **Table 3**

Sacrum	Polymicrobial infected ulcer	Usually a decubitus (pressure) ulcer (or "bed sore") in patients with prolonged immobility; may be complicated by underlying osteomyelitis
Dermatomal distribution	Shingles (Zoster or Herpes zoster) (VZV)	Occurs usually in older adults; onset many years after initial VZV infection (chickenpox); painful vesicular lesions with subsequent ulceration and crusting; in immunocompromised hosts, lesions may present in multiple dermatomes and disseminate to CNS and other organs[10]
Skin folds	Candidiasis (Candida spp)	See preceding comments
	Tinea corporis (ringworm; T rubrum, T mentagrophytes, and Microsporum audouinii)	See specific body sites with tinea,[24,25] noted above

Abbreviations: CNS, central nervous system; DM, diabetes mellitus; HPV, human papilloma virus; HSV, herpes simplex virus; MRSA, methicillin-resistant S aureus; VZV, varicella zoster virus.

of infectious skin lesions is the dermatomal distribution of painful vesicles caused by VZV in shingles (see **Table 2**).

For infections that occur by direct inoculation, the anatomic site of a lesion also may be a useful clue in narrowing the differential diagnosis. For example, fish tank granuloma, caused often by *Mycobacterium marinum*, is commonly on the hands or upper extremities, where lacerations of the skin occur in the course of doing work in a fish tank or another site with water.[28] Similarly, sporotrichosis, usually caused by the fungus *S schenckii*, often occurs on the upper extremities because injuries from stems or thorns tend to occur on the hands or arms during gardening.

Thus, the initial anatomic location of a skin lesion and its evolution over time must be considered carefully in conjunction with the history of host characteristics, exposures, and behaviors (considered later in this article) to narrow the differential diagnosis, optimally before diagnostic laboratory tests are sent.

ENVIRONMENTAL EXPOSURES AND BEHAVIORS ASSOCIATED WITH SPECIFIC SKIN AND SOFT TISSUE INFECTION PATHOGENS

Like all infectious diseases, SSTIs occur only when host, pathogen, and environmental factors are aligned to predispose an individual to infection. Some pathogens have a distinctive geographic distribution. Sometimes duration of time elapsed after a particular exposure until the onset of symptoms may suggest a pathogen by its typical incubation period. The morphology of the skin lesion, the progression of the lesion over time, or the anatomic distribution of the lesion may provide important evidence to support a diagnosis. Certain recent behaviors can also provide clues in discerning a likely pathogen, such as sports participation, travel, interaction with animals, injection drug use, sexual activity, occupation, hiking, fishing, camping, gardening, farming, or swimming. A wide variety of environmental exposures as well as behaviors known to increase the risk of specific SSTI syndromes are summarized in **Table 3**.

Many pathogens are associated with water exposure, and distinctive groups of pathogens are known to cause infections in swimming pools, hot tubs, fresh pond or lake water, and salt water. In and around swimming pools, certain pathogens are transmitted from person to person directly or indirectly via fomites, such as molluscum contagiosum virus and human papilloma virus (HPV). Bacteria such as *P aeruginosa* and nontuberculous mycobacteria (especially *M marinum*) are common pathogens in pools as well as hot tubs. These infections are particularly common when swimming pools are not maintained properly.[26] Sea water exposures to injured skin are common in those with occupational exposures, such as fishermen, lobstermen, crabbers, and oystermen, as well as recreational visitors to the beach and boaters. Pathogens of the greatest concern are the rapid-growing *M marinum*, *Aeromonas* spp, and *Pseudomonas* spp. In warm seawater, typical in the Gulf of Mexico, the dangerous bacterial pathogen *Vibrio vulnificus* is found, which is associated with necrotizing SSTIs. Also if consumed in raw or undercooked seafood it can cause sepsis and death, with a greater risk of systemic symptoms and poor outcomes in those with previous liver disease.[26,65] In freshwater ponds and lakes, the pathogens that may cause SSTIs depend on interaction with animals and fish in the water, whether the water is stagnant, and the geographic location of the water.[41] Certain pathogens are associated with aquaculture; for example, tilapia farming places workers at risk of *Streptococcus iniae* SSTIs, whereas fishing and cleaning fish puts people at risk of distinctive *Erysipelothrix* infections. Fish tank cleaning, ichthyotherapy, and footbath use in nail salons and spas pose the risk of nontuberculous mycobacterial infections (see **Table 3**).

Table 3
Behaviors and environmental exposures that predispose to selected skin and soft tissue infections

Exposure or Behavior	Disease/Type of Lesion	Frequent Pathogens	Comments that May Guide Development of Differential Diagnosis
Swimming pools, hot tubs	Hot tub folliculitis	Pseudomonas aeruginosa; Aeromonas spp	Pruritic, folliculitislike papulopustules appearing 8–48 h after exposure to hot tubs, showers, baths, saunas, synthetic sponges, water slides, swimming pool inflatables, or pools with poor maintenance[26]
	Molluscum contagiosum ("Water warts")	Molluscum contagiosum virus	Pox virus infection associated with swimming pools; pearly white or skin-colored papules and nodules; may have a central umbilication[39,40]
	Tinea pedis (Athlete's foot)	Dermatophytes (Trichophyton rubrum)	May be transmitted by direct contact or from contact with shower floors, pool decks, pools, or other fomites[39,40]
	Warts	HPV	Direct contact with swimming pool environments; plantar warts may be from foot shower surface contact[39]
	Free-living amebic skin infection	Acanthamoeba spp and Balamuthia mandrillaris	After exposure of injured skin to fresh water, hot tubs, hot-spring spas, swimming pools, or soil; occurs worldwide; skin lesions may be erythematous plaques or ulceronecrotic with an eschar; usually are papulonodular with purulent drainage[29]
	Hot foot syndrome	P aeruginosa	Swimming pools; wading pools; most common in children; microabscesses with painful, erythematous plantar

(continued on next page)

Table 3
(continued)

Exposure or Behavior	Disease/Type of Lesion	Frequent Pathogens	Comments that May Guide Development of Differential Diagnosis
			nodules developing into pustular lesions after swimming pool exposure; may be related to microabrasions from floor of pool; often on soles of feet[39]
	Swimmer's ear	P aeruginosa or Staphylococcus aureus	Otitis externa after swimming; may be complicated by sequelae of otorrhea or hearing loss[39]
	Swimming pool granuloma; fish tank granuloma (or fish fancier's granuloma)	Mycobacterium marinum or Mycobacterium scrofulaceum	Fish tanks, fresh or salt water bathing, hot tubs, or swimming pool exposure; fish, snails, shellfish, dolphins, and water fleas may serve as vectors; often verrucous nodules or plaques 6 wk after infection; may be sporotrichoid in distribution[28,39]
Seawater/ Salt water	GNB skin infections	Aeromonas spp, Escherichia coli, Klebsiella pneumoniae, P aeruginosa, Proteus spp, and Shewanella spp	Folliculitis, cellulitis, or skin abscesses; bullous lesions are less common and are associated especially with Shewanella spp[26]
	Mycobacterial infections	M marinum	After minor cuts, cleaning aquariums, working in sea water, after a crab bite, or after sea urchin spine or crustacean injury; incubation 1 wk to several mo; red-violet, verrucous, raised patches sometimes with sporotrichoid spread are typical; often with yellow, purulent

Exposure	Organism	Comments
		discharge; may progress to deeper tissue infections if not treated; seen in skin divers, boaters, and dolphin trainers; diagnosis often delayed[26,28]
Warm saltwater	Vibrio spp infections Vibrio vulnificus	Usually with water exposure following a puncture wound; hemorrhagic bullae, and ulcers with tissue necrosis; may progress to necrotizing fasciitis, ecthyma gangrenosum, sepsis or death; more common in men; in the United States, especially after exposure to the Gulf of Mexico[41]
Fresh water	Freshwater animal or fish bites, exposure with minor trauma — Aeromonas spp (especially Aeromonas hydrophila); Plesiomonas shigelloides; and other GNB	Leech, fish, snake, or alligator bites; appearance similar to cellulitis around bite site; Aeromonas spp infections may also occur after other minor skin trauma in fresh water and may progress to necrotizing fasciitis if not treated promptly; A hydrophila also causes gastroenteritis[41]
	Exposure to water after flooding — Aeromonas spp (especially A hydrophila)	See preceding comments; associated with SSTIs after a tsunami in water-exposed populations[42]
	Crab fishing — Edwardsiella tarda	Skin abscess after marine injuries; more commonly in warm weather[26,41]

(continued on next page)

Table 3
(continued)

Exposure or Behavior	Disease/Type of Lesion	Frequent Pathogens	Comments that May Guide Development of Differential Diagnosis
	Buruli ulcer	*Mycobacterium ulcerans*	Exposure to rivers, ponds, swamps, marshes, and other bodies of water most commonly in western and central Africa, Australia, New Guinea, Malaysia, Suriname, Mexico, Peru, Japan, and China; initially painless plaques that progress to nodules with tissue destruction caused by a toxin (polyketide), and then deep ulcers develop with undermined borders; often on extremities after a minor skin abrasion or insect bite; if untreated, there is risk of progression to contractures, joint involvement, limb deformities, and osteonecrosis; more common in children and most common on the lower extremities[28]
	Pythiosis ("swamp cancer")	*Pythium insidiosum*	After boating or fishing or in agricultural workers contacting stagnant or swampy water; oomycete that causes painful, nodular ulcerations that develop into necrotizing hemorrhagic plaques; especially in immunocompromised hosts; in Thailand and rarely North America[43]

Achlorophyllous algae	Prototheca wickerhamii and Prototheca zopfii	Exposure to ponds, other stagnant fresh water, or aquariums; rare cause of ulcerative or papulonodular lesions after minor trauma; central and southern United States; especially in immunocompromised hosts[26]
Free-living amebae	Acanthamoeba spp and B mandrillaris	Exposure of injured skin to fresh water, hot tubs, hot-spring spas, swimming pools, or soil; worldwide; erythematous plaques or ulceronecrotic lesions with an eschar, although usually a papulonodular lesion with purulent drainage; usually in immunocompromised hosts[29]
Melioidosis (Whitmore disease)	Burkholderia pseudomallei	Ulcer, nodule, or skin abscess developing after exposure to water; infection can also result from inhalation of contaminated dust or direct exposure to soil and may affect any organ in the body; most common in southeast Asia (especially Thailand, Malaysia, and Singapore) and northern Australia[44]
Swimmer's itch (Clam digger's itch or Schistosome dermatitis)	Larvae of the fluke Schistosomatidae, from bird excrement	Freshwater lake swimming in states surrounding Great Lakes; also widespread worldwide outside of the United States; 3–5-mm erythematous papules; usually >20 lesions that resolve in 4–7 d; most common in June to July[26,39]

(continued on next page)

Table 3
(continued)

Exposure or Behavior	Disease/Type of Lesion	Frequent Pathogens	Comments that May Guide Development of Differential Diagnosis
Fish		*Erysipelothrix rhusiopathiae*	Exposure during fishing and filleting of fish with minor skin injuries; causes erysipelas with painful, throbbing, and pruritic lesions appearing 1–2 d after exposure[37]
		Streptococcus iniae	Tilapia farming or preparation of fish from fresh or brackish water; causes impetigo and cellulitis[41]
		Chromobacterium violaceum	Stagnant fresh or brackish water; often following a fish bite in subtropical regions including southern United States; can progress to sepsis in patients with CGD; wound may have a bluish, purulent discharge or disseminated abscesses may occur[41]
Farms	Primary cutaneous listeriosis	*Listeria monocytogenes*	Veterinarians and farmers exposed to live calf births; impetiginous lesions, typically on the hands and arms[30]
	Cutaneous anthrax	*Bacillus anthracis*	From soil exposure to anthrax spores or animal exposures; animal hide workers; most common in Africa, Asia, and Eastern Europe; lesion is a painless, pruritic papule that turns into a vesicle then ruptures and forms an ulcer with a dark, black eschar without purulence; may cause lymphadenopathy; organism also used as a bioweapon[45]

Gardening	Fungal infections	Sporothrix schenckii	Occurs from minor abrasions or deeper puncture wounds from wood or other plants; often gardening and rose bush thorn injuries; uncommonly follows a cat bite (especially caused by Sporothrix brasiliensis in Brazil); classically lesions are initially a small, painless nodule and progress to a larger, raised lesions that may ulcerate and form an eschar; additional lesions following lymph vessels may develop serially up the arm with lymphangitic streaking; often associated with lymphadenopathy[46]
Skin contact, often in congregate settings	Scabies	Sarcoptes scabei var. hominis	These mites spread in schools, health care facilities, homeless shelters, homes, and other congregate settings; in superficial epidermis, eggs hatch and mature, causing a maculopapular rash that may also rarely be vesicular with especially nocturnal pruritis; raised, serpiginous tracts of the adult burrows may commonly appear in the intertriginous areas; in immunocompromised hosts, lesions may advance to thick, hyperkeratotic crusts in crusted (also known as Norwegian) scabies[29]
	Skin abscesses	S aureus (MRSA or MSSA)	Spread associated with contact sports, household contact, health care settings, jails and prisons, IVDU, hemodialysis, and other settings[5,13,47]

(continued on next page)

Table 3
(continued)

Exposure or Behavior	Disease/Type of Lesion	Frequent Pathogens	Comments that May Guide Development of Differential Diagnosis
	Herpes	HSV	From direct skin-to-skin contact in sports, household contacts, and sexual contact[47]
	Tinea capitis	*Microsporum audouinii*	Spreads often among children in daycare or school by direct contact[24,40,48]
Hunting/Camping	Tularemia (rabbit fever, deer fly fever)	*Francisella tularensis*	In the United States (Arkansas, Missouri, South Dakota, and Oklahoma) or elsewhere in the northern hemisphere; high fever (often up to 104°F) with ≥1 painful, erythematous, ulcerating 25-mm to 4-cm papule with ragged edges and a necrotic base at the site of inoculation, usually on the upper extremity; often with lymphadenopathy and eschar formation; later, if disseminated disease, tularemids (macular, maculopapular, nodular, acneiform, papulovesicular, or plaquelike lesions) appear on extensor extremity surfaces; transmitted by several arthropod vectors including ticks; can also be spread by direct skin contact with infected animals (eg, rabbits, cats, coyotes), consumption of contaminated water, or inhalation of dust; common in the spring and summer overall, but hunters typically face higher risk in fall and early winter[49,50] (see **Fig. 10**)

Nail salons/footbaths; body piercing; acupuncture	Tick-borne infections; Mycobacterial furuncles	Mycobacterium marinum, M ulcerans, Mycobacterium fortuitum, rarely Mycobacterium abscessus or other rapid-growing mycobacteria	See comments that follow. Especially with pedicures or using ichthyotherapy in spas; 3–12-wk incubation period; erythematous papules and later fluctuant violaceous furuncles sometimes with ulceration (cause scarring); also may cause infections at sites of body piercing, acupuncture, mesotherapy, or plastic surgery[28]
Intravenous drug use (IVDU)	Clostridial infections	Clostridium spp	From black tar heroin contaminated with bacterial spores; skin lesions are necrotizing and may advance to necrotizing fasciitis and wound botulism (if infection with Clostridium botulinum)[51]
	Anthrax	B anthracis	Heroin use; spores enter skin, are engulfed by macrophages, and germinate; painless, pruritic papule that becomes vesicular, then ruptures and forms an ulcer with a dark, black eschar with no purulence; often lymphadenopathy; usually deeper, local infections from IVDU lack typical eschar, and the deep adipose tissue is necrosed with no purulence[45,52]
	Skin abscess ("syringe abscess")	S aureus (MRSA and MSSA)	High-risk group[53] due to shared equipment for injection, as well as close physical contact; since 2000 particular risk for the USA300 CA-MRSA strain in the United States and Canada[51,54,55]

(continued on next page)

Table 3
(continued)

Exposure or Behavior	Disease/Type of Lesion	Frequent Pathogens	Comments that May Guide Development of Differential Diagnosis
	Infection with oral or environmental flora	*Eikenella corrodens*, other oral flora, Group A streptococcus, or *P aeruginosa*	From licking needles, storing bagged drugs in the mouth, or use of tap or toilet water in preparation of injected drugs; high risk of bacteremia and its complications[51]
Soil/Sand	Cutaneous larva migrans (creeping eruption)	*Gnathostoma* spp, *Ancylostoma caninum*, *Ancylostoma braziliense*, or *Uncinaria stenocephala*	Infection by direct inoculation of hookworm or other nematode larvae from walking with bare feet or sandals in soil or at beaches; can also occur on other areas of skin (from sitting or lying down) in contact with soil or sand; after infection, patients develop a small, pruritic, red papule and then a serpiginous track with intense pruritis as the larva burrows into the epidermis; lesions may persist for months; each pathogen has a distinctive geographic distribution; although the condition may occur worldwide, it is most common in the tropics, especially in developing countries[29,56], outbreaks have been reported in the United States after rainy periods in the region stretching from the mid-Atlantic

Condition	Organism	Comments
Clostridial infection	Clostridium spp	states to Texas; beach soccer (Spain) and volleyball (Brazil) are risk factors[47] Often necrotizing infections, and soil exposure, especially with a puncture wound, raises concern for tetanus (Clostridium tetani) and wound botulism (C botulinum)
Bacillus infections	Bacillus spp, including B anthracis	Cutaneous infections (cellulitis with marked edema) and may progress to disseminated anthrax; see previously for clinical description[45]
Melioidosis (Whitmore disease)	B pseudomallei	See preceding comments
Mycetoma/Madura foot	Bacterial or fungal infection	Most common in the mycetoma belt between south latitude 15° and north latitude 30°; usually multiple, chronic, draining sinuses are present[57]
Tungiasis	Tunga penetrans	Infection in the stratum granulosum of skin by a sand flea (which is sometimes called a jigger or chigoe flea) after walking with bare feet in sandy soil; in the tropics and subtropics, especially in Central or South America; subcutaneous nodules develop, causing pain, erythema, and pruritis; can be complicated by bacterial superinfection[29]
Tattoos — Cellulitis or abscess	S aureus; Streptococcus spp, P aeruginosa, Clostridium spp	Must consider mycobacteria, fungi, parasites, and syphilis in the differential diagnosis; sources include pathogens colonizing the tattooist, the ink, the water used to (continued on next page)

Table 3
(continued)

Exposure or Behavior	Disease/Type of Lesion	Frequent Pathogens	Comments that May Guide Development of Differential Diagnosis
	Mycobacterial furuncles	*M marinum* and other rapidly growing mycobacteria	dilute the ink, the needles, and the skin of the recipient[58]
Human bite	Bacterial infection	*S aureus*, CONS, *Streptococcus anginosus*, *Streptococcus oralis*, *E corrodens*, other human oral flora	See preceding comments
			Polymicrobial infection is common, as is infection with several anaerobic bacteria[59]
Animal exposures	Dog bite	Polymicrobial, often including *Pasteurella canis* or *Pasteurella multocida*, *Streptococcus* spp, and *Staphylococcus* spp	Cellulitis, abscess, or lymphangitis; often present as nonpurulent wounds. *Capnocytophaga canimorsus* can cause SSTI and sepsis, purpura fulminans, gangrene, infective endocarditis, and meningitis, especially in immunocompromised and asplenic patients; *Capnocytophaga cynodegmi* has a similar presentation; risk of tetanus (*C tetani*), and therefore consider tetanus vaccination if time of last vaccination was >10 y prior or not known[59,60]
	Cat bite	Polymicrobial, often including *Pasteurella* spp, *Streptococcus* spp, and *Staphylococcus* spp	May penetrate deep to tendons or bone; can lead to abscess or cellulitis; nonpurulent infections are common; risk of tetanus (see preceding comments)[59,60]
	Rat bite fever	*Streptobacillus moniliformis*, *Spirillum minus*	Occurs in North America; 3–10 d after a rat bite, fever, headache, and

			myalgias are common; then maculopapular, petechial, pustular, or vesicular rash of extremities, face, and trunk may appear 2–4 d later; usually the bite site heals before systemic symptoms begin; the bite site may then go on to ulcerate[61]
Sexual contact	Syphilis	Treponema pallidum	In primary syphilis, the classic lesion is the chancre, a painless, indurated ulcer with raised borders appearing 9–90 d after infection, often on the genitalia or near the rectum; it can appear as a linear chancre without an ulcer, and rarely a painful ulcer; the primary lesion resolves within several days with therapy and in 3–6 wk if not; secondary and tertiary syphilis have a myriad of dermatologic manifestations and have recently been reviewed[32]
	Herpes	HSV	See preceding comments; genital HSV infections are sexually transmitted[10]
	Genital warts	HPV	Sexually transmitted disease resulting in chronic infection of skin in the genital, peritoneal, or perirectal region; painless, verrucous lesions; often flesh-colored brown or pink; sometimes in large clusters[62]
Tick bites	Spotted fevers	Rickettsia conorii, other Rickettsia spp	Rhipicephalus spp or Haemaphysalis spp tick bites may transmit R conorii conorii causing Mediterranean spotted fever (also known as

(continued on next page)

Table 3
(continued)

Exposure or Behavior	Disease/Type of Lesion	Frequent Pathogens	Comments that May Guide Development of Differential Diagnosis
			Boutonneuse spotted fever); approximately 6 d after bite: fever, chills, headache, arthralgias, and myalgias with a single eschar (*tache noire*) without lymphadenopathy, accompanied by a generalized maculopapular rash; self-limited after 2–3 wk; endemic in southern Europe (especially Sicily) and Africa. Similar spotted fever syndromes are caused by specific *Rickettsia* spp, each with a limited geographic distribution around the world[49]
	African tick bite fever	*Rickettsia africae*	6–7 d after an *Amblyomma* spp tick bite, fever with multiple eschars (~50%) with a vesicular or maculopapular rash and sometimes aphthous stomatitis develops; in sub-Saharan Africa or the Caribbean; associated with game hunting, safaris, sports, and volunteerism; usually November to April[63]
	Rocky Mountain Spotted Fever (RMSF)	*Rickettsia rickettsiae*	Approximately 5 d after a *Dermacentor andersoni* (western United States) or *Dermacentor variabilis* (eastern United States) tick bite; morbilliform rash then a maculopapular rash starting on palms and soles and progressing to hands, feet, and trunk 2–4 d after onset of a fever and headache (80%), myalgias, nausea, and

		abdominal pain; sometimes purpuric lesions and petechiae; April to September; in all US states, but cases concentrated in Arkansas, Virginia, Missouri, North Carolina, and Tennessee; other tick vectors in Mexico and Central and South America; Flinders Island spotted fever (*Rickettsia honei*) is similar to RMSF in travelers to Flinders Island, Tasmania, Thailand, and Texas[49,64]
Tularemia	*F tularensis*	See preceding comments; can be transmitted by ticks and other arthropods[49,50]
Tick-borne relapsing fever	*Borrelia parkeri*, *Borrelia hermsii*, or *Borrelia turicatae*	Episodic fever syndrome (eg, 3 d of fever followed by 1 wk without), and often a macular rash and an eschar approximately 1 wk after an *Orinithodoros parkeri*, *Orinithodoros hermsi*, or *Orinithodoros turicata* tick bite. Skin lesions with a variety of presentations may occur later (20%); *B parkeri* and *B hermsii* high risk is only at 1500–8000-foot elevation in US coniferous forests in California, Washington, and Colorado in June to September; *O turicata* bites at lower elevations, biting in fall and winter, especially in Texas; risk factors: hiking, living in a rural dwelling, or spelunking (for *O turicata*)[49]

(continued on next page)

Table 3
(continued)

Exposure or Behavior	Disease/Type of Lesion	Frequent Pathogens	Comments that May Guide Development of Differential Diagnosis
Sports	Diving suit folliculitis or dermatitis	P aeruginosa (especially serotypes O:10 and O:6)	Neoprene wetsuits in scuba divers; can prevent infection by showering after diving[39]
	Bacterial skin abscess	S aureus (in US often CA-MRSA)	Associated with football, soccer, weightlifting, rugby, wrestling, fencing, hockey, and basketball; associated with physical contact during play, skin trauma, sharing equipment, or locker room transmission[47]
	Herpes	HSV	Wrestling (herpes gladiatorum), judo, sumo, and rugby (herpes rugbiorum); from direct skin-to-skin contact; see preceding comments[47]
	Dermatophyte infections (Tinea corporis)	Trichophyton spp	Erythematous, squamous medallion pattern with a distinct margin and sometimes pruritis; associated with judo and wrestling (tinea gladiatorum) from skin-to-skin contact[47]
	Warts	HPV	Swimming; contact sports from skin-to-skin contact; plantar warts may results from shower floor exposure[39]; see preceding comments
	Cellulitis	Group A streptococcus	Soccer, football, and rugby; direct skin-to-skin contact[47]

	Aeromonas spp	Mud football or rugby, resulting from soil and water exposure during play[40,41]
Cutaneous larva migrans	Gnathostoma spp, Ancylostoma caninum, A. braziliense, or U stenocephala	Reported in beach sports, such as beach soccer (Spain) and volleyball (Brazil); see preceding for clinical presentation[47]
Insect exposures Myiasis	Human botfly Dermatobia hominis (Mexico to South America); new world screwworm Cochliomyia hominivorax (Central, South America and Florida keys); Tumbu fly Cordylobia spp (sub-Saharan Africa)	Fly larvae embedded in the skin, mature over 5–10 wk as they grow larger; may form small pustules developing into larger, tender furuncles with drainage of serosanguinous fluid or may be in larger wounds (wound myiasis); left untreated, the insect will burrow out from the skin; usually tropical and subtropical regions[29]
Cutaneous leishmaniasis	Leishmania spp	Infection by the protozoon Leishmania spp promastigotes from bite of a sandfly (biting midges, belonging to the Phlebotomus or Lutzomyia families), causing most commonly a single, painful, papulonodular lesion with later ulceration with an indurated, raised border and satellite lesions; lymphadenopathy may develop after 1–2 wk; diffuse cutaneous leishmaniasis shows multifocal, nodular lesions that may not ulcerate; less commonly there can be a verrucous or sporotrichoid pattern; most common in Afghanistan, Algeria, Brazil, Colombia, Peru, and the Middle East[29]

(continued on next page)

Table 3
(continued)

Exposure or Behavior	Disease/Type of Lesion	Frequent Pathogens	Comments that May Guide Development of Differential Diagnosis
	Rickettsialpox	*Rickettsia akari*	Transmitted by the bite of a larval or adult mouse mite; the reservoir for the pathogen is likely the mouse; between 1 d and several weeks later, a painless 1–1.5 cm, erythematous papule develops at the site of the bite that then ulcerates, and an eschar (*tache noire*) develops that leaves a scar; multiple eschars may occur but are rare; regional lymphadenopathy is common; approximately 7 d later, fever, chills, myalgias, photophobia, diaphoresis, and headache are common, which last approximately a week; approximately 48–72 h after the onset of fever, a transient whole-body papulovesicular rash that spares palms and soles and heals without scarring is common; occurs in the United States, Russia, Korea, and Africa[64]

Abbreviations: CA-MRSA, community-associated methicillin-resistant *Staphylococcus aureus*; CGD, chronic granulomatous disease; CONS, coagulase-negative *Staphylococcus* species; GNB, gram-negative bacilli; HPV, human papilloma virus; HSV, herpes simplex virus; IVDU, intravenous drug user; MSSA, methicillin-susceptible *S aureus*; MRSA, methicillin-resistant *S aureus*; SSTI, skin and soft tissue infection; VZV, varicella zoster virus.

ntravenous drug use (IVDU) has been associated frequently with abscesses of the skin, most commonly caused by S aureus but also by mouth flora and contaminants of water used to prepare drugs for injection.[51] These SSTIs can progress to more invasive infections, so it is essential to treat them promptly. More rarely, bacterial spores contaminate drugs themselves, especially heroin, and may lead to a distinctive SSTI caused by Bacillus anthracis or Clostridium spp[51,52,66] (see **Table 3**). Anthrax is a bacterial skin infection that can be caused by direct inoculation of B anthracis spores by IVDU; however, it is also contracted from exposure to contaminated animals or soil. The inoculation lesion in people with exposure to soil, farming, or handling of animals or animal hides is a painless, pruritic papule that evolves into a vesicle that ruptures and ulcerates with formation of a dark (coal-colored, hence the name "anthrax") eschar with edematous borders (**Fig. 9**). The appearance of the typical anthrax skin lesion in IVDU differs from this (see **Table 3**).

Walking barefoot in soil or sand places a person at risk for certain pathogens that differ by geographic region of the world. Among the most common causes of skin disease after travel to the tropics is hookworm-related cutaneous larva migrans. It is caused by penetration of the skin (most commonly on the foot or other parts of the body in contact with sand or soil) from cat or dog nematode larvae, usually while walking on contaminated lake and ocean beaches or soils of tropical and subtropical countries.[29,67]

Dog and cat bites are common worldwide and are associated with polymicrobial SSTIs often including Pasteurella spp, Streptococcus spp, and Staphylococcus spp, as well as anaerobic bacteria (see **Table 3**). In dog, cat, and other mammalian bites, infection with Capnocytophaga spp may cause potentially fatal purpura fulminans.[60,68] Rat bites may transmit Streptobacillus moniliformis, resulting in a systemic syndrome, rat bite fever, with an ulcerating lesion at the site of the bite and an extensive violaceous rash.[61,68] Bites of reptiles can transmit a number of pathogens, but commonly result in cellulitic SSTIs caused by Aeromonas spp.[68] Exposure to armadillos in the southeastern United States may pose a risk of leprosy.[69]

Sexual contact may lead to a host of sexually transmitted diseases. The most common associated with a local SSTI in the genital region are syphilis, HPV (genital warts), and HSV. These have distinctive clinical presentations after the initial infection (see **Table 3**). Syphilis, if left untreated, may progress to secondary and then tertiary

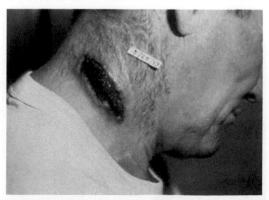

Fig. 9. Typical eschar of cutaneous anthrax with visible edema surrounding the lesion. (*From* the Public Health Image Library, CDC. ID #1934 PHIL CDC. https://phil.cdc.gov/Details.aspx?pid=1934.)

disease. Secondary syphilis has a myriad of skin manifestations that are beyond the scope of this review.[32]

Insect bites in travelers and others can serve as the portal of entry for SSTIs, which present with a broad spectrum of clinical manifestations. Common resultant cutaneous bacterial infections include impetigo, erysipelas, and ecthyma, of which *S aureus* and *Streptococcus* spp are the most frequent causes.[67]

Many tick-borne pathogens, particularly the *Rickettsia*, cause systemic infectious syndromes, including *Rickettsia rickettsiae* (Rocky Mountain spotted fever [RMSF]), several subspecies of *Rickettsia conorii* (rickettsial spotted fevers), and *Rickettsia africae* (African tick-bite fever). However, they also may result in a host of dermatologic manifestations both from direct inoculation of a pathogen and later, disseminated rashes[49] (see **Table 3**). Clues to making a diagnosis in patients with a skin lesion and possible recent tick exposures come from travel history, known exposure to ticks, the species of tick causing a bite (if available), the presence of one (*R conorii*) or more (*R africae*) eschars or their absence (*R rickettsiae*), and the interval between a tick bite and emergence of an eschar[49,70] (see **Table 3**). Tularemia (rabbit fever), which can be transmitted by ticks, has a distinctive geographic distribution and is associated with hunting and other outdoors activities. The inoculation lesion starts as a painful papule, usually on the hands or arms, that often ulcerates with a ragged border (**Fig. 10**). Although not included in **Table 3**, plague, caused by the bipolar staining, gram-negative bacterium *Yersinia pestis*, can present as an SSTI after exposure to flea bites in regions of endemic plague foci with small mammal (prairie dogs, marmots, mice, chipmunks, voles, and rabbits) reservoirs, present in Africa, Asia (including southeastern Russia), and the western United States.[71]

Participation in team sports or shared locker room and shower use can be risk factors for pathogen transmission by direct skin-to-skin contact or by shared fomites or surfaces.[47] Direct transmission of HSV (herpes gladiatorum) and dermatophytes (tinea gladiatorum) are well known risks of wrestling, for example.[47] Transmission of MRSA by shared towels, bars of soap, or razors for cosmetic shaving in locker rooms has been observed in outbreaks on football teams.[72] Shared equipment has been identified as a route of transmission of MRSA from person to person in fencing,[73] and scuba divers are at risk of *P aeruginosa* folliculitis from using neoprene wetsuits.[39]

This review does not address all dermatologic infections that occur around the world, but it instead focuses on the more common etiologies and also on representative infections associated with specific environmental exposures. Recent literature

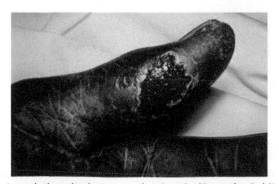

Fig. 10. Tularemia inoculation site lesion on the thumb. (*From* the Public Health Image Library, CDC. ID #1344 PHIL CDC. https://phil.cdc.gov/Details.aspx?pid=1344.)

reviews can be consulted for a more thorough differential diagnosis depending on travel and specific exposures.

HOST FACTORS AND INCREASED RISK FOR SPECIFIC PATHOGENS

There are a multitude of health conditions that increase the risk for SSTIs. The most common of these are listed in **Table 4**. Approximately 40% to 70% of patients with primary immune deficiencies will develop recurrent SSTIs.[74] Recurrent and difficult-to-treat mucocutaneous candidiasis during infancy can be a presenting sign of T-cell deficiency, including severe combined immunodeficiency (SCID) and DiGeorge syndrome. Patients with hyper–immunoglobulin (Ig)E syndrome have recurrent skin abscesses, usually from *S aureus*. These have been described as "cold abscesses," as they present with minimal inflammation and are less tender than expected. Chronic granulomatous disease (CGD) often manifests in early childhood with dermatitis, followed by recurrent folliculitis, furunculosis, and impetigo. Leukocyte adhesion deficiency results in recurrent cutaneous abscesses and pyoderma gangrenosum due to *S aureus*, *Serratia* spp, *Klebsiella* spp, *Enterobacter* spp, *Proteus* spp, and *P aeruginosa*.[74]

For patients receiving immunosuppressive drugs following solid organ or bone marrow transplantation, the likely etiology of SSTIs varies based on chronicity. Typically, wound infections, pyoderma, or the reactivation of herpes viruses occur during the first month after transplantation; in months 2 to 5 opportunistic infections and reactivation of VZV predominate. After 6 months, as immunosuppression is reduced, the spectrum of pathogens approaches that of the general population; mycoses and HPV infections predominate.[83] Cutaneous HPV is a consequence of immunosuppression in bone marrow transplant recipients and has been shown to increase the risk for skin cancer.[84] Interestingly, pemphigus vulgaris seems to be protective against SSTIs in kidney transplant recipients, which may be due to T-helper 1 and 2 cytokines in perilesional skin.[85]

SSTIs are common complications of cancer and anticancer therapy. Ecthyma gangrenosum (EG) is a macular or vesicular lesion that evolves into an area with central necrosis in immunocompromised patients with cancer. In a review of EG, *P aeruginosa* was detected in 123 cases (73.65%) of which only 72 (58.5%) had septicemia; other bacterial etiologies were detected in 29 cases (17.35%), and fungi were detected in 15 cases (9%).[86] EG can occur anywhere on the body, but the most commonly affected areas include the extremities, trunk, face, axillae, and anogenital region. Gram-positive and gram-negative bacteria, *Candida* spp, *Cryptococcus neoformans*, HSV, VZV, cytomegalovirus, *Toxoplasma gondii*, and *Acanthamoeba* have all been identified as etiologies of SSTIs in patients with malignancies.[76] Diagnosis is often challenging, and tissue biopsy and culture are often necessary.

Recurrent SSTIs are frequent in people with diabetes mellitus and can occur even before the diagnosis is made. Elevated serum glucose predisposes to SSTIs.[80] Also, the skin pH of diabetic patients is higher than in nondiabetic patients, which promotes bacterial and fungal colonization.[87] Diabetic neuropathy can make mechanical trauma painless, thereby facilitating microbial entry (see **Table 2**). MRSA colonization is more frequent among diabetic patients, which is a particular problem in diabetic foot infections.[88] Malignant otitis externa (MOE), usually caused by *P aeruginosa*, involves infection and damage of the bones of the ear canal and at the base of the skull. MOE usually begins painlessly, then progresses to an earache with purulent discharge. Microangiopathy and pH alterations due to hyperglycemia play important roles in the pathogenesis of MOE.[89] Thus, optimizing glycemic control is an important strategy to prevent SSTIs in diabetic patients.

Table 4
Host risk factors for skin and soft tissue infections

Host Characteristic	Specific Risk or Pathogen	References
Immune deficiency	*CGD: Staphylococcus aureus, Burkholderia cepacia, Aspergillus spp;* causes granulomas and lymph node suppuration	Lehman,[74] 2014
	Hyper-IgE syndrome: recurrent skin abscesses	
	Asplenia: infection with *Capnocytophaga canimorsus* or *Capnocytophaga cynodegmi* after dog bite	
	Solid organ transplantation: chronologic variation, see text	
Recurrent abscesses or furunculosis	MRSA colonization	Demos et al,[75] 2012
Malignancy	*Pseudomonas aeruginosa* ecthyma gangrenosum	Gandhi et al,[76] 2014
Hidradenitis suppurativa	Can become secondarily infected, particularly with staphylococcal abscess formation; smoking	Sabat et al,[77] 2020
Human immunodeficiency virus infection	MRSA, HPV, *Cryptococcus neoformans,* Kaposi sarcoma, *Bartonella henselae* or *Bartonella quintana* (bacillary angiomatosis), *Histoplasma capsulatum, Blastomyces dermatitidis, Coccidioides immitis*	Crum-Cianflone et al,[78] 2012
Postsurgery	MRSA, gram-negative bacilli	Mueck & Kao,[79] 2017
Diabetes mellitus	MRSA colonization	Lima et al,[80] 2017
Smoking	Higher risk for postoperative infections	Huttunen et al,[81] 2011
Chronic limb ischemia	Infections can be polymicrobial	Dryden et al,[82] 2015
Foreign travel	Hookworm-related cutaneous larva migrans, insect bites, myiasis, cutaneous leishmaniasis, African tick bite fever, tick-borne relapsing fever, for example, see **Table 3**	Hochedez & Caumes,[67] 2008

Abbreviations: CGD, chronic granulomatous disease; HPV, human papilloma virus; Ig, immunoglobulin; MRSA, methicillin-resistant *Staphylococcus aureus.*

Patients with human immunodeficiency virus (HIV) infection have a high incidence of CA-MRSA SSTIs. Possible biological reasons for this include innate immune factors, low CD4+ lymphocyte counts, and detectable HIV viral loads.[78] SSTIs remain a significant problem in outpatients living with HIV, although rates appear to have declined by approximately 40% between 2009 and 2014.[90] Other skin infections associated with HIV include Kaposi sarcoma, bacillary angiomatosis caused by *Bartonella quintana* or *Bartonella henselae*, and lesions resulting from disseminated infections with fungi such as *C neoformans*, *Blastomyces dermatitidis*, *Coccidioides immitis*, and *Histoplasma capsulatum*.

DIAGNOSTIC TESTING APPROACHES FOR SKIN AND SOFT TISSUE INFECTIONS

The approach to choosing laboratory tests to diagnose an SSTI rests on the differential diagnosis prepared from evaluation of the history and physical examination of a patient. For most putative common bacterial SSTIs, such as skin abscesses, impetigo, pyomyositis, and folliculitis, culture of any drainage from the infected soft tissue site usually is adequate to identify the causative pathogen or pathogens. Care should be taken to obtain a culture sample without contamination by commensal skin flora. In the case of a skin abscess, culture of fluid from needle drainage or of fluid expressed at the time of an incision and drainage procedure is optimal and recommended.[6] In SSTIs caused by group A streptococcus, the pathogen can usually be grown in routine bacterial culture if there is purulent drainage present, but if not, an elevated antistreptolysin-O antibody titer supports the diagnosis.

Certain bacterial SSTI pathogens can be cultured but require specialized techniques to identify them in a laboratory. For example, *Capnocytophaga canimorsus* is a bacterial species that causes SSTIs after a dog bite, and because it is an encapsulated organism, risk of progression to a life-threatening syndrome is great for asplenic patients. Culture from a human SSTI requires blood or chocolate agar supplemented with a CO_2-enriched atmosphere.[68] If this organism is suspected, the clinician may need to alert the clinical microbiology laboratory to perform the necessary cultures.

When cultures are not possible or if they are negative and when the presentation suggests a specific pathogen, polymerase chain reaction (PCR)-based tests, antigen detection assays, or serologic tests are sometimes useful.

Serology or direct or indirect immunofluorescence assays are often used to infer infection caused by fastidious bacterial organisms, such as *Bartonella* spp and rickettsia, as the cause of an infected skin lesion in the appropriate clinical setting. Infection with *B henselae*, the cause of cat-scratch disease, can be diagnosed serologically using an indirect immunofluorescent assay.[49] For *R rickettsiae*, the etiologic agent of RMSF, an indirect immunofluorescence assay of biopsied tissue specimens is 90% sensitive 10 to 14 days after the onset of illness. A fourfold rise in antibody titers taken 3 weeks apart confirms the diagnosis. A PCR assay of a skin or organ biopsy specimen also can be used to detect *R rickettsiae*.[64] *R conorii*, the etiology of Mediterranean spotted fever and other spotted fever syndromes, is usually diagnosed with a serologic test or PCR assay on tissue. Similar specific assays are available for *R africae*. For *Rickettsia akari* (the cause of rickettsialpox), an indirect fluorescent antibody assay and complement fixation assay are available to measure acute and convalescent antibodies. A fourfold increase, or greater than 1:64 dilution of IgG, is considered diagnostic.[64]

For certain bacterial pathogens, serology is used more often than culture because culture poses specific logistical difficulties. For example, *Francisella tularensis*, the cause of tularemia, can be readily grown in culture from a tissue specimen, but if grown, it requires special infection control precautions in the clinical laboratory, as it can readily spread to cause an outbreak of tularemia in laboratory personnel. *F tularensis* serologic testing can be used as an alternative to culture; if there is an infection, we expect a >1:20 antibody titer or a fourfold increase in titer from acute to convalescent sera as well as a single titer greater than 1:160.[50] There are similar laboratory safety concerns in the diagnosis of an anthrax soft tissue infection caused by *B anthracis*.[91]

Many fungal pathogens causing SSTIs can often be grown in culture in the laboratory. *Candida* spp grow readily. *Malassezia furfur*, the causative agent of tinea versicolor, grows optimally with the addition of lipids to the culture media, and olive oil is sometimes used for this purpose. *Aspergillus* spp, *Mucor* spp, and *Rhizopus* spp, relatively rare causes of fungal SSTIs, usually in immunocompromised hosts, can also be cultured and are often identified morphologically after culture or histologically in tissue on microscopy. Serologic testing is used to detect certain other fungal pathogens, including *B dermatitidis* and *H capsulatum*, which may disseminate to the skin from the blood. Antigen tests for *Histoplasma* are available from blood and urine, whereas for *C neoformans* (a rare cause of skin infection mostly in immunocompromised hosts) antigen tests are available from blood and cerebrospinal fluid.

Borrelia spp, like other spirochetes, are difficult to culture. For *Borrelia parkeri*, *Borrelia hermsii*, or *Borrelia turicatae*, causes of relapsing fever, the organisms can be seen on Giemsa- or Wright-stained peripheral blood smear during fever. Serologic tests are also available.[49,92] Syphilis is diagnosed using serologic tests (Rapid Plasma Reagin [RPR], venereal disease research laboratory [VDRL]), a direct fluorescent treponemal antibody test (FTA-ABS), nucleic acid amplification test, or dark field microscopy on a swab sample obtained from a primary chancre, which is usually teaming with organisms.[32]

Suspected mycobacterial skin infections are often diagnosed by a culture of biopsied material from the site of an SSTI on appropriate acid-fast bacilli (AFB) nutrient broth or agar. Whether or not cultures grow a pathogen, histology on a biopsy specimen with a Fite stain or the Kinyoun or Ziehl-Neelsen carbol fuchsin stain for AFB may reveal the presence of the organism. Species identification can then be performed by commercial PCR tests or for some species, gene probe assays. Alternatively 16S ribosomal RNA sequencing on tissue may reveal the species. Some species, such as *Mycobacterium ulcerans* (the cause of Buruli ulcer), are difficult to culture, particularly in resource-limited settings where it is most common, and thus Buruli ulcer is usually diagnosed clinically.[28]

Insect parasites often can be diagnosed after removal by gross evaluation or by light microscopy. For example, scabies is diagnosed clinically or the organism can be examined microscopically. Tungiasis, an infection by a sand flea, *Tunga penetrans*, is diagnosed clinically or by stereoscopic microscopy of the expelled flea.[29] Amebic skin infections, which are rare but can occur worldwide after exposure to fresh water, can also be diagnosed under light microscopy, which shows the typical double-walled cysts and trophozoites of *Acanthamoeba* spp or *Balamuthia mandrillaris*. Periodic acid–Schiff and Grocott methenamine silver stains may be useful in identifying these species in tissue. *Acanthamoeba* spp can be cultured from a clinical specimen in tap water with an overlay of *E coli*. A PCR assay also is available to identify the amebae in tissue specimens.[29]

Cutaneous leishmaniasis is often diagnosed with skin scrapings or biopsies showing macrophages with phagocytosed *Leishmania* amastigotes on microscopy after hematoxylin and eosin staining or, alternatively, with histochemical stains. Culture of *Leishmania* is possible but difficult. Hamster inoculation has also been used diagnostically. PCR assays can demonstrate the presence of the parasite in biopsied tissue.[29]

Radiographic studies can be used to identify the extent and location of SSTIs. For uncomplicated bacterial SSTIs, such as skin abscesses and cellulitis, imaging in most cases is not indicated. Plain x-ray films in the setting of an SSTI may identify gas in subcutaneous or deeper soft tissues, which would raise concern for gas-forming organisms, suggesting the presence of anaerobic bacterial pathogens. Compared with x-rays, however, CT and MRI scans provide better definition of abscess cavities, necrotic soft tissues that may require debridement, involvement of a bone or joint in an infectious process, or evidence of inflammation in soft tissues not visible or palpable on the physical examination. CT and MRI scans are useful in the diagnosis of myositis if it is suspected but cannot be identified on soft tissue ultrasound examination.[93] CT or ultrasound are also useful in directing needle drainage or biopsy procedures to sample infected soft tissues for diagnostic studies and for therapeutic drainage of deep abscesses (eg, pyomyositis). Interestingly, certain characteristics of skin abscesses seen on ultrasound are associated with MRSA infection.[94]

SUMMARY

The approach to a patient suspected of having an SSTI is complex. These infections may be caused by numerous bacterial, viral, fungal, or parasitic pathogens. Diagnosis begins with an extensive history and physical examination, which enables the clinician to develop a targeted differential diagnosis based on exposures, behaviors, and contacts as well as past medical history, combined with the anatomic location of skin lesions, their time of onset relative to exposures, their morphology on examination, and their evolution over time. Laboratory and radiographic tests are then often useful in confirming a diagnosis.

CLINICS CARE POINTS

- The approach to a patient with a putative SSTI requires careful attention to history, physical examination, and laboratory studies to develop a narrow differential diagnosis
- Past exposures to insects, arthropods, domesticated or wild animals, fish, salt or fresh water, beaches, soil, or spas may provide clues to the etiology of an SSTI
- Travel itineraries often help to narrow a differential diagnosis for an SSTI
- Behaviors such as drug use, sexual activity, hunting, fishing, hiking, swimming, gardening, or obtaining a tattoo place individuals at risk for encountering specific pathogens that cause SSTIs
- The anatomic location of skin lesions on the body and their evolution over time may guide the choice of laboratory or radiographic tests to confirm a diagnosis of an SSTI

DISCLOSURE

M.Z. David has served as a consultant to GSK and to Baxter. R.R. Watkins has served on the speakers' bureau and received grant support from Allergan.

REFERENCES

1. Miller LG, Eisenberg DF, Liu H, et al. Incidence of skin and soft tissue infections in ambulatory and inpatient settings, 2005-2010. BMC Infect Dis 2015;15:362.
2. Edelsberg J, Taneja C, Zervos M, et al. Trends in US hospital admissions for skin and soft tissue infections. Emerg Infect Dis 2009;15:1516-8.

3. Talan DA, Krishnadasan A, Gorwitz RJ, et al. Comparison of *Staphylococcus aureus* from skin and soft-tissue infections in US emergency department patients, 2004 and 2008. Clin Infect Dis 2011;53:144–9.

4. Morgan E, Hohmann S, Ridgway JP, et al. Decreasing incidence of skin and soft-tissue infections in 86 US emergency departments, 2009-2014. Clin Infect Dis 2019;68:453–9.

5. Moffarah AS, Al Mohajer M, Hurwitz BL, et al. Skin and soft tissue infections. Microbiol Spectr 2016;4(4).

6. Stevens DL, Bisno AL, Chambers HF, et al. Practice guidelines for the diagnosis and management of skin and soft tissue infections: 2014 update by the Infectious Diseases Society of America. Clin Infect Dis 2014;59:e10–52.

7. Brink AJ, Richards GA. The role of multidrug and extensive-drug resistant Gamnegative bacteria in skin and soft tissue infections. Curr Opin Infect Dis 2020;33:93–100.

8. Esposito S, De Simone G, Gioia R, et al. Deep tissue biopsy vs. superficial swab culture, including microbial loading determination, in the microbiological assessment of skin and soft tissue infections (SSTIs). J Chemother 2017;29:154–8.

9. Bystritsky R, Chambers H. Cellulitis and soft tissue infections. Ann Intern Med 2018;168:ITC17–32.

10. Ramdass P, Mullick S, Farber HF. Viral skin diseases. Prim Care 2015;42:517–67.

11. Sachdeva M, Gianotti R, Shah M, et al. Cutaneous manifestations of COVID-19: report of three cases and a review of literature. J Dermatol Sci 2020;98(2):75–81.

12. Gunaydin SD, Arikan-Akdagli S, Akova M. Fungal infections of the skin and soft tissue. Curr Opin Infect Dis 2020;33:130–6.

13. Clebak KT, Malone MA. Skin infections. Prim Care 2018;45(3):433–54.

14. Bowen AC, Tong SY, Chatfield MD, et al. The microbiology of impetigo in indigenous children: associations between *Streptococcus pyogenes, Staphylococcus aureus*, scabies, and nasal carriage. BMC Infect Dis 2014;14:727.

15. Weng QY, Raff AB, Cohen JM, et al. Costs and consequences associated with misdiagnosed lower extremity cellulitis. JAMA Dermatol 2017;153:141–6.

16. Clarke MC, Cheng AC, Pollard JG, et al. Lessons learned from a randomized controlled trial of short-course intravenous antibiotic therapy for erysipelas and cellulitis of the lower limb (Switch Trial). Open Forum Infect Dis 2019;6:ofz335.

17. Sullivan T, de Barra E. Diagnosis and management of cellulitis. Clin Med (Lond) 2018;18:160–3.

18. Singh J, Johnson RC, Schlett CD, et al. Multi-body-site microbiome and culture profiling of military trainees suffering from skin and soft tissue infections at Fort Benning, Georgia. mSphere 2016;1:e00232-16.

19. McKinnell JA, Huang SS, Eells SJ, et al. Quantifying the impact of extranasal testing of body sites for methicillin-resistant *Staphylococcus aureus* colonization at the time of hospital or intensive care unit admission. Infect Control Hosp Epidemiol 2013;34(2):161–70.

20. Gaver-Wainwright MM, Zack RS, Foradori MJ, et al. Misdiagnosis of spider bites: bacterial associates, mechanical pathogen transfer, and hemolytic potential of venom from the hobo spider, *Tegenaria agrestis* (Araneae: Agelenidae). J Med Entomol 2011;48:382–8.

21. Chauhan S, Jain S, Varma S, et al. Tropical pyomyositis (myositis tropicans): current perspective. Postgrad Med J 2004;80(943):267–70.

22. Morgan MS. Diagnosis and management of necrotising fasciitis: a multiparametric approach. J Hosp Infect 2010;75:249–57.

23. Al-Qurayshi Z, Nichols RL, Killackey MT, et al. Mortality risk in necrotizing fasciitis: national prevalence, trend, and burden. Surg Infect (Larchmt) 2020. https://doi.org/10.1089/sur.2019.277.
24. Woo TE, Somayaji R, Haber RM, et al. Diagnosis and management of cutaneous tinea infections. Adv Skin Wound Care 2019;32:350–7.
25. Gupta AK, Chaudhry M, Elewski B. Tinea corporis, tinea cruris, tinea nigra, and piedra. Dermatol Clin 2003;21(3):395–400.
26. Ayi B. Infections acquired via fresh water: from lakes to hot tubs. Microbiol Spectr 2015;3(6). https://doi.org/10.1128/microbiolspec.IOL5-0019-2015.
27. Botting AM, McIntosh D, Mahadevan M. Paediatric pre- and post-septal periorbital infections are different diseases. a retrospective review of 262 cases. Int J Pediatr Otorhinolaryngol 2008;72:377–83.
28. Franco-Paredes C, Marcos LA, Henao-Martínez AF, et al. Cutaneous mycobacterial infections. Clin Microbiol Rev 2018;32(1):e00069-18.
29. Norgan AP, Pritt BS. Parasitic infections of the skin and subcutaneous tissues. Adv Anat Pathol 2018;25:106–23.
30. Godshall CE, Suh G, Lorber B. Cutaneous listeriosis. J Clin Microbiol 2013;51:3591–6.
31. Esposito S, Principi N. Hand, foot and mouth disease: current knowledge on clinical manifestations, epidemiology, aetiology and prevention. Eur J Clin Microbiol Infect Dis 2018;37:391–8.
32. Çakmak SK, Tamer E, Karadağ AS, et al. Syphilis: a great imitator. Clin Dermatol 2019;37:182–91.
33. Lappin E, Ferguson AJ. Gram-positive toxic shock syndromes. Lancet Infect Dis 2009;9:281–90.
34. Petersen E, Kantele A, Koopmans M, et al. Human monkeypox: epidemiologic and clinical characteristics, diagnosis, and prevention. Infect Dis Clin North Am 2019;33:1027–43.
35. Read RC. *Neisseria meningitidis* and meningococcal disease: recent discoveries and innovations. Curr Opin Infect Dis 2019;32:601–8.
36. Madison-Antenucci S, Kramer LD, Gebhardt LL, et al. Emerging tick-borne diseases. Clin Microbiol Rev 2020;33:e00083-18.
37. Vairo F, Haider N, Kock R, et al. Chikungunya: epidemiology, pathogenesis, clinical features, management, and prevention. Infect Dis Clin North Am 2019;33:1003–25.
38. Hagedorn JC, Wessells H. A contemporary update on Fournier's gangrene. Nat Rev Urol 2017;14:205–14.
39. Tlougan BE, Podjasek JO, Adams BB. Aquatic sports dermatoses: part 1. in the water: freshwater dermatoses. Int J Dermatol 2010;49:874–85.
40. Stürchler DA. Exposure: a guide to sources of infections. Washington (DC): ASM Press; 2006.
41. Diaz JH. Skin and soft tissue infections following marine injuries and exposures in travelers. J Travel Med 2014;21:207–13.
42. Hiransuthikul N, Tantisiriwat W, Lertutsahakul K, et al. Skin and soft-tissue infections among tsunami survivors in southern Thailand. Clin Infect Dis 2005;41:e93–6.
43. Permpalung N, Worasilchai N, Chindamporn A. Human pythiosis: emergence of fungal-like organism. Mycopathologia 2019. https://doi.org/10.1007/s11046-019-00412-0.
44. Gassiep I, Armstrong M, Norton R. Human melioidosis. Clin Microbiol Rev 2020;33:e00006-19.

45. Sweeney DA, Hicks CW, Cui X, et al. Anthrax infection. Am J Respir Crit Care Med 2011;184:1333–41.
46. Barros MB, de Almeida Paes R, Schubach AO. *Sporothrix schenckii* and sporotrichosis. Clin Microbiol Rev 2011;24:633–54.
47. Grosset-Janin A, Nicolas X, Saraux A. Sport and infectious risk: a systematic review of the literature over 20 years. Med Mal Infect 2012;42:533–44.
48. Haedersdal M, Stenderup J, Møller B, et al. An outbreak of tinea capitis in a child care centre. Dan Med Bull 2003;50:83–4.
49. Dana AN. Diagnosis and treatment of tick infestation and tick-borne diseases with cutaneous manifestations. Dermatol Ther 2009;22:293–326.
50. Carvalho CL, Lopes de Carvalho I, Zé-Zé L, et al. Tularaemia: a challenging zoonosis. Comp Immunol Microbiol Infect Dis 2014;37:85–96.
51. Kaushik KS, Kapila K, Praharaj AK. Shooting up: the interface of microbial infections and drug abuse. J Med Microbiol 2011;60(Pt 4):408–22.
52. Ramsay CN, Stirling A, Smith J, et al. An outbreak of infection with *Bacillus anthracis* in injecting drug users in Scotland. Euro Surveill 2010;15:19465.
53. Monk AB, Curtis S, Paul J, et al. Genetic analysis of *Staphylococcus aureus* from intravenous drug user lesions. J Med Microbiol 2004;53(Pt 3):223–7.
54. Gilbert M, MacDonald J, Gregson D, et al. Outbreak in Alberta of community-acquired (USA300) methicillin-resistant *Staphylococcus aureus* in people with a history of drug use, homelessness or incarceration. CMAJ 2006;175:149–54.
55. Bassetti S, Hoffmann M, Bucher HC, et al. Infections requiring hospitalization of injection drug users who participated in an injection opiate maintenance program. Clin Infect Dis 2002;34:711–3.
56. Feldmeier H, Schuster A. Mini review: hookworm-related cutaneous larva migrans. Eur J Clin Microbiol Infect Dis 2012;31:915–8.
57. Lichon V, Khachemoune A. Mycetoma: a review. Am J Clin Dermatol 2006;7:315–21.
58. Serup J, Carlsen KH, Sepehri M. Tattoo complaints and complications: diagnosis and clinical spectrum. Curr Probl Dermatol 2015;48:48–60.
59. Rothe K, Tsokos M, Handrick W. Animal and human bite wounds. Dtsch Arztebl Int 2015;112:433–43.
60. Talan DA, Citron DM, Abrahamian FM, et al. Bacteriologic analysis of infected dog and cat bites. Emergency Medicine Animal Bite Infection Study Group. N Engl J Med 1999;340:85–92.
61. Elliott SP. Rat bite fever and *Streptobacillus moniliformis*. Clin Microbiol Rev 2007;20:13–22.
62. Sendagorta-Cudós E, Burgos-Cibrián J, Rodríguez-Iglesias M. Genital infections due to the human papillomavirus. Infecciones genitales por el virus del papiloma humano. Enferm Infecc Microbiol Clin 2019;37:324–34.
63. Frean J, Grayson W. South African tick bite fever: an overview. Dermatopathology (Basel) 2019;6:70–6.
64. Blanton LS. The rickettsioses: a practical update. Infect Dis Clin North Am 2019;33:213–29.
65. Baker-Austin C, Oliver JD, Alam M, et al. *Vibrio spp.* infections. Nat Rev Dis Primers 2018;4:8.
66. Berger T, Kassirer M, Aran AA. Injectional anthrax - new presentation of an old disease. Euro Surveill 2014;19:20877.
67. Hochedez P, Caumes E. Common skin infections in travelers. J Travel Med 2008;15:252–62.

68. Abrahamian FM, Goldstein EJ. Microbiology of animal bite wound infections. Clin Microbiol Rev 2011;24:231–46.
69. Oliveira IVPM, Deps PD, Antunes JMAP. Armadillos and leprosy: from infection to biological model. Rev Inst Med Trop Sao Paulo 2019;61:e44.
70. Wood H, Artsob H. Spotted fever group rickettsiae: a brief review and a Canadian perspective. Zoonoses Public Health 2012;59(Suppl 2):65–79.
71. Vallès X, Stenseth NC, Demeure C, et al. Human plague: an old scourge that needs new answers. PLoS Negl Trop Dis 2020;14:e0008251.
72. Kazakova SV, Hageman JC, Matava M, et al. A clone of methicillin-resistant *Staphylococcus aureus* among professional football players. N Engl J Med 2005;352:468–75.
73. Centers for Disease Control and Prevention. Methicillin-resistant *Staphylococcus aureus* infections among competitive sports participants—Colorado, Indiana, Pennsylvania, and Los Angeles County, 2000-2003. MMWR Morb Mortal Wkly Rep 2003;52:793–5.
74. Lehman H. Skin manifestations of primary immune deficiency. Clin Rev Allergy Immunol 2014;46:112–9.
75. Demos M, McLeod MP, Nouri K. Recurrent furunculosis: a review of the literature. Br J Dermatol 2012;167:725–32.
76. Gandhi M, Brieva JC, Lacouture ME. Dermatologic infections in cancer patients. Cancer Treat Res 2014;161:299–317.
77. Sabat R, Jemec GBE, Matusiak Ł, et al. Hidradenitis suppurativa. Nat Rev Dis Primers 2020;6:18.
78. Crum-Cianflone NF, Grandits G, Weintrob A, et al. Skin and soft tissue infections among HIV-infected persons in the late combination antiretroviral therapy era. Int J STD AIDS 2012;23:507–11.
79. Mueck KM, Kao LS. Patients at high-risk for surgical site infection. Surg Infect (Larchmt) 2017;18:440–6.
80. Lima AL, Illing T, Schliemann S, et al. Cutaneous manifestations of diabetes mellitus: a review. Am J Clin Dermatol 2017;18:541–53.
81. Huttunen R, Heikkinen T, Syrjänen J. Smoking and the outcome of infection. J Intern Med 2011;269:258–69.
82. Dryden M, Baguneid M, Eckmann C, et al. Pathophysiology and burden of infection in patients with diabetes mellitus and peripheral vascular disease: focus on skin and soft-tissue infections. Clin Microbiol Infect 2015;21(Suppl 2):S27–32.
83. Ulrich C, Hackethal M, Meyer T, et al. Skin infections in organ transplant recipients. J Dtsch Dermatol Ges 2008;6:98–105.
84. Hampras SS, Locke FL, Chavez JC, et al. Prevalence of cutaneous viral infections in incident cutaneous squamous cell carcinoma detected among chronic lymphocytic leukemia and hematopoietic stem cell transplant patients. Leuk Lymphoma 2018;59:911–7.
85. Sharquie KE, Noaimi AA, Al-Jobori AA. Skin tumors and skin infections in kidney transplant recipients vs. patients with pemphigus vulgaris. Int J Dermatol 2014; 53:288–93.
86. Vaiman M, Lazarovitch T, Heller L, et al. Ecthyma gangrenosum and ecthyma-like lesions: review Article. Eur J Clin Microbiol Infect Dis 2015;34:633–9.
87. Yosipovitch G, Tur E, Cohen O, et al. Skin surface pH in intertriginous areas in NIDDM patients. possible correlation to candidal intertrigo. Diabetes Care 1993;16:560–3.

88. Stacey HJ, Clements CS, Welburn SC, et al. The prevalence of methicillin-resistant *Staphylococcus aureus* among diabetic patients: a meta-analysis. Acta Diabetol 2019;56:907–21.
89. Rubin Grandis J, Branstetter BFT, Yu VL. The changing face of malignant (necrotising) external otitis: clinical, radiological, and anatomic correlations. Lancet Infect Dis 2004;4:34–9.
90. Hemmige V, Arias CA, Pasalar S, et al. Skin and soft tissue infection in people living with human immunodeficiency virus in a large, urban, public healthcare system in Houston, Texas, 2009-2014. Clin Infect Dis 2020;70:1985–92.
91. Zasada AA. Detection and identification of *Bacillus anthracis*: from conventional to molecular microbiology methods. Microorganisms 2020;8:125.
92. Talagrand-Reboul E, Boyer PH, Bergström S, et al. Relapsing fevers: neglected tick-borne diseases. Front Cell Infect Microbiol 2018;8:98.
93. Simpfendorfer CS. Radiologic approach to musculoskeletal infections. Infect Dis Clin North Am 2017;31:299–324.
94. Gaspari RJ, Blehar D, Polan D, et al. The Massachusetts abscess rule: a clinical decision rule using ultrasound to identify methicillin-resistant *Staphylococcus aureus* in skin abscesses. Acad Emerg Med 2014;21:558–67.

Cellulitis

Rachel J. Bystritsky, MD

KEYWORDS

- Cellulitis • Skin and soft tissue infection • Erysipelas

KEY POINTS

- Cellulitis is caused predominantly by gram-positive organisms, most frequently beta-hemolytic streptococci.
- Cellulitis is a clinical diagnosis made on the basis of history and clinical examination.
- Bilateral cellulitis is uncommon and should prompt consideration of alternative diagnoses.
- Cellulitis should be distinguished from purulent skin and soft tissue infections because the latter require incision and drainage.
- In patients presenting with evidence of cellulitis that is rapidly progressive or associated with severe sepsis, necrotizing fasciitis should be considered.

INTRODUCTION

Cellulitis is an acute spreading infection of the skin involving the deep dermis and subcutaneous fat. Cellulitis may be classified as purulent or nonpurulent; purulent cellulitis is defined as cellulitis associated with a pustule, abscess, or purulent drainage. In contrast to nonpurulent cellulitis, however, purulent cutaneous infections are treated primarily with drainage, and antimicrobial treatment is adjunctive. Purulent cellulitis, therefore, may be conceptualized better as inflammation surrounding the primary focus of infection.[1] Erysipelas is defined classically as an infection involving the superficial skin and lymphatics but also may refer to cellulitis involving the face only or may be used synonymously with cellulitis. The distinction between erysipelas and cellulitis is becoming less important because they cannot always be reliably distinguished clinically and increasing evidence suggests a large overlap between these 2 entities.[2,3] US guidelines do not distinguish erysipelas from (nonpurulent) cellulitis in terms of recommended antimicrobials and management.[1] In the preantibiotic era, the mortality rate for cellulitis and erysipelas was greater than 10%,[4] which was reduced greatly with the introduction of sulfonamides in the 1930s and penicillin in the 1940s.[5]

Department of Medicine, Infectious Diseases, University of California-San Francisco, 350 Parnassus, Rm 808B, UCSF Box 0654, San Francisco, CA 94117, USA
E-mail address: Rachel.bystritsky@ucsf.edu

Infect Dis Clin N Am 35 (2021) 49–60
https://doi.org/10.1016/j.idc.2020.10.002
0891-5520/21/© 2020 Elsevier Inc. All rights reserved.

id.theclinics.com

EPIDEMIOLOGY

Cellulitis is a common infection; however, population-based estimates of incidence are limited because it is not a publicly reportable condition. Although there are no specific data on cellulitis as an individual entity, a retrospective analysis of claims-based data from 50 million commercially insured persons between the ages of 18 years and 65 years in the United States between 2005 and 2010 found that the incidence of cellulitis/abscess or erysipelas was 27 cases/1000 patient years in the inpatient and ambulatory settings, higher than the incidence of pneumonia and urinary tract infection combined.[6]

Cellulitis can occur at any age but is most common in middle-aged and older adults.[7,8] In temperate climates, cellulitis occurs more frequently in summer months.[8] Specific risk factors include prior episodes of cellulitis, presence of wounds or ulcers, tinea pedis, chronic edema/lymphedema, venous insufficiency, excoriating skin disease, and obesity.[9–11] Although some studies have suggested that incidence may be higher in men,[8,10,11] others have shown no difference by sex.[12]

MICROBIOLOGY

Because of the difficulty of obtaining a microbiological diagnosis in cellulitis, the exact frequency of certain pathogens, including the relative frequency of streptococci and Staphylococcus aureus in nonpurulent infections, is uncertain. Beta-hemolytic streptococci are thought to cause the vast majority of cases of cellulitis. One 1989 microbiological study of direct immunofluorescence staining of skin biopsy specimens identified streptococci in 96% of specimens from patients with erysipelas and 73% of specimens from patients with cellulitis.[13] More recent studies using serologic testing for streptococci and blood cultures have found that in the majority of episodes of cellulitis, streptococci can be confirmed as the etiologic agent,[14–16] with 96% of episodes responding to beta-lactam antibiotics,[15] suggesting that methicillin-resistant Staphylococcus aureus (MRSA) is not a frequent cause of these infections. One systematic review of patients with cellulitis and positive skin aspirate or skin biopsy cultures found that Staphylococcus aureus was the most common isolated organism (50%–51%).[17] Only 16% of patients, however, had positive skin aspirate or biopsy cultures. Clinical trials investigating the addition of trimethoprim-sulfamethoxazole to cephalexin for the treatment of uncomplicated cellulitis have found the addition of MRSA coverage did not result in a significant improvement in the clinical cure rate,[18,19] supporting the limited contribution of MRSA in cellulitis. Studies examining cellulitis-associated bacteremia support beta-hemolytic streptococci as the most common etiology.[3] Surprisingly, gram-negative organisms appear to account for a larger proportion of cellulitis-associated bacteremia than Staphylococcus aureus (14% vs 11%, respectively).[3] This may reflect a greater propensity for bacteremia in gram-negative cellulitis, which likely occurs with greater frequency in immunocompromised hosts. Of beta-hemolytic streptococci, the most frequently implicated groups are group A (Streptococcus pyogenes) and group G (predominantly Streptococcus dysgalactiae) followed by groups B and C.[14,16] Purulent skin and soft tissue infections, including abscess, most commonly are caused by Staphylococcus aureus with a significant proportion being methicillin resistant.[20,21]

Other pathogens may be implicated with specific exposures (**Table 1**). In immunosuppressed hosts, infection with uncommon pathogens is more frequent (skin and soft tissue infections in immunocompromised hosts are reviewed elsewhere in this issue). In diabetic patients with uncomplicated cellulitis, the microbiology is similar to those without diabetes, with gram-positive organisms predominating.[22] Certain anatomic

Table 1	
Exposures and associated pathogens	
Human bite	*Eikenella corrodens*, viridans group streptococci, anaerobes
Cat bite	*Pasteurella multocida*
Dog bite	*Pasteurella multocida, Capnocytophaga canimorsus*
Rat bite	*Streptobacillus moniliformis*
Laceration occurring in fresh water	*Aeromonas hydrophila*
Laceration occurring in brackish water	*Vibrio* species
Fish handling	*Erysipelothrix rhusiopathiae*

Adapted from Bystritsky R, Chambers H. Cellulitis and soft tissue infections. *Annals of Internal Medicine.* 2018;168(3):ITC17-ITC31; with permission.

variants of cellulitis may be associated with particular pathogens. Historically, orbital and buccal cellulitis in young children commonly was caused by *Haemophilus influenzae* type B, but this has become exceedingly rare since the advent of the conjugated vaccine.[23] Recurrent group B streptococcal vulvar and inguinal cellulitis has been described following radical hysterectomy and radiation therapy.[24–26]

CLINICAL PRESENTATION

Cellulitis typically presents with acute onset of skin erythema, swelling, tenderness, and warmth.

The lower extremities are the most common site of infection, but any area of skin can be involved. Anatomic variants include orbital cellulitis, vulvar or inguinal cellulitis after pelvic radiation or radical pelvic surgery, and abdominal wall cellulitis in morbidly obese individuals. Bilateral lower extremity involvement is uncommon and should prompt consideration of an alternative diagnosis. Lymphangitis (proximal extension of tender red streaking) and tender regional lymph nodes may be observed. Bullae, petechiae, and ecchymoses also may develop. Skin may become dimpled around hair follicles creating a peau d'orange appearance secondary to edema of the skin. Systemic manifestations, such as fevers, chills or malaise, when present, are suggestive of more severe infection. Erysipelas, when distinguished from cellulitis, is characterized by sharp demarcation of involved skin.

EVALUATION

Cellulitis is a clinical diagnosis made on the basis of clinical history and physical examination. Evaluation of the patient should focus on establishing the severity of illness, assessing for factors that may predispose to specific pathogens or recurrent infection, and identifying purulent foci of infection, which will influence antimicrobial choice and may necessitate drainage. Many conditions may mimic cellulitis and misdiagnosis is common, representing an estimated 30% of cellulitis diagnoses.[27] Mimics of skin and soft tissues are reviewed elsewhere in this issue.

Necrotizing fasciitis, an aggressive infection of the deep soft tissue that spreads along fascial planes, should be considered in the differential diagnosis for patients presenting with severe cellulitis or systemic toxicity. Signs that suggest the presence of necrotizing fasciitis include rapidly progressive spread of cutaneous findings, pain out of proportion to physical examination, crepitus, bullae, dusky skin discoloration, and hypotension. These signs are not sensitive for the diagnosis of necrotizing fasciitis and may be late findings.[28] Necrotizing fasciitis is a surgical emergency and a high index of suspicion for this diagnosis, therefore, is critical.

Laboratory testing is not necessary for uncomplicated cellulitis but may be useful for evaluating the severity of illness. Leukocytosis is reported in 30% to 50% of patients presenting to the emergency department or admitted to the hospital with cellulitis.[29–32] Inflammatory markers often are elevated, but this is a nonspecific finding.[29–31] The Laboratory Risk Indicator for Necrotizing Fasciitis (LRINEC) score was developed in the early 2000s to assist in distinguishing necrotizing fasciitis from other soft tissue infections, including cellulitis using readily available laboratory parameters.[33] Subsequent prospective studies, however, of the scoring system have demonstrated poor sensitivity.[34] The LRINEC score, therefore, should not be used to rule out necrotizing fasciitis when this diagnosis is suspected clinically; maintaining a high index of clinical suspicion remains critical.

Superficial swabs, skin biopsy, and needle aspirate cultures are not recommended routinely for (nonpurulent) cellulitis. Skin swabs and superficial wound cultures are discouraged because they are unreliable for identifying the causative organism and cannot distinguish pathogens from colonizers. Skin biopsy or needle aspirate should be considered in patients with significant immunosuppression, unusual exposures (animal bites and immersion injury) or if the patient has failed to respond to antimicrobial therapy. For infections associated with a purulent focus, cultures of purulent fluid should be obtained prior to antimicrobial therapy, although in mild typical cases without a history of recurrence treatment without obtaining cultures may be reasonable.[1]

Blood cultures typically are not indicated in uncomplicated cellulitis but should be considered in patients with immersion injuries, neutropenia, malignancy on chemotherapy, severe cell-mediated immune deficiency,[1] or signs of systemic toxicity. Blood cultures are positive in less than 10% of patients, with cellulitis with reports ranging from 1% to 10%.[29,35–40] These studies are subject to significant selection bias because only patients evaluated in the emergency department and hospital setting for whom blood cultures were collected are included.

Radiologic studies are not required in the routine evaluation of cellulitis but can be useful in identifying drainable fluid collections and assessing necrotizing infection or associated osteomyelitis (**Table 2**). Deep venous ultrasound commonly is used for patients with cellulitis to rule out deep vein thrombosis, but the yield typically is low,[41,42] and compression ultrasound should be reserved for cases in which the diagnosis of cellulitis is in doubt. On the other hand, point-of-care soft tissue ultrasound is simple and low cost; it can be useful in identifying superficial abscesses[43] and is more sensitive than computerized tomography (CT).[44] Imaging for the presence of abscess

Table 2 Imaging[a]	
Ultrasound	Preferred test to exclude underlying abscess, may demonstrate signs suggestive of necrotizing fasciitis
Plain films	Presence of gas suggestive of necrotizing fasciitis (insensitive), may be used to evaluate for associated osteomyelitis (less sensitive than MRI)
CT	Possible role for evaluation for necrotizing fasciitis
MRI	Most sensitive for signs of necrotizing fasciitis, less specific

[a] Not generally required for uncomplicated cellulitis.

should be considered if examinations findings are equivocal or the patient is failing therapy.

Imaging studies also can be helpful in identifying necrotizing infections including necrotizing fasciitis. Plain film radiographs may show gas along fascial planes but are insensitive for the diagnosis of necrotizing fasciitis,[45,46] and findings may not be present until late in the course of disease. CT is more sensitive than plain films for necrotizing fasciitis,[45,47,48] although these studies generally are limited by small numbers of cases. Magnetic resonance imaging (MRI) appears to have enhanced sensitivity for the diagnosis of necrotizing fasciitis,[48,49] but specificity is imperfect and positive findings may be seen in other non-necrotizing infections and noninfectious conditions. Ultrasonography has been investigated as a means of evaluation for possible necrotizing fasciitis[41,50–52]; however, an experienced operator is necessary and performance characteristics have not been well validated, and there is, therefore, insufficient evidence to support its routine use. If there is clinical suspicion for necrotizing fasciitis, surgical exploration should not be delayed while awaiting imaging.

Clinical examination also should evaluate for the presence of predisposing factors, such as fissuring, wounds, maceration, tinea pedis, chronic venous insufficiency, and lymphedema, because such factors may predispose to recurrent infection and should be treated.

MANAGEMENT
Antimicrobial Therapy

Because an etiologic organism is identified infrequently in cellulitis, most treatment is empirical. A majority of patients with uncomplicated cellulitis can be treated with oral antimicrobials. Because most nonpurulent cellulitis is caused by beta-hemolytic streptococci, initial therapy for mild cases should target these organisms. Acceptable regimens for oral therapy include penicillin VK and amoxicillin. Some clinicians choose to include methicillin-susceptible *Staphylococcus aureus* (MSSA) coverage in their initial regimen; options include amoxicillin-clavulanate, dicloxacillin, cephalexin, and clindamycin (although clindamycin resistance increasingly has been recognized in both beta-hemolytic streptococci[53–58] and *S aureus*,[53,54] with geographic variation). MRSA coverage generally is unnecessary for nonpurulent cellulitis. Two randomized controlled trials have shown no differences in clinical outcomes with addition of trimethoprim-sulfamethoxazole to cephalexin for the treatment of uncomplicated cellulitis without a purulent focus.[18,19] Both trials excluded hospitalized and immunocompromised patients and 1 excluded patients with diabetes and peripheral vascular diseases.[19] Guidelines recommend consideration of MRSA coverage for patients whose cellulitis is associated with injection drug use, purulent drainage, evidence of MRSA infection elsewhere, and nasal colonization with MRSA.[1] One small study suggested that MRSA nasal colonization was associated with MRSA infection for those patients admitted with cellulitis who developed purulence, although this study was limited by the small number of patients included with MRSA nasal carriage.[59] Other studies have shown, however, that rates of MRSA nasal colonization are comparable between patients admitted with cellulitis and controls[60] and MRSA nasal carriage has not been shown to predict improved treatment response with addition of anti-MRSA coverage in patients with cellulitis.[19] For patients with purulent infections (eg abscess, carbuncle, and furuncle), an agent with MRSA activity should be chosen (**Table 3**). Oral anti-MRSA agents include trimethoprim-sulfamethoxazole, doxycycline, clindamycin, and linezolid, which ideally should be chosen based on local susceptibility

Table 3
Antimicrobials commonly used for treatment of cellulitis

Antibiotic	Standard Dosing[a]
Streptococci	
Amoxicillin	500 mg PO, 3 times a day
Penicillin VK	500 mg PO, 4 times a day
Penicillin G	2–4 million units IV, every 4–6 h
Streptococci and MSSA	
Amoxicillin-clavulanate	875/125 mg PO, twice a day
Dicloxacillin	500 mg PO, 4 times a day
Cephalexin	500 mg PO, 4 times a day
Cefazolin	1g IV, every 8 h
Ceftriaxone	1-2g IV, every 24 h
Nafcillin	1-2g IV, every 4 h
Streptococci and MSSA/MRSA	
Clindamycin	300 mg PO, 3 times a day[b]
Trimethoprim-sulfamethoxazole	1–2 double-strength tablet, PO, twice a day[b]
Linezolid	600 mg PO or IV, twice a day
Tedizolid	200 mg PO or IV, twice a day
Delafloxacin	450 mg PO, twice a day
Vancomycin	15 mg/kg IV, every 12 h
Daptomycin	4mg/kg IV, every 24 h
Ceftaroline	600 mg IV, every 12 h
Dalbavancin	One dose of 1500 mg IV, over 30 min
Oritavancin	One dose of 1200 mg IV, over 3 h

[a] Dosing may vary by weight and renal function.
[b] Treatment with low-dose clindamycin and trimethoprim-sulfamethoxazole (eg 150–300 mg every 6 hours to 8 hours or 1 double-strength tablet, twice a day, respectively) has been associated with clinical failure in patients with BMI greater than or equal to 40.[62]

profiles. Newer oral agents include tedizolid, delafloxacin, and omadacycline,[61] which have been approved for skin and soft tissue infections and provide MRSA coverage but should be reserved for scenarios where other agents cannot be used. Delafloxacin is a novel fluoroquinolone,[63] which is active against even ciprofloxacin and levofloxacin resistant strains of MRSA.[64] For patients with exposure histories suggesting infection with an unusual pathogen, empiric regimens should include coverage targeting the organisms suggested by the exposure history.

Streptococcus pyogenes commonly is believed to be resistant to trimethoprim-sulfamethoxazole, resulting in the frequent use of the combination of a beta-lactam plus trimethoprim-sulfamethoxazole when there is suspicion for staphylococcal infection in nonpurulent cellulitis. The presence of thymidine in culture media, however, which allows streptococci to bypass inhibition of folate metabolism by sulfonamides reduces in vitro susceptibility to these agents. When cultured on thymidine depleted media, however, in vitro susceptibility to trimethoprim-sulfamethoxazole can be demonstrated.[65] Recent clinical trials suggest that trimethoprim-sulfamethoxazole monotherapy may be effective in the treatment of uncomplicated skin and soft tissue infections. A retrospective cohort of outpatients with cellulitis with or without abscess found trimethoprim-sulfamethoxazole was associated with improved cure rates compared with cephalexin (and no statistically significant difference with clindamycin) in the subgroup with cellulitis without abscess.[66] One recent randomized controlled trial comparing clindamycin to trimethoprim-sulfamethoxazole for the treatment of uncomplicated skin and soft tissue infections showed similar outcomes between both treatment groups. More than half of participants enrolled had cellulitis without associated abscess and no difference in outcomes was seen in the cellulitis-only subgroup.[67]

Patients without evidence of sepsis, altered mental status, or hemodynamic instability can be managed as outpatients. Hospitalization is recommended if there is concern for deep or necrotizing infection, if the patient is severely immunocompromised, or if outpatient therapy has failed.[68] For patients with moderate nonpurulent cellulitis (defined as presence of systemic signs of infection, without evidence of sepsis), intravenous (IV) therapy is indicated. Penicillin G, cefazolin, ceftriaxone, and clindamycin all are acceptable options.[1] Many clinicians choose to include coverage for MSSA for moderate cellulitis requiring parenteral therapy. Patients with risk factors for MRSA, as listed previously, or purulent infection should receive an agent covering MRSA. Broad-spectrum IV therapy, including coverage for MRSA and gram-negative organisms, should be considered for patients with severe or rapidly progressive infection or in the setting of severe immunocompromise. Clindamycin should be added for patients in whom necrotizing fasciitis or streptococcal toxic shock syndrome is suspected. If an etiologic agent is recovered, antibiotics should be narrowed accordingly. For patients requiring parenteral therapy but declining hospitalization, dalbavancin[69] and oritavancin[70] are lipoglycopeptides with broad-spectrum gram-positive coverage, including MRSA; their long terminal half-lives allow them to be given as a single IV dose.

Symptoms of cellulitis may get worse within the first 24 hours to 48 hours after starting treatment but should then begin to improve. Failure to improve after 48 hours to 72 hours should prompt consideration of resistant pathogens or an alternative diagnosis.

Duration of therapy for uncomplicated cellulitis typically is 5 days, which has been shown to have similar cure rates to 10 day courses of therapy for patients whose cellulitis had improved by day 5 of treatment.[71] If the infection has not improved within this time frame, treatment should be extended. The recommended duration of therapy for neutropenic patients with bacterial skin and soft tissue infections is 7 days to 14 days.[1]

Adjunctive Treatments

For purulent infections, incision and drainage should be performed. For cellulitis involving the extremities, the affected limb should be elevated to facilitate drainage and hasten resolution. Underlying conditions that predispose to cellulitis, such as interdigital toe space maceration or fissuring, chronic venous stasis or lymphedema, or tinea pedis, should be treated to prevent recurrences.

Antimicrobial Prophylaxis for Recurrent Cellulitis

For patients with frequent recurrences of cellulitis (defined as 3–4 episodes per year[1]), despite attempts to manage predisposing conditions, antimicrobial prophylaxis can be considered. Erythromycin, intramuscular penicillin, and oral penicillin VK have been studied as potential options for prophylaxis.[72–74] Penicillin generally is preferred given superior tolerability. A meta-analysis of 5 trials (including erythromycin and penicillin) found a 69% decrease in risk of recurrent cellulitis compared with placebo as well as an increased time to next episode.[73] Economic analysis of penicillin prophylaxis has demonstrated cost-effectiveness.[75] Protective effects of prophylaxis do not appear to last once antibiotics are discontinued.

SUMMARY

Cellulitis is a common infection of the skin and subcutaneous tissue caused predominantly by gram-positive organisms, most frequently beta-hemolytic streptococci. Risk factors include prior episodes of cellulitis, cutaneous lesions, tinea pedis, and chronic edema. Cellulitis is a clinical diagnosis and presents with localized skin erythema, edema, warmth, and tenderness. Uncomplicated cellulitis can be managed in the outpatient setting with oral antibiotics. Imaging often is not required but can be helpful in identifying occult fluid collections and evaluating for necrotizing infection. Indications for admission and parenteral therapy include signs and symptoms of sepsis, systemic toxicity, rapid progression, failure of oral therapy, and severe immunocompromise. Recurrent cellulitis is common, and predisposing conditions should be assessed for and treated at the time of initial diagnosis. For patients with frequent recurrences despite management of underlying conditions, antimicrobial prophylaxis can be effective.

CLINICS CARE POINTS

- Cellulitis is caused predominantly by gram-positive organisms, most frequently beta-hemolytic streptococci.
- Cellulitis is a clinical diagnosis made on the basis of history and clinical examination.
- Bilateral cellulitis is uncommon and should prompt consideration of alternative diagnoses.
- Cellulitis should be distinguished from purulent skin and soft tissue infections as the latter require incision and drainage.
- Uncomplicated cellulitis can be treated as an outpatient with oral antibiotics.
- Indications for hospitalization include sepsis, concern for deep or necrotizing infection, infection in severely immunocompromised patients, and failure of outpatient therapy,
- In patients presenting with evidence of cellulitis that is rapidly progressive or associated with severe sepsis, necrotizing fasciitis should be considered.

DISCLOSURE

The authors have nothing to disclose.

REFERENCES

1. Stevens DL, Bisno AL, Chambers HF, et al. Practice guidelines for the diagnosis and management of skin and soft tissue infections: 2014 update by the infectious diseases society of America. Clin Infect Dis 2014;59(2). https://doi.org/10.1093/cid/ciu296.
2. Bläckberg A, Trell K, Rasmussen M. Erysipelas, a large retrospective study of aetiology and clinical presentation. BMC Infect Dis 2015;15(1):1–6.
3. Gunderson CG, Martinello RA. A systematic review of bacteremias in cellulitis and erysipelas. J Infect 2012;64(2):148–55.

4. Hoyne AL, Wolf AA, Prim L. Fatality rates in the treatment of 998 erysipelas patients. J Am Med Assoc 1939;113(26):2279–81.
5. Spellberg B, Talbot GH, Boucher HW, et al. Antimicrobial agents for complicated skin and skin-structure infections: justification of noninferiority margins in the absence of placebo-controlled trials. Clin Infect Dis 2009. https://doi.org/10.1086/600296.
6. Miller LG, Eisenberg DF, Liu H, et al. Incidence of skin and soft tissue infections in ambulatory and inpatient settings, 2005-2010. BMC Infect Dis 2015;15(1):1–8.
7. Abramowicz S, Rampa S, Allareddy V, et al. The burden of facial cellulitis leading to inpatient hospitalization. J Oral Maxillofac Surg 2017;75(8):1656–67.
8. Marcelin JR, Challener DW, Tan EM, et al. Incidence and effects of seasonality on nonpurulent lower extremity cellulitis after the emergence of community-acquired methicillin-resistant staphylococcus aureus. Mayo Clin Proc 2017. https://doi.org/10.1016/j.mayocp.2017.04.008.
9. Quirke M, Ayoub F, McCabe A, et al. Risk factors for nonpurulent leg cellulitis: a systematic review and meta-analysis. Br J Dermatol 2017;177(2):382–94.
10. Dupuy A, Benchikhi H, Roujeau JC, et al. Risk factors for erysipelas of the leg (cellulitis): case-control study. BMJ 1999;318(7198):1591–4.
11. Bjornsdottir S, Gottfredsson M, Thorisdottir AS, et al. Risk factors for acute cellulitis of the lower limb: a prospective case-control study. Clin Infect Dis 2005;41(10):1416–22.
12. McNamara DR, Tleyjeh IM, Berbari EF, et al. Incidence of lower-extremity cellulitis: a population-based study in Olmsted County, Minnesota. Mayo Clin Proc 2007;82(7):817–21.
13. Bernard P. Streptococcal cause of erysipelas and cellulitis in adults. Arch Dermatol 1989;125(6):779.
14. Bruun T, Oppegaard O, Kittang BR, et al. Etiology of cellulitis and clinical prediction of streptococcal disease: a prospective study. Open Forum Infect Dis 2016;3(1):1–9.
15. Jeng A, Beheshti M, Li J, et al. The role of β-hemolytic streptococci in causing diffuse, nonculturable cellulitis: a prospective investigation. Medicine 2010;89(4):217–26.
16. Eriksson B, Jorup-Rönström C, Karkkonen K, et al. Clinical and bacteriologic spectrum and serological aspects. Clin Infect Dis 1996;23(5):1091–8.
17. Chira S, Miller LG. Staphylococcus aureus is the most common identified cause of cellulitis: a systematic review. Epidemiol Infect 2010;138(3):313–7.
18. Moran GJ, Krishnadasan A, Mower WR, et al. Effect of cephalexin plus trimethoprim-sulfamethoxazole vs cephalexin alone on clinical cure of uncomplicated cellulitis: a randomized clinical trial. JAMA 2017;317(20):2088–96.
19. Pallin DJ, Binder WD, Allen MB, et al. Clinical trial: comparative effectiveness of cephalexin plus trimethoprim-sulfamethoxazole versus cephalexin alone for treatment of uncomplicated cellulitis: a randomized controlled trial. Clin Infect Dis 2013;56(12):1754–62.
20. Moran GJ, Krishnadasan A, Gorwitz RJ, et al. Methicillin-resistant S. aureus infections among patients in the emergency department. N Engl J Med 2006. https://doi.org/10.1056/NEJMoa055356.
21. Jenkins TC, Knepper BC, Moore SJ, et al. Microbiology and initial antibiotic therapy for injection drug users and non-injection drug users with cutaneous abscesses in the era of community-associated methicillin-resistant staphylococcus aureus. Acad Emerg Med 2015;22(8):993–7.

22. Jenkins TC, Knepper BC, Jason Moore S, et al. Comparison of the microbiology and antibiotic treatment among diabetic and nondiabetic patients hospitalized for cellulitis or cutaneous abscess. J Hosp Med 2014. https://doi.org/10.1002/jhm.2267.

23. Fisher RG, Benjamin DK. Facial cellulitis in childhood: a changing spectrum. South Med J 2002. https://doi.org/10.1097/00007611-200207000-00004.

24. Chmel H, Hamdy M. Recurrent streptococcal cellulitis complicating radical hysterectomy and radiation therapy. Obstet Gynecol 1984;63(6):862–4.

25. Binnick AN, Klein RB, Baughman RD. Recurrent erysipelas caused by group b streptococcus organisms. Arch Dermatol 1980;116(7):798–9.

26. Bystritsky R, Chambers H. Cellulitis and soft tissue infections. Ann Intern Med 2018;168(3):ITC17–31.

27. Weng QY, Raff AB, Cohen JM, et al. Costs and consequences associated with misdiagnosed lower extremity cellulitis. JAMA Dermatol 2017;153(2):141–6.

28. Kiat HJ, En Natalie YH, Fatimah L. Necrotizing fasciitis: how reliable are the cutaneous signs? J Emerg Trauma Shock 2017. https://doi.org/10.4103/JETS.JETS_42_17.

29. Hook EW, Hooton TM, Horton CA, et al. Microbiologic evaluation of cutaneous cellulitis in adults. Arch Intern Med 1986;146(2):295–7.

30. Krasagakis K, Valachis A, Maniatakis P, et al. Analysis of epidemiology, clinical features and management of erysipelas. Int J Dermatol 2010;49(9):1012–7.

31. Lazzarini L, Conti E, Tositti G, et al. Erysipelas and cellulitis: clinical and microbiological spectrum in an Italian tertiary care hospital. J Infect 2005;51(5):383–9.

32. Raff AB, Weng QY, Cohen JM, et al. A predictive model for diagnosis of lower extremity cellulitis: a cross-sectional study. J Am Acad Dermatol 2017;76(4):618–25.e2.

33. Wong CH, Khin LW, Heng KS, et al. The LRINEC (Laboratory Risk Indicator for Necrotizing Fasciitis) score: A tool for distinguishing necrotizing fasciitis from other soft tissue infections. Crit Care Med 2004. https://doi.org/10.1097/01.CCM.0000129486.35458.7D.

34. Hsiao CT, Chang CP, Huang TY, et al. Prospective validation of the laboratory risk indicator for necrotizing fasciitis (LRINEC) score for necrotizing fasciitis of the extremities. PLoS ONE 2020;15(1):1–11.

35. Ko LN, Garza-Mayers AC, John JS, et al. Clinical usefulness of imaging and blood cultures in cellulitis evaluation. JAMA Intern Med 2018. https://doi.org/10.1001/jamainternmed.2018.0625.

36. Perl B, Gottehrer NP, Raveh D, et al. Cost-effectiveness of blood cultures for adult patients with cellulitis. Clin Infect Dis 1999;29(6):1483–8.

37. Lasa JS, Recalde MLF, Finn BC, et al. Bacteriemia en pacientes internados con celulitis. Medicina (B Aires) 2012;72(4):298–304.

38. Lee C, Kunin C, Chang C, et al. Development of a prediction model for bacteremia in hospitalized adults with cellulitis to aid in the efficient use of blood cultures: A retrospective cohort study. BMC Infect Dis 2016;16(1). https://doi.org/10.1186/s12879-016-1907-2.

39. Ho PWL, Pien FD, Hamburg D. Value of cultures in patients with acute cellulitis. South Med J 1979;72(11):1402–3.

40. Paolo WF, Poreda AR, Grant W, et al. Blood culture results do not affect treatment in complicated cellulitis. J Emerg Med 2013;45(2):163–7.

41. Tayal VS, Hasan N, Norton HJ, et al. The effect of soft-tissue ultrasound on the management of cellulitis in the emergency department. Acad Emerg Med 2006. https://doi.org/10.1197/j.aem.2005.11.074.

42. Glover JL, Bendick PJ, Mattos MA, et al. Appropriate indications for venous duplex ultrasonographic examinations. Surgery 1996;120(4):725–31.
43. Squire BT, Fox JC, Anderson C. Abscess: Applied bedside sonography for convenient evaluation of superficial soft tissue infections. Acad Emerg Med 2005;12(7):601–6.
44. Gaspari R, Dayno M, Briones J, et al. Comparison of computerized tomography and ultrasound for diagnosing soft tissue abscesses. Crit Ultrasound J 2012; 4(1):1–7.
45. Fernando SM, Tran A, Cheng W, et al. Necrotizing soft tissue infection: diagnostic accuracy of physical examination, imaging, and lrinec score: a systematic review and meta-analysis. Ann Surg 2019;269(1):58–65.
46. Goh T, Goh LG, Ang CH, et al. Early diagnosis of necrotizing fasciitis. Br J Surg 2014;101(1):119–25.
47. Wysoki MG, Santora TA, Shah RM, et al. Necrotizing fasciitis: CT characteristics. Radiology 1997;203(3):859–63.
48. Schmid MR, Kossmann T, Duewell S. Differentiation of necrotizing fasciitis and cellulitis using MR imaging. AJR Am J Roentgenol 1998;170(3):615–20.
49. Kim KT, Kim YJ, Lee JW, et al. Can necrotizing infectious fasciitis be differentiated from nonnecrotizing infectious fasciitis with MR imaging? Radiology 2011. https://doi.org/10.1148/radiol.11101164.
50. Oelze L, Wu S, Carnell J. Emergency ultrasonography for the early diagnosis of necrotizing fasciitis: a case series from the ED. Am J Emerg Med 2013;31(3):5–7.
51. Wronski M, Slodkowski M, Cebulski W, et al. Necrotizing fasciitis: early sonographic diagnosis. J Clin Ultrasound 2011;39(4):236–9.
52. Yen ZS, Wang HP, Ma HM, et al. Ultrasonographic screening of clinically-suspected necrotizing fasciitis. Acad Emerg Med 2002;9(12):1448–51.
53. Cornaglia G, Ligozzi M, Mazzariol A, et al. Rapid increase of resistance to erythromycin and clindamycin in streptococcus pyogenes in Italy, 1993-1995. Emerg Infect Dis 1996;2(4):339–42.
54. Chen I, Kaufisi P, Erdem G. Emergence of erythromycin- and clindamycin-resistant Streptococcus pyogenes emm 90 strains in Hawaii. J Clin Microbiol 2011;49(1):439–41.
55. Megged O, Assous M, Weinberg G, et al. Inducible clindamycin resistance in beta-hemolytic streptococci and streptococcus pneumoniae. Isr Med Assoc J 2013;15(1):27–30.
56. de Muri GP, Sterkel AK, Kubica PA, et al. Macrolide and clindamycin resistance in group a streptococci isolated from children with pharyngitis. Pediatr Infect Dis J 2017;36(3):342–4.
57. Walsh SR, Ferraro MJ, Durand ML. Clindamycin-resistant Streptococcus pyogenes: report of a case. Diagn Microbiol Infect Dis 2004;49(3):223–5.
58. Lewis JS, Lepak AJ, Thompson GR, et al. Failure of clindamycin to eradicate infection with beta-hemolytic streptococci inducibly resistant to clindamycin in an animal model and in human infections. Antimicrobial Agents Chemother 2014;58(3):1327–31.
59. Hsu MS, Liao CH, Fang CT. Role of nasal swab culture in guiding antimicrobial therapy for acute cellulitis in the era of community-acquired methicillin-resistant Staphylococcus aureus: a prospective study of 89 patients. J Microbiol Immunol Infect 2019;52(3):494–7.
60. Eells SJ, Chira S, David CG, et al. Non-suppurative cellulitis: risk factors and its association with Staphylococcus aureus colonization in an area of endemic

community-associated methicillin-resistant S. aureus infections. Epidemiol Infect 2011;139(4):606–12.

61. O'Riordan W, Green S, Scott Overcash J, et al. Omadacycline for acute bacterial skin and skin-structure infections. N Engl J Med 2019;380(6):528–38.

62. Halilovic J, Heintz BH, Brown J. Risk factors for clinical failure in patients hospitalized with cellulitis and cutaneous abscess. J Infect 2012;65(2):128–34.

63. Pullman J, Gardovskis J, Farley B, et al. Efficacy and safety of delafloxacin compared with vancomycin plus aztreonam for acute bacterial skin and skin structure infections: a Phase 3, double-blind, randomized study. J Antimicrob Chemother 2017;72(12):3471–80.

64. McCurdy S, Lawrence L, Quintas M, et al. In vitro activity of delafloxacin and microbiological response against fluoroquinolone-susceptible and nonsusceptible staphylococcus aureus isolates from two phase 3 studies of acute bacterial skin and skin structure infections. Antimicrobial Agents Chemother 2017; 61(9):1–8.

65. Bowen AC, Lilliebridge RA, Tong SY, et al. Is Streptococcus pyogenes resistant or susceptible to trimethoprim-sulfamethoxazole? J Clin Microbiol 2012;50(12):4067–72.

66. Khawcharoenporn T, Tice A. Empiric outpatient therapy with trimethoprim-sulfamethoxazole, cephalexin, or clindamycin for cellulitis. Am J Med 2010;123(10):942–50.

67. Miller LG, Daum RS, Buddy Creech C, et al. Clindamycin versus trimethoprim-sulfamethoxazole for uncomplicated skin infections. N Engl J Med 2015;372(12):1093–103.

68. Gunderson CG, Cherry BM, Fisher A. Do patients with cellulitis need to be hospitalized? a systematic review and meta-analysis of mortality rates of inpatients with cellulitis. J Gen Intern Med 2018;33(9):1553–60.

69. Boucher HW, Wilcox M, Talbot GH, et al. Once-weekly dalbavancin versus daily conventional therapy for skin infection. N Engl J Med 2014. https://doi.org/10.1056/NEJMoa1310480.

70. Corey GR, Loutit J, Moeck G, et al. Single intravenous dose of oritavancin for treatment of acute skin and skin structure infections caused by gram-positive bacteria: Summary of safety analysis from the phase 3 SOLO studies. Antimicrobial Agents Chemother 2018. https://doi.org/10.1128/AAC.01919-17.

71. Hepburn MJ, Dooley DP, Skidmore PJ, et al. Comparison of short-course (5 days) and standard (10 days) treatment for uncomplicated cellulitis. Arch Intern Med 2004;164(15):1669–74.

72. Kremer M, Zuckerman R, Avraham Z, et al. Long-term antimicrobial therapy in the prevention of recurrent soft-tissue infections. J Infect 1991;22(1):37–40.

73. Dalal A, Eskin-Schwartz M, Mimouni D, et al. Interventions for the prevention of recurrent erysipelas and cellulitis. Cochrane Database Syst Rev 2017;2017(6). https://doi.org/10.1002/14651858.CD009758.pub2.

74. Thomas K. Prophylactic antibiotics for the prevention of cellulitis (erysipelas) of the leg: results of the U.K. dermatology clinical trials network's PATCH II trial. Br J Dermatol 2012. https://doi.org/10.1111/j.1365-2133.2011.10586.x.

75. Mason JM, Thomas KS, Crook AM, et al. Prophylactic antibiotics to prevent cellulitis of the leg: economic analysis of the patch I & II trials. PLoS ONE 2014; 9(2):1–7.

Distinguishing Cellulitis from Its Noninfectious Mimics: Approach to the Red Leg

Briana M. Garcia, BS[a], Carla Cruz-Diaz, MD[b],
Ritesh Agnihothri, MD[b], Kanade Shinkai, MD, PhD[b],*

KEYWORDS

- Cellulitis • Mimics • Pseudocellulitis • Red leg

KEY POINTS

- Misdiagnosis of cellulitis is common; roughly one-third of patients diagnosed with cellulitis are ultimately found to have a noninfectious diagnosis (pseudocellulitis).
- The term pseudocellulitis includes many inflammatory and noninflammatory skin diseases that mimic the clinical appearance of cellulitis.
- Cellulitis is a diagnostic challenge because there is no test or imaging modality that can ultimately confirm or rule it out from consideration.
- There are certain clinical characteristics, laboratory test abnormalities, and diagnostic algorithms that should be considered when evaluating a person suspected of having cellulitis to aid in the confirmation of cellulitis or an alternative noninfectious diagnosis.

INTRODUCTION

Cellulitis is a common clinical diagnosis in the outpatient, emergency, and inpatient settings, accounting for 2.3 million Emergency Department (ED) visits and 10% of all infectious disease (ID)-related hospital admissions annually in the United States.[1] Untreated cellulitis may lead to complications that include extensive tissue damage, necrosis, disseminated infection, septic shock, and death.[2] However, in a cross-sectional study, Weng and colleagues[1] found that 30.5% of cases of "red leg" were misdiagnosed as cellulitis. Pseudocellulitis is a broad term encompassing a spectrum of inflammatory and noninflammatory dermatoses involving the lower extremity that are misdiagnosed as cellulitis.

The misdiagnosis of cellulitis as pseudocellulitis has important clinical implications for patients and health care systems. Of patients with pseudocellulitis, 66% was admitted to the hospital for presumed cellulitis, 92% received unnecessary antibiotics,

[a] University of California San Francisco School of Medicine, 513 Parnassus Avenue, San Francisco, CA 94143, USA; [b] Department of Dermatology, University of California San Francisco, 1701 Divisadero Street, 3rd Floor, San Francisco, CA 94115, USA
* Corresponding author.
E-mail address: kanade.shinkai@ucsf.edu

Infect Dis Clin N Am 35 (2021) 61–79
https://doi.org/10.1016/j.idc.2020.10.001
0891-5520/21/© 2020 Elsevier Inc. All rights reserved.

id.theclinics.com

and 84% had a final diagnosis not requiring hospital admission. Weng and colleagues[1] estimate that 50,000 to 130,000 unnecessary hospitalizations may result from a misdiagnosis as well as $194 to $515 million in avoidable health care spending, 44,000 patients receiving unnecessary antibiotics, and 9000 nosocomial infections in the United States annually. Nearly 1 in 3 of these cases of pseudocellulitis experienced an iatrogenic complication (eg, nosocomial infection, antibiotic-related *Clostridium difficile* colitis, and rarely, anaphylaxis) directly attributed to unnecessary admission and treatment of pseudocellulitis. These findings are corroborated by other studies finding similar rates of misdiagnosed pseudocellulitis.[3] Therefore, the accurate diagnosis of cellulitis versus one of its many mimics is crucial to prevent harm as a result of both overtreatment of cellulitis and the undertreatment of pseudocellulitis.

Cellulitis is a common infection of the deep dermis and subcutaneous tissue, clinically characterized as an acute infection that displays cardinal signs of inflammation, including redness (rubor), swelling (tumor), tenderness (dolor), and warmth (calor) (**Fig. 1**).[4] In patients with darker skin tones, erythema may be more subtle and therefore difficult to perceive (**Fig. 2**).[5] It is a well-demarcated, irregularly bordered superficially spreading skin infection without an underlying collection of pus, and it is typically unilateral.[6,7] It is often caused by streptococci, which sometimes reside in the interdigital toe spaces.[6]

History of trauma in the affected area as well as leukocytosis and tachycardia is supportive of the diagnosis, and some patients will have a fever.[4,7] Predisposing factors include a prior episode of cellulitis, older age, obesity, immunosuppression, new medications, new travel or outdoor exposure, poor hygiene, and comorbidities (diabetes, history of cancer, peripheral vascular disease, lymphedema, history of saphenous venectomy, edema, and inflammatory skin diseases, such as interdigital intertrigo, tinea pedis, allergic contact dermatitis, atopic dermatitis, and stasis dermatitis).[6]

OTHER SKIN AND SOFT TISSUE INFECTIONS

Other skin and soft tissue infections must be differentiated from cellulitis, including abscess, erysipelas, necrotizing fasciitis, and pyomyositis.

Abscess represents a fluctuant collection of pus within the dermis or subcutaneous space, and it may be distinguished from cellulitis through ultrasound visualization. Because abscesses are walled-off areas of infection, they are primarily treated with incision and drainage. Of note, abscess and cellulitis may occur together.[8]

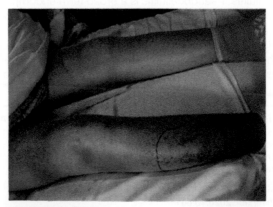

Fig. 1. Unilateral presentation of cellulitis.

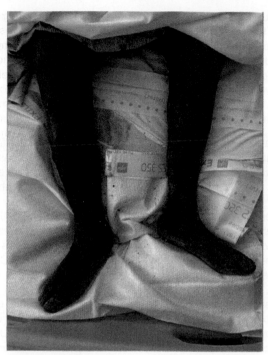

Fig. 2. Bilateral presentation of venous stasis dermatitis with erythema, overlying verrucous changes, and edema bullae. Note that the erythema may be more subtle in appearance in patients with darker skin types.

Erysipelas is considered a subtype of cellulitis affecting the superficial dermis and lymphatics in contrast to cellulitis, which involves deeper reticular dermis and subcutaneous fat. On examination, erysipelas typically has more clearly delineated borders as compared with cellulitis and may appear as a raised, shiny, or waxy plaque.[6]

Necrotizing fasciitis is a rare, rapidly progressive infection of the skin and subcutaneous soft tissue that extends down to and spreads along the fascial plane. It is often polymicrobial, sometimes with gas-producing bacteria causing crepitus on examination. The rash may begin in 1 location and spread to large areas of the body within a few hours. Classically, it is associated with pain out of proportion to the clinical examination because of involvement of the neurovascular bundle lying in the fascial plane; early in infection, the skin changes can mimic those of cellulitis, whereas later in the infection, there are typically dramatic color changes (deep erythema, violaceous changes), bullae, and eventually necrotic changes, crepitus, and anesthesia. Most cases follow minor trauma to the skin; cardiovascular disease and diabetes portend the highest risk.[9] The loss of key neurovasculature in the fascia owing to infection ultimately results in anesthesia of the skin, and also loss of vascular access to deliver antibiotics to the infected tissue, thus requiring surgical debridement. Antibiotics are still used in cases of necrotizing fasciitis for control of infection at surgical margins.

Pyomyositis is a bacterial infection that leads to the collection of purulent material within muscle (psoas, gluteus, quadriceps). Because of the depth of infection, very few cutaneous changes are seen in early pyomyositis, with eventual woody induration, fluctuance, or overlying cutaneous erythema eventually developing. It is most commonly due to *Staphylococcus aureus* infection and occurs primarily in patients who are immunosuppressed, use injection drugs, or have diabetes mellitus.[9] There is also tropical form that affects children or younger adults.

Osteomyelitis occurs when infection deep to the muscle spreads to the bone. Osteomyelitis is often due to the presence of a chronic, nonhealing ulcer with bacterial superinfection that spreads into the bone. It may also occur as a complication of severe or long-standing cellulitis.[8]

INITIAL APPROACH TO THE RED LEG

When evaluating a patient with a red leg, it is important to look for factors that might suggest an alternate noninfectious cause (ie, pseudocellulitis). As a general rule, chronic onset, recurrent nature, presence of scale, slowly progressive course, bilateral presentation, and unsuccessful treatment with antibiotics are highly suggestive of pseudocellulitis.[9,10]

Fever and systemic symptoms are not reliable markers of cellulitis; however, their absence should also prompt consideration of alternative diagnoses. About 30% to 80% of patients with lower-limb cellulitis are afebrile.[6] Leukocytosis and elevated inflammatory markers (eg, erythrocyte sedimentation rate [ESR], C-reactive protein [CRP]) may suggest a diagnosis of cellulitis, although they are also not reliable diagnostic criteria, as they occur in only 35% to 50% and 60% to 95% of patients, respectively; therefore, their absence is less helpful in ruling out cellulitis.[6] Clinical decision-making tools to improve the diagnosis of cellulitis are being developed based on small preliminary studies, including the ALT-70 and NEW HAvUN scores. These aggregate multiple laboratory tests and clinical data points into scores that predict a diagnosis of cellulitis, yet their performance is not yet validated and has not yet been tested across a variety of practice settings. Based on small, single-center studies, the ALT-70 score has a sensitivity of 61.3% and specificity of 70.9% for cellulitis versus pseudocellulitis, and the NEW HAvUN score has a sensitivity of 100% and specificity of 95% in distinguishing cellulitis from venous stasis dermatitis.[2] Although no single test, symptom, or score has emerged as a single diagnostic tool, all of these factors could be considered in the evaluation of each case of cellulitis versus pseudocellulitis.

There is a wide array of inflammatory and noninflammatory conditions that should be considered within the broad category of pseudocellulitis (**Figs. 3–5, Table 1**). Many of these conditions are associated with key morphologic clues (eg, the presence of scale, verrucous changes), other associated features (eg, nail changes, pruritis, systemic involvement, associated conditions), and other sites of involvement that guide the differential diagnosis. Although imaging, laboratory tests, and biopsy are not typically diagnostic for cellulitis, these diagnostic modalities may be quite helpful in identifying a specific diagnosis within the category of pseudocellulitis.

DISCUSSION: A REVIEW OF THE DIAGNOSTIC METHODS

Cellulitis is considered a largely clinical diagnosis, and laboratory tests that are typically helpful in diagnosing infection, including bacterial swab and blood cultures, may be negative in cellulitis.[2] Punch biopsy samples may be cultured successfully, but this is not routinely performed and is typically only used if patients are known to be at risk for specific pathogens, for example, because of known animal or water exposure.[2] The recognition of the high incidence of misdiagnoses has prompted several research groups to develop and validate diagnostic algorithms and techniques that might improve the accuracy of cellulitis diagnosis.[2] These approaches include thermal imaging, clinical prediction models (eg, ALT-70, NEW HAvUN, and Visually based Computerized Diagnostic Decision Support System [VCDDSS]), and

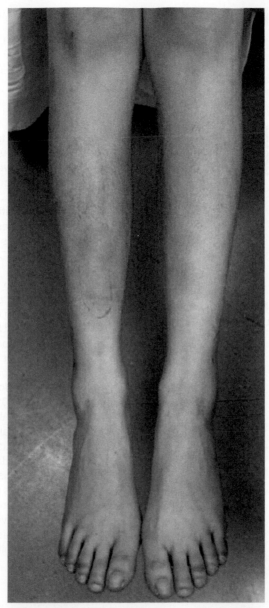

Fig. 3. Bilateral presentation of erythema nodosum.

procalcitonin testing, the efficacy of which has been reported in small, largely prelim-inary studies.[2]

A. Thermal imaging: Because skin warmth is characteristic of cellulitis, signaling acute inflammation, thermal imaging has been tested in the comparison of sus-pected cellulitis to the contralateral site on the body. There are thermal cameras that can be attached to smartphone cameras. In patients with a final diagnosis

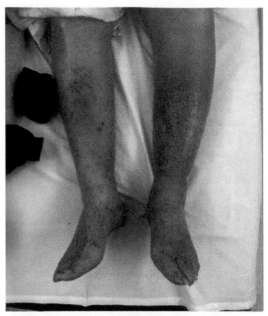

Fig. 4. Bilateral (left > right) presentation of venous stasis dermatitis.

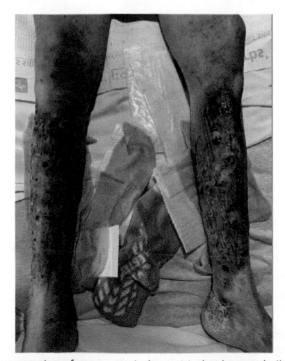

Fig. 5. Bilateral presentation of venous stasis dermatitis that is secondarily infected (as suggested by the numerous areas of crusting).

Table 1
Comprehensive differential diagnosis of pseudocellulitis

Broad Category (Vascular, Inflammatory, or Malignancy)	Diagnosis	Subtype (If Relevant)	Morphology	Diagnostic Markers/ Recommended Testing	Associated Features	Histopathology Findings	Management
Vascular	Venous stasis dermatitis		Pink, scaly and edematous plaques involving the distal lower leg and ankle ± red to brown mottled pigmentation	Duplex ultrasonography: useful for assessing venous reflux and obstruction; skin biopsy rarely necessary	Longstanding venous hypertension and insufficiency can lead to lipodermatosclerosis (see later discussion), other signs of venous insufficiency: edema, varicose veins, vascular blebs	Mild spongiosis, proliferation of superficial dermal vessels, extravasated erythrocytes, abundant hemosiderin (especially in the deeper dermis), and fibrosis	Compressive therapy, leg elevation, topical glucocorticoids
	Acute inflammatory edema		Blanchable, erythematous, and edematous plaques affecting fluid-dependent areas and sparing skin folds, may appear pseudovesicular	Physical examination and associated features	Evidence of edema due to fluid overload or organ dysfunction (cardiac, renal, or liver), low albumin, elevated BMI	Marked papillary dermal edema with an inflammatory infiltrate consisting of scattered neutrophils and lymphocytes with varying numbers of admixed histiocytes, including pale edemaphages with bubbly cytoplasm	Reassurance and discontinuation of antibiotics if started for concern of cellulitis. Helpful interventions include management of fluid overload, compression, frequent repositioning, and increased mobility.
	Phlegmasia[a]		Edema, pain, and violaceous discoloration or skin mottling, 2 types: white (alba) and blue (cerulea dolens)	Doppler ultrasound	Venous gangrene, pulmonary embolism, shock	Nonspecific inflammatory changes	Anticoagulation therapy, thrombolysis, thrombectomy, fasciotomy

(continued on next page)

Table 1
(continued)

Broad Category (Vascular, Inflammatory, or Malignancy)	Diagnosis	Subtype (If Relevant)	Morphology	Diagnostic Markers/ Recommended Testing	Associated Features	Histopathology Findings	Management
	Deep vein thrombosis[a]		Unilateral extremity swelling, erythema, or tenderness	Ultrasound: highly specific and sensitive test	A palpable cord may be appreciated in the calf	N/A	Anticoagulation therapy
	Thrombophlebitis		Erythematous, tender, palpable, indurated, cordlike venous segments	Doppler ultrasound	Migratory form associated with malignancy (Trousseau syndrome), up to 40% cases concurrent DVT	Nonnecrotizing inflammation of superficial veins, distinguished from arterial structures by discontinuous wreath arrangement of muscular layers	NSAIDs, LMWH, local heat, elevation, compressive therapy, ambulation, ± anticoagulation
	Small vessel vasculitis		Palpable purpura; may become papulonodular, vesicular, bullous, pustular, or ulcerated; subcutaneous edema	ESR, complement levels, CBC with differential to look for eosinophils and leukocytosis; biopsy	Fever, malaise, arthralgia, myalgia	Angiocentric, segmental inflammation, endothelial cell swelling, fibrinoid necrosis	Removal of offending agent, topical corticosteroid/ antibiotics, systemic corticosteroids, NSAIDs, dapsone, immunosuppression
	Lymphedema		Unilateral > bilateral edematous extremity; early pitting edema and erysipelas; later nonpitting with overlying fibrosis, epidermal hyperplasia, and verrucous hyperkeratosis	Isotopic lymphoscintigraphy; radiocontrast lymphangiography; MRI > CT demonstrates honeycomb pattern of subcutaneous tissue	Swollen toes with upturned nails, thickening of skin over digits (Kaposi-Stemmer sign)	Edema, fibroadipose deposition, archlike elevations of endothelial cells from connective tissue bed with corresponding opening of lymph vessel lumen to the tissue bed	Compressive therapy, leg elevation, massage

	Hematoma	Erythematous to purpuric swollen plaque; may be warm but without lymphangitic streak	Imaging in coordination with the radiologist may help look for findings that may distinguish between a soft tissue infection and a hematoma	Tenderness to palpation. Presence of risk factors: use of anticoagulation medications or intrinsic coagulopathy	May show extravasation of red blood cells into dermis	Surgical evacuation and debridement of necrotic tissue if present, empiric antibiotics if unable to evacuate hematoma as it may be a nidus for infections
	Diabetic myonecrosis[a]	Swelling, exquisite tenderness, induration	Creatine kinase, ESR, CRP; MRI hyperintensity in affected subcutaneous and muscular tissues	Poor glycemic control	Muscle necrosis, edema, replacement of necrotic muscle fibers by fibrous tissue, lymphocytic infiltration	Rest, analgesia, glycemic control
Inflammatory	*Neutrophilic dermatoses:* Pyoderma gangrenosum, Sweet syndrome, and necrotizing Sweet syndrome — Pyoderma gangrenosum	Initial lesion is usually a pustule or violaceous papule that develops into an ulcer with undermined borders	Diagnosis of exclusion; history, physical examination, laboratories or imaging studies that suggest an underlying associated systemic disease, in addition to skin biopsy for histologic examination and tissue cultures	Pain associated with lesions, pathergy, or an associated systemic disease, such as inflammatory bowel disease, arthritis, monoclonal gammopathies, and other hematologic disorders	Nonspecific, but may include epidermal ulceration with a superficial and deep dermal neutrophilic (or suppurative) infiltrate; stains for organisms will be negative	Corticosteroids, anti-neutrophilic agents, immunosuppressants, and treatment of underlying systemic disease
	Sweet syndrome	Erythematous and edematous papules or plaques	Laboratories demonstrating leukocytosis and elevated inflammatory markers, although in cases associated with malignancies cytopenias may be seen instead	Abrupt onset of cutaneous lesions associated with fever, leukocytosis, arthralgias, and other systemic symptoms	Dermal edema accompanied by a dense neutrophilic infiltrate, with minimal or no vasculitic changes	Corticosteroids, potassium iodide, immunosuppressants, and treatment of hematologic disease if present

(continued on next page)

Table 1
(continued)

Broad Category (Vascular, Inflammatory, or Malignancy)	Diagnosis	Subtype (If Relevant)	Morphology	Diagnostic Markers/ Recommended Testing	Associated Features	Histopathology Findings	Management
		Necrotizing variant	Erythematous and edematous plaques that may rapidly evolve with purpura and necrosis, mimicking necrotizing fasciitis	Blood cultures and skin biopsy for histologic evaluation and tissue cultures	Sepsis-like signs, such as fever, leukocytosis, tachycardia, hypotension, and organ failure. A lack of response or clinical worsening with antibiotics and surgical interventions are a diagnostic clue	Diffuse subcutaneous and dermal neutrophilic infiltrate, associated with leukocytoclasia and edema; necrosis may extend to fascia or muscle; stains for organisms will be negative	Systemic steroids will provide dramatic improvement of skin lesions and systemic symptoms
	Well's		Edematous and brightly erythematous plaques	Skin biopsy confirms clinical suspicion; CBC with differential may show peripheral eosinophilia	Significant pruritus, burning, or pain	Dermal eosinophils and eosinophilic material adherent to collagen bundles	Topical/systemic corticosteroids, antineutrophilic agents
	Gout		Single joint that is warm, erythematous, tender ± edema; first metatarsophalangeal joint of knee most commonly	Plain radiograph of affected joint; biopsy or aspirate with polarizing microscopy; serum uric acid level is not sensitive nor specific for this diagnosis	Nodules in tophaceous gout: vary in size, yellow to tan in color. Commonly on rims of ears, distal toe/finger joints, the Achilles tendon, or the olecranon bursae	Granulomatous reaction surrounding amorphous gray acellular material. Alcohol fixed: brown, needle-shaped crystals	Urate-lowering therapy, anti-inflammatory and antineutrophilic medications. Limit alcohol and high-purine foods
	Contact dermatitis		Erythematous papules, vesicles. Chronic cases can develop lichenification and fissures	Patch testing		Parakeratosis, spongiosis, vesiculation. Eosinophils and edema in the superficial dermis	Topical/systemic steroids, phototherapy, immunosuppressants, allergen avoidance
	Radiation recall (Gemcitabine-associated pseudocellulitis)		Well-demarcated within borders of prior treatment field, ranges from simple erythema to desquamation and necrosis	None	Lung, oral mucosa, gastrointestinal, genitourinary, muscle, and central nerve involvement	Vasodilation, inflammatory mediator infiltrate	Topical/systemic corticosteroids

Panniculitis					
Lipodermatosclerosis	Erythematous, indurated, and tender plaques usually on medial lower leg, over malleolus	Physical examination and evaluation for signs of venous insufficiency; incisional biopsy of most proximal edge if needed	Inverted champagne bottle appearance in chronic form	Septal and lobular panniculitis with lipomembranous changes	Leg elevation and consistent compression; systemic options, such as danazol and pentoxifylline may be considered
Erythema nodosum	Erythematous, tender, subcutaneous nodules usually over bilateral pretibial areas	Testing for most common causes (eg, streptococcal infection, tuberculosis, sarcoidosis): CBC, sed rate, antistreptolysin O titers, chest radiograph; incisional skin biopsy	Patients may have fever, arthralgias, and malaise, or features associated with the underlying cause	Classically, a septal panniculitis with edematous septae, lymphocytic infiltrate, and neutrophils in early lesions	Bed rest, NSAIDs, potassium iodide, colchicine, and immuno-suppressants
Erythema induratum (nodular vasculitis)	Erythematous nodules or plaques, usually on posterior lower legs (calves)	Tuberculin skin test or interferon gamma release assay to exclude tuberculosis; incisional skin biopsy	May be associated with tuberculosis or idiopathic, associated with drugs, or other infections	Lobular or mixed panniculitis with a mixed inflammatory infiltrate and medium vessel vasculitis in most cases	Treatment of underlying cause, and in nontuberculous cases, use of NSAIDs, potassium iodide, and immuno-suppressants
Systemic lupus erythematosus	Tender subcutaneous nodules most commonly located on upper arms and face, and less so on distal extremities	Positive ANA, anti-dsDNA, or anti-RNP, lymphopenia on CBC with differential count, hypocomplementemia, and elevated sed rate; incisional biopsy	Discoid lupus lesions, arthralgias, and Raynaud phenomenon	Predominantly lobular panniculitis with a lymphoplasmacytic infiltrate (can be confused with subcutaneous panniculitis-like T-cell lymphoma)	Antimalarial drugs, systemic steroids in initial phase and immuno-suppressants
Pancreatic	Erythematous nodules over extremities, presenting as single lesions or crops, that can ulcerate or discharge oily material	Pancreatic enzymes (amylase, lipase, and/or tryptase), imaging studies to evaluate for pancreatic pathologies, incisional skin biopsy	May be accompanied by fever, abdominal pain, or arthritis	Mixed panniculitis with "ghost cells" (anuclear lipocytes) and fat necrosis with saponification	Treatment of underlying pancreatic disease

(continued on next page)

Table 1
(continued)

Broad Category (Vascular, Inflammatory, or Malignancy)	Diagnosis	Subtype (If Relevant)	Morphology	Diagnostic Markers/Recommended Testing	Associated Features	Histopathology Findings	Management
		Alpha-1-antitrypsin (AAT) deficiency	Usually painful and ulcerated subcutaneous nodules that may have an oily discharge	Measurement of AAT serum levels, and if low, assessment of AAT variant or phenotype; incisional biopsy	Symptoms associated with AAT deficiency, such as chronic liver disease with cirrhosis, emphysema, and pancreatitis	Lobular or mixed panniculitis with neutrophils causing dissolution of collagen and resulting in a characteristic liquefactive necrosis	Systemic replacement of AAT enzyme
		Cold injury (eg. equestrian panniculitis)	Erythematous to violaceous, tender plaques usually on upper lateral thighs. Lesions may be pruritic and sometimes necrotic	History and physical examination; incisional biopsy if needed	History of horse riding, usually while wearing tight-fitting clothes, during the cold	Lobular panniculitis with a periadnexal lymphohistiocytic infiltrate predominantly located at the dermal-subcutaneous border	Avoidance of tight fitting or uninsulated pants while riding in the cold temperatures. Very potent topical steroids may be used for symptomatic relief
	Pustular psoriasis		Clusters of 2- to –3-mm pustules on a background of erythema	Calcium, monitor for electrolyte disturbances	May appear systemically ill	Subcorneal pustules with collections of neutrophils within stratum corneum	Remove any precipitating cause, supportive measures, oral retinoids and immuno-suppressants, skin-directed therapy
	Insect bite hypersensitivity		Small punctum with surrounding erythema and swelling ± vesicles/bullae. Papular urticarial lesions may be seen with certain arthropod bites	Skin scraping and microscopic examination for scabies mites; high index of clinical suspicion or patient recollection of a bite or sting	Pain, burning, pruritus	Dense wedge-shaped perivascular lymphoid infiltrate with eosinophils	Symptomatic relief with anti-inflammatory agents and oral antihistamines, combined with reduction/elimination of further arthropod bites

Erythema migrans	Red macule, or thin edematous plaques	High clinical index of suspicion in an endemic area + characteristic examination or laboratory test evaluation; *Borrelia burgdorferi* C6 peptide antibody assay (best first test) vs 2-tier serologic testing with enzyme immunoassay to detect immunoglobulin M (IgM) and IgG antibodies. If positive, immunoblot for IgM/IgG antibodies to multiple individual components of the spirochete	Skin lesions typically asymptomatic or minimally pruritic	Superficial and deep perivascular infiltrate, plasma cells. Eosinophils prominent adjacent to bite location. Warthin-Starry stain highlight organism	Oral antibiotics: regimen, duration, and route depending on prophylaxis, early localized disease, mild/severe disseminated, or late disease
Charcot foot	Swollen, warm, erythematous foot with mild to modest pain	Radiographs (low sensitivity for early detection); MRI and bone scan (more sensitive)	Preserved or exaggerated arterial blood flow, musculoskeletal deformity	Degenerating fibrillary remains of cartilage, reactive bone that is, structurally disorganized	Foot immobilization, protective weight-bearing, surgical correction
Malignancy Subcutaneous panniculitis-like T-cell lymphoma	Solitary or multiple subcutaneous nodules	Laboratory tests may reveal cytopenias or abnormal liver function tests; hemophagocytic syndrome may be seen in rare cases. Skin biopsy is recommended	Constitutional symptoms, such as fever, weight loss, and fatigue, may be present	An infiltrate mimicking a lobular panniculitis, composed of pleomorphic T cells that rim adipocytes; necrosis and cytophagocytosis are common	Chemotherapy, immunosuppressive regimens (eg, prednisone and cyclosporine), or radiation for single lesions
Angiosarcoma	Ranges from bruiselike patches to bluish or reddish papules, nodules, or plaques, on a lymphedematous extremity	Skin biopsy	History of congenital lymphedema of affected extremity, acquired lymphedema secondary to venous stasis or morbid obesity, or history of lymph node dissection or radiation	Anastomosing dilated vessels, usually of lymphatic origin in cases associated with lymphedema, lined by endothelial cells with hyperchromatic nuclei	Surgical resection and radiation; amputation may also be considered

(continued on next page)

Table 1
(continued)

Broad Category (Vascular, Inflammatory, or Malignancy)	Diagnosis	Subtype (If Relevant)	Morphology	Diagnostic Markers/ Recommended Testing	Associated Features	Histopathology Findings	Management
	Metastases		Inflammatory carcinoma (or carcinoma erysipeloids) is characterized by erythema, edema, warmth, and a well-demarcated edge, for which it mimics erysipelas	Skin biopsy or clinical diagnosis in a patient with a known metastatic tumor (most likely breast, but has been associated with other tumors)	Skin is usually more indurated than in a soft tissue infection; firm papules or nodules may also be present within erysipeloid plaque suggesting cancer rather than infection	Tumor cells within dilated dermal vessels	Presence of cutaneous metastases carries a poor prognosis; in addition to treatment of underlying malignancy if feasible, symptomatic or palliative treatment targeted to skin lesions may be needed

Abbreviations: BMI, body mass index; CBC, complete blood count; CT, computed tomography; DVT, deep vein thrombosis; LMWH, low-molecular-weight heparin; N/A, not applicable; NSAIDs, nonsteroidal anti-inflammatory drugs.

a A condition that may lead to chronic morbidity and/or mortality and should always be considered and ruled out.

of cellulitis, the affected site's skin temperature was 3.7°C warmer than the corresponding unaffected site (confidence interval [CI] 2.7–4.8°C, P<.00001). Ultimately, a temperature difference of 0.47°C or greater conferred 96.6% sensitivity but only 45.5% specificity.[11]

B. Clinical prediction models are in development, although they have only been subject to limited small-scale studies, and none are strongly validated to date. These include the following:

- ALT-70: The ALT-70 score predicts the diagnosis of lower-extremity cellulitis based on the results of a cross-sectional review of 259 patients admitted with a diagnosis of lower-extremity cellulitis from a single large academic hospital. In patients with "true cellulitis" (ie, having the same admission and discharge diagnosis), 4 variables were most strongly associated with cellulitis: asymmetry (unilateral involvement), leukocytosis (>10,000), tachycardia (≥90 bpm), and age ≥70 years old. Each variable is assigned several points based on predictive value such that asymmetry = 3 points, leukocytosis = 1 point, tachycardia = 1 point, and age ≥70 = 2 points. With a score of 0 to 2 points, there is a ≥83.3% likelihood of pseudocellulitis. More than or equal to 5 points indicates a ≥82.2% likelihood of true cellulitis.[7] This model was also tested in a small prospective study of 67 patients that compared classification measures and accuracy for the ALT-70 model, thermal imaging (as described above), and both of these modalities combined. The ALT-70 score outperformed thermal imaging, and there was a marginal additional benefit to the combination of ALT-70 and thermal imaging. Ultimately, the small cohort size and single-center designs of these studies significantly limit their generalizability, and the ALT-70 score method requires further validation.

- NEW HAvUN Score System: This is a predictive index of 7 factors that were found to be associated with true cellulitis in a retrospective analysis of 57 patients, 20 of whom had cellulitis and the remainder with venous stasis dermatitis. The factors include new onset (<72 hours), erythema, warmth or fever (>38°C), history of trauma, ache and tenderness, unilaterality, number of white blood cells (>10,000). Analysis of cases meeting ≥4 criteria was 100% sensitive and 95% specific for the diagnosis of cellulitis versus venous stasis dermatitis.[12]

- VCDDSS (ie, VisualDx): VisualDx is a clinical decision support application that allows users to input their clinical findings and then suggests a differential diagnosis accordingly. In 1 study, in cases misdiagnosed by the ED teams, the VCDDSS included the correct diagnosis in the initial differential diagnosis more frequently than the admitting team. Although this VCDDSS is likely to also include cellulitis in the differential diagnosis, it may have utility in reminding care providers to consider alternative diagnoses of cellulitis.[13]

C. Procalcitonin: Procalcitonin is an inflammatory response protein that, when elevated, suggests a diagnosis of bacterial infection and guides the use of antibiotic therapy. It has been validated in patients with acute respiratory infections (ie, pneumonia) and sepsis. In the algorithm based on trial protocols, a level ≥0.25 ng/mL suggests higher probability of bacterial infection and indication for antibiotic therapy.[14] Its use has been suggested but has not been validated for use in cellulitis. One study found that procalcitonin levels are not elevated in limb cellulitis; therefore, the study investigators concluded, procalcitonin cannot be used to confirm the diagnosis or use of antibiotics in cellulitis.[15]

Ultimately, none of these clinical prediction models performs strongly enough to be sufficient for diagnosis of lower-extremity cellulitis. They remain largely unvalidated and are therefore not yet widely used in current practice.[2] The NEW HAvUN and ALT-70 scores have limited evidence for their predictive value, and when paired with other pieces of information (clinical evidence, dermatology consult, ID consult), these may provide useful guidance in clinical decision making.

DISCUSSION: ROLE OF SPECIALTY CONSULTATION
Early Dermatology Consultation

The involvement of a specialist in skin and soft tissue infections, such as a dermatologist or an ID specialist, may be important to improve patient- and health care-related outcomes. In a prospective study of patients seen in the ED and in the inpatient setting, with a presumed diagnosis of cellulitis, early consultation by a dermatologist led to a reduction of inappropriate antibiotic use and to a lower rate of hospitalization.[16] Evaluation by a dermatologist carried a change of diagnosis from cellulitis in 39/136 (33.6%) of patients evaluated. The most common final diagnoses were stasis dermatitis (23.1%), contact dermatitis (15.4%), and other variants of dermatitis (10.3%). Dermatology consultation also resulted in antibiotic discontinuation and avoidance of admission to the ED observation unit or the inpatient setting in 92.9% and 85% of evaluated patients, respectively.

A retrospective review of inpatient dermatology consultations of 4 academic medical centers also confirmed the high prevalence of misdiagnoses of cellulitis and demonstrated that involving dermatology in the care of these patients could improve diagnostic accuracy and decrease unnecessary use of antibiotics. Strazzula and colleagues[17] reviewed 74 cases of patients with a diagnosis of cellulitis consulted to the inpatient dermatology service and found that 55 (74.2%) of these patients had been misdiagnosed and did not have cellulitis. The most common final diagnoses were stasis dermatitis (30.91%), contact dermatitis (14.55%), and inflammatory tinea (9.09%). Importantly, a total of 21/55 (38.18%) patients had more than 1 cutaneous condition as found by the dermatologist's examination.

Intervention by a dermatologist has not only proven to be beneficial in the inpatient setting but also in the outpatient diagnosis of cellulitis. In a nonblinded randomized clinical trial, Arakaki and colleagues[18] evaluated 29 patients diagnosed as having cellulitis by their primary care physician (PCP). All of these patients were subsequently evaluated by a dermatologist, and their diagnoses were recorded. After randomization to receive care by their PCP (one-third of patients) or by a dermatologist (two-thirds of patients), only 10% of patients in the dermatologist cohort had true cellulitis and received antibiotics versus 66% of patients in the PCP managed cohort; only 3 of 9 patients in the PCP cohort had true cellulitis, yet all received antibiotics. Although limited by a small sample size, this study adds to the evidence demonstrating that evaluation by a dermatologist may help in discerning patients with true cellulitis from those with pseudocellulitis, in turn improving patient care by providing a correct course of treatment, and avoiding incorrect use of antibiotics.

Because cellulitis is very common and contributes to a high burden of health care dollars as well as patient morbidity, making a correct diagnosis is paramount. Dermatology consultation when available may prove to be a cost-effective intervention that decreases unnecessary hospitalization and improves patient care. Patients with cellulitis may have associated risk factors and physical examination findings that are indistinguishable from those of patients with pseudocellulitis.[13] Expert dermatologic consultation may be needed early in the evaluation of a patient with suspected cellulitis to potentially result in better outcomes.

Early Infectious Diseases Consultation

Evaluation by ID specialists may also improve the diagnostic accuracy and appropriate management of patients with pseudocellulitis. In a study comparing patients referred to an ED specialist with patients referred to an ID specialist for intravenous antibiotic treatment of cellulitis, 40% (54/136) of patients seen by ID were given a diagnosis other than cellulitis, compared with only 11% (16/149) of patients evaluated by an ED specialist.[19] Another important finding of this study was that among those given an alternative diagnosis by an ID specialist, 61% were given an infectious diagnosis.[19] These patients with a different infectious diagnosis may benefit from further therapeutic interventions, such as aspiration and drainage, or from different antibiotic selection or duration.

In efforts to reduce factors influencing cellulitis recurrence, modifiable risk factors have been identified. Jain and colleagues[19] found that the most commonly identified risk factors were venous stasis (38%), tinea pedis (24%), and active diabetic foot ulcer (19%). These patients may benefit from addressing these underlying causes to prevent the recurrence of cellulitis, which include management with nonbacterial therapy.

Jain and colleagues also found that among the patients diagnosed with actual cellulitis, 26% (21/82) of patients were treated for an underlying risk factor by the ID specialist, compared with 3/133 (2%) of patients treated by an ED specialist ($P = .001$). This trend possibly demonstrates a failure to identify underlying risk factors from the ED specialist, which if unaddressed may contribute to recurrence of cellulitis. Consultation of an ID specialist was also associated with a lower rate of disease recurrence (hazard ratio [HR], 0.06; 95% CI, 0.009 to 0.33; $P = .003$), lower rate of hospitalization (HR, 0.11; 95% CI, 0.02–0.62; $P = .01$), and earlier narrowing of antimicrobial therapy ($P = .001$) in comparison to ED specialists.[19]

Thus, involvement of an ID specialist upon making a presumed diagnosis of cellulitis could improve patient outcomes by reducing the rate of misdiagnosis, resulting in adequate therapy in addition to reducing rates of hospitalizations, which may expose patients to further morbidity.

SUMMARY

Misdiagnosis of inflammatory skin diseases as cellulitis places patients at risk for adverse events secondary to hospital-acquired infections and suboptimal outcomes, in addition to unnecessary health care system expenditure. Cellulitis remains a clinical diagnosis, with no single test able to make the diagnosis. Given the broad differential diagnosis for cellulitis and its mimics, it is helpful to use a standardized diagnostic algorithm that takes into consideration a patient's vital signs, laboratory test findings, skin findings, and distribution of skin involvement. Early consideration of alternative diagnoses is important for timely and accurate diagnosis especially in cases whereby atypical signs or symptoms are noted, or if a patient fails to respond to appropriate therapy. Involvement of dermatologists in the care of patients suspected of having cellulitis may optimize high-value diagnosis and management.[20,21]

CLINICS CARE POINTS

- Given the high rate of misdiagnosis, it is important to maintain a broad differential diagnosis when evaluating a patient with suspected cellulitis.[1]
- Certain characteristics should prompt consideration of noncellulitic causes of a "red leg," including chronic onset, slowly progressive course, bilateral presentation, and unsuccessful

treatment with antibiotics.[9,10] Skin biopsy may be useful to confirm the diagnosis of pseudocellulitis.

- Although fever, leukocytosis, and elevated inflammatory markers may not be present in cellulitis, absence of a fever, leukocytosis, and elevated inflammatory markers should also prompt a thorough consideration of pseudocellulitis.[6]
- Early involvement of Dermatology and Infectious Disease specialists may improve the sensitivity and specificity of a cellulitis diagnosis.[13,16–19]

DISCLOSURE

The authors have nothing to disclose.

REFERENCES

1. Weng QY, Raff AB, Cohen JM, et al. Costs and consequences associated with misdiagnosed lower extremity cellulitis. JAMA Dermatol 2017;153(2):141–6.
2. Edwards G, Freeman K, Llewelyn MJ, et al. What diagnostic strategies can help differentiate cellulitis from other causes of red legs in primary care? BMJ 2020; 368. https://doi.org/10.1136/bmj.m54.
3. Hirschmann JV, Raugi GJ. Lower limb cellulitis and its mimics: part II. Conditions that simulate lower limb cellulitis. J Am Acad Dermatol 2012;67(2):177.e1-9 [quiz: 185–6].
4. Patel M, Lee SI, Thomas KS, et al. The red leg dilemma: a scoping review of the challenges of diagnosing lower-limb cellulitis. Br J Dermatol 2019;180(5):993–1000.
5. Rabin RC. Dermatology has a problem with skin color. The New York Times 2020. Available at: https://www.nytimes.com/2020/08/30/health/skin-diseases-black-hispanic.html. Accessed September 3, 2020.
6. Hirschmann JV, Raugi GJ. Lower limb cellulitis and its mimics: part I. Lower limb cellulitis. J Am Acad Dermatol 2012;67(2):163.e1-12.
7. Raff AB, Weng QY, Cohen JM, et al. A predictive model for diagnosis of lower extremity cellulitis: a cross-sectional study. J Am Acad Dermatol 2017;76(4): 618–25.e2.
8. Raff AB, Kroshinsky D. Cellulitis: a review. JAMA 2016;316(3):325–37.
9. Fitzpatrick TB, Kang S. Fitzpatrick's dermatology. 9th edition. New York: McGraw-Hill Education; 2019. Available at: http://ucsf.summon.serialssolutions.com/2.0.0/link/0/ eLvHCXMwY2AwNtIz0EUrE5ItLFIsjU0TTYH RnWKcnGximmaZbJ6abGxmnpqU-Br6lztHVODDUPDwStFQHvqm_NLk4TS8zJRe-NxnzsMTSZNA0MFguwNNF3xDY iwbtq2Y2NTBhYWAF9iMjo6C9MWBfDJg8oafuwPigrfMgW5BqFTdBBtZU0FYDI-Qam1DxhBg5f6DS3ClOkW2ZJVQH48Pxs9WKFFFDpCb5ntlKUQdbNNcTZQxdk WDx07CU-CdiiMAYdkWUsxsAC7M-nSjAomFgaJ5klmhsbJSUbmJiYJ1mkp-KaamFqYmaeZmFsmpqVKMohhN0MKI4Q0AxewHreEjAzIMLCUFJWmykK8JQc NAgAo6mvw.
10. Keller EC, Tomecki KJ, Alraies MC. Distinguishing cellulitis from its mimics. Cleve Clin J Med 2012;79(8):547–52.
11. Ko LN, Raff AB, Garza-Mayers AC, et al. Skin surface temperatures measured by thermal imaging aid in the diagnosis of cellulitis. J Invest Dermatol 2018;138(3): 520–6.
12. Ezaldein HH, Waldman A, Grunseich K, et al. Risk stratification for cellulitis versus noncellulitic conditions of the lower extremity: a retrospective review of the NEW HAvUN criteria. Cutis 2018;102(1):E8–12.

13. David CV, Chira S, Eells SJ, et al. Diagnostic accuracy in patients admitted to hospitals with cellulitis. Dermatol Online J 2011;17(3):1. Avaialble at: https://escholarship.org/uc/item/9gn050rr. Accessed August 28, 2020.
14. Durkin M. Procalcitonin: promise and pitfalls. Avaialble at: https://acphospitalist.org/archives/2018/08/procalcitonin-promise-and-pitfalls.htm. Accessed August 28, 2020.
15. Brindle RJ, Ijaz A, Davies P. Procalcitonin and cellulitis: correlation of procalcitonin blood levels with measurements of severity and outcome in patients with limb cellulitis. Biomarkers 2019;24(2):127–30.
16. Li DG, Xia FD, Khosravi H, et al. Outcomes of early dermatology consultation for inpatients diagnosed with cellulitis. JAMA Dermatol 2018;154(5):537–43.
17. Strazzula L, Cotliar J, Fox LP, et al. Inpatient dermatology consultation aids diagnosis of cellulitis among hospitalized patients: a multi-institutional analysis. J Am Acad Dermatol 2015;73(1):70–5.
18. Arakaki RY, Strazzula L, Woo E, et al. The impact of dermatology consultation on diagnostic accuracy and antibiotic use among patients with suspected cellulitis seen at outpatient internal medicine offices: a randomized clinical trial. JAMA Dermatol 2014;150(10):1056–61.
19. Jain SR, Hosseini-Moghaddam SM, Dwek P, et al. Infectious diseases specialist management improves outcomes for outpatients diagnosed with cellulitis in the emergency department: a double cohort study. Diagn Microbiol Infect Dis 2017;87(4):371–5.
20. Ko LN, Garza-Mayers AC, St John J, et al. Effect of dermatology consultation on outcomes for patients with presumed cellulitis: a randomized clinical trial. JAMA Dermatol 2018;154(5):529–36.
21. Levell NJ, Wingfield CG, Garioch JJ. Severe lower limb cellulitis is best diagnosed by dermatologists and managed with shared care between primary and secondary care. Br J Dermatol 2011;164(6):1326–8.

Staphylococcal Skin and Soft Tissue Infections

Timothy J. Hatlen, MD[a,b,c,d],*, Loren G. Miller, MD, MPH[a,c,d,e]

KEYWORDS

- Cellulitis with abscess • Purulent cellulitis • Suppurative cellulitis
- Staphylococcus aureus skin infection
- Acute bacterial skin and skin structure infections

KEY POINTS

- *Staphylococcus aureus* is the most common cause of purulent skin and soft tissue infections, both abscess and purulent cellulitis; most patients with *these* infections can be managed as outpatients with low rates of complication.
- After incision and drainage, antibiotic treatment for uncomplicated abscess is generally recommended, regardless of abscess size.
- Empiric therapy of purulent skin and soft tissue infections should include coverage for methicillin-resistant *S aureus*.
- For nonpurulent skin and soft tissue infections, there is no evidence that methicillin-resistant *S aureus* coverage improves outcomes.
- No one agent has proven superiority for treatment of *S aureus* skin and soft tissue infection; antibiotic choice should consider disease severity, infection location, host comorbidities, safety, tolerability, availability, and cost.

INTRODUCTION

Staphylococcus aureus, a ubiquitous pathogen, is the most common bacteria involved in purulent acute bacterial skin and skin structure infections (ABSSSI)[1]. Over the years, different terms have been have used to describe what is now referred by the US Food and Drug Administration (FDA) for registrational clinical trials as ABSSSI.[2] In this review, ABSSSI infections will be referenced as skin and soft tissue infections (SSTI), because this term or "skin infection" is more commonly used in clinical care and the medical literature.

---

[a] Division of Infectious Diseases, Harbor-UCLA Medical Center, Torrance, CA, USA; [b] Division of HIV, Harbor-UCLA Medical Center, Torrance, CA, USA; [c] Lundquist Institute for Biomedical Innovation at Harbor-UCLA Medical Center, Torrance, CA, USA; [d] David Geffen School of Medicine at UCLA, Los Angeles, CA, USA; [e] Harbor-UCLA Medical Center, 1000 West Carson Street, Box 466, Torrance, CA 90509, USA
* Corresponding author. 1124 West Carson Street, CDCRC #204, Torrance, CA 90502.
E-mail address: Timothy.hatlen@lundquist.org

Infect Dis Clin N Am 35 (2021) 81–105
https://doi.org/10.1016/j.idc.2020.10.003   id.theclinics.com
0891-5520/21/© 2020 Elsevier Inc. All rights reserved.

S aureus-SSTI (SA-SSTI) can manifest in a wide range of severity, from a mild, self-limiting folliculitis to a severe, life-threating necrotizing soft tissue infection. Recognized as a common commensal organism of the skin, the interplay of the host defense, pathogen virulence factors, and environmental conditions (eg, surgical wounds) all are significant factors of progression to clinical disease. This focused review on SA-SSTI emphasizes diagnostic and treatment algorithms.

PATHOGENICITY

S aureus is a gram-positive bacteria with diverse pathophysiological properties and virulence factors in SSTI (**Fig. 1**).[3,4] Highlighted elsewhere in this article are a few important virulence factors that may explain the success of *S aureus* as a pathogen.

Colonization

Preexisting colonization by *S aureus* is clearly a risk factor of *S aureus* infection in hospitalized patients.[5–7] However, among community-onset SA-SSTI, often patients have

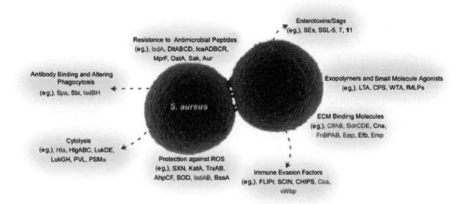

Fig. 1. Virulence factors of *S aureus*. *S aureus* virulence molecules. *S aureus* can produce multiple types of molecules that contribute to virulence and pathogenesis. Many of these molecules have been linked to the pathogenesis of abscesses (*red text*). AhpCF, alkyl hydroperoxide reductase subunits C and F; Aur, aureolysin; BsaA, glutathione peroxidase; CHIPS, chemotaxis inhibitory protein of staphylococcus; Clf, clumping factor; Cna, collagen adhesin; Coa, coagulase; CPS, capsule; Eap, extracellular adherence protein; Efb, extracellular fibrinogen binding protein; FLIPr, formyl peptide receptor-like 1 inhibitory protein; fMLP, N-formyl-methionyl-leucyl-phenylalanine; FnBPAB, fibronectin binding protein A and B; Hla, a-hemolysin; HlgABC, gamma-hemolysin subunits A, B, and C; IcaADBCR, intercellular adhesin subunits A, D, B, C, and R; Isd, iron-regulated surface determinant; KatA, catalase; LTA, lipoteichoic acid; Luk, leukocidin; MprF, multiple peptide resistance factor; OatA, O-acetyltransferase A; PSM, phenol-soluble modulin; PVL, Panton-Valentine leukocidin; ROS, reactive oxygen species; Sak, staphylokinase; Sbi, staphylococcal IgG-binding protein; SCIN, staphylococcal complement inhibitor; SdrCDE, Ser-Asp rich fibrinogen/bone sialoprotein-binding protein subunits C, D, and E; SE, staphylococcal enterotoxin; SOD, superoxide dismutase; Spa, staphylococcal protein A; SSL, staphylococcal superantigen-like protein; SXN, staphyloxanthin; TrxAB, thioredoxin (TrxA) and thioredoxin reductase (TrxB); vWbp, von Willebrand factor binding protein; WTA, wall techoic acid. (*From* Kobayashi SD, Malachowa N, DeLeo FR. Pathogenesis of Staphylococcus aureus abscesses. *Am J Pathol.* 2015;185(6):1518-1527; with permission.)

no demonstrable preexisting colonization with *S aureus*, suggesting direct inoculation or bypassing of the colonization step.[5,7] Overall *S aureus* colonization in the general population is often cited to be around 30% to 40% with nares swabs; however, the addition of extranares surveillance cultures increases the observed colonization prevalence by approximately one-third.[5,7–9] Virulence factors, such as the *speG*, a gene product of the arginine catabolic mobile element locus, and phenol-soluble modulins, are examples of mechanisms that protect *S aureus* against epithelial cell produced defense proteins as well as function to lyse human cells, facilitating adherence and colonization.[10]

Immune Evasion

The primary host defense mechanism against *S aureus* is orchestrated by the neutrophil response. Upon disruption by *S aureus* of the keratinocyte physical barrier, a sequence of proinflammatory cell signaling leads to neutrophil recruitment. *S aureus* inhibits this response and downstream actions of the neutrophils through a variety of virulence molecules that limit polymorphonuclear cell diapedesis (eg, staphylococcal superantigen-like protein 5 and 11, chemotaxis inhibitory protein, SA complement inhibitor), block phagocytosis (protein A or cell wall modifications blocking opsonization), or advert conventional apoptotic pathways of the polymorphonuclear, thus limiting clearance of *S aureus* and promoting invasion.[4]

USA300 Community Methicillin-Resistant S aureus

In the early 2000s, in the United States, SA-SSTI incidence increased significantly and was attributed to the concurrent rise of a new clonal lineage of methicillin-resistant *S aureus* (MRSA), USA300 (**Fig. 2**A, B).[11–13] USA300 possesses a number of virulence factors, but their exact role in infection is controversial. Panton Valentine leukocidin, a toxin that lyses leukocytes, has been strongly associated with abscess development.[14] However, linkage of increased virulence to Panton Valentine leukocidin has been debated because, for example, higher levels of production of Panton Valentine leukocidin do not always correlate clinically with increased disease severity.[15] Additional factors associated with enhanced virulence of the USA300 include alpha-hemolysin, phenol-soluble modulins, as well as genetic factors conferring increased resistance (*speG* gene), which are beyond the scope of this discussion.

Epidemiology and Microbiology

The majority of SSTI presenting to clinical care are cellulitis or abscess, 95% of which are managed in the ambulatory setting.[13] *S aureus* and beta-hemolytic streptococci are the most common pathogens in culture confirmed cases.[16] US hospitalizations from 2001 to 2009 for SA-SSTI increased by 123% (from 57 to 117 per 100,000 people), a change closely associated with emergence of the USA300 clone.[11] Overall, complications related to SSTI are infrequent. However, among patients ill enough to require hospitalization, 23% have complications that include suppurative lymphadenitis, myositis, necrotizing fasciitis, gangrene, osteomyelitis, bacteremia, endocarditis, and septicemia. The highest rates of complications are seen with -device or graft-associated infections (44%), decubitus ulcer (35%), and surgical site infections (24%).[13] Concurrent *S aureus* bacteremia in hospitalized patients with SA-SSTI is reported in up to 6.2% of cases.[17]

Identifying a gold standard microbiologic diagnosis of nonpurulent (nonsuppurative) cellulitis has been difficult. Biopsy and aspiration of nonpurulent cellulitis recover organisms in less than 20% of cases.[18] Serology, blood cultures, and clinical response to empiric beta-lactam monotherapy suggest that beta-hemolytic streptococci are the

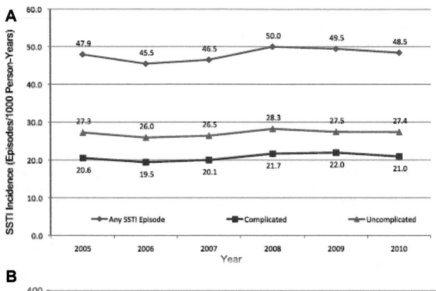

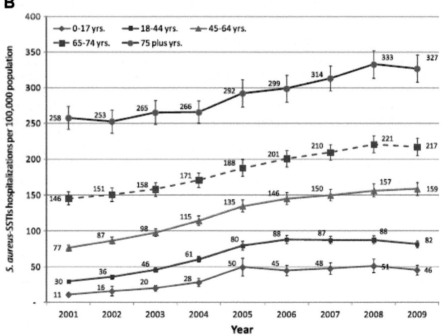

Fig. 2. Incidence of SA-SSTI. (*A*) Incidence of SSTIs by severity from 2005 through 2010. Note: 95% confidence interval bars are not included, because the confidence intervals are very narrow and would not be visible in figure. (*B*) Incidence of *S aureus* SSTI hospitalizations by age group in the United States, 2001 to 2009. (*From* [*A*] Miller LG, Eisenberg DF, Liu H, et al. Incidence of skin and soft tissue infections in ambulatory and inpatient settings, 2005-2010. *BMC Infect Dis*. 2015;15:362; and [*B*] Suaya JA, Mera RM, Cassidy A, et al. Incidence and cost of hospitalizations associated with Staphylococcus aureus skin and soft tissue infections in the United States from 2001 through 2009. *BMC Infect Dis*. 2014;14:296; with permission.)

primary cause of nonpurulent cellulitis (see the section on Nonpurulent Skin Infection elsewhere in this article).[19] However, determination of the bacterial etiology of SSTI based on data collected from large cohorts is limited by use of ICD-9 billing codes, which lump abscess and cellulitis together, and by absence of microbiological data. Culture data may only be available for a subset of those with purulent disease. For example, in a US cohort of nearly 650,000 SSTIs (including purulent and nonpurulent) from 2006 to 2009, only 23% had culture data. Of that subset, 81% had S aureus isolated (50% MRSA and 50% methicillin-susceptible S aureus [MSSA]).[16] In another series of purulent SSTI presenting to the emergency department in 2008, more than 75% of culture isolates were S aureus, of which 79% were MRSA.[12]

Epidemiologically, MRSA is classified as health care-associated hospital onset, health care-associated community onset, and community-associated (CA) MRSA. The clinical usefulness of these categories is unclear. Typically, CA-MRSA causes SSTI; however, outcomes of hospitalized patients with CA-MRSA and health care-associated community onset/health care-associated hospital onset MRSA are similar.[20] We believe, given numerous reports of "community" strains causing health care infections, and vice versa, distinctions between CA-MRSA and health care-associated community onset/health care-associated hospital onset MRSA strains and infections are no longer clinically relevant and have only epidemiologic significance.[21] In contrast, differentiating between MSSA and MRSA is clinically important given (i) therapeutic superiority of a beta-lactam compared with vancomycin in severe MSSA infections and (ii) patients with MRSA may be candidates for decolonization protocols.[22,23]

Commonly observed S aureus SSTI risk factors are outlined in **Box 1**. The most common associations are previous S aureus infection or colonization, recent exposure in a health care facility, or skin-to-skin contact with a colonized individual in the community.[24–26]

CLINICAL SPECTRUM OF SKIN AND SOFT TISSUE DISEASE

Historically, SSTI has been classified into categories of primary pyoderma (including impetigo, furuncles, and carbuncles) or soft tissue infections, separated into erysipelas and cellulitis with or without abscess.[27] Definitions and nomenclature often overlap. For example, erysipelas to some providers is cellulitis of the epidermal layer

---

Box 1
Risk factors for S aureus skin and skin structure infection

Risk Factors Associated with MRSA SSTI[24–26]

- Ethnicity (African Americans, Hispanic compared with Caucasian)
- Socioeconomic lower quintile
- Previous colonization or S aureus infection
- Exposure: hospital, long-term care facility, household contacts
- Contact activities, such as daycare children, contact sports, military
- Comorbidities: diabetes, peripheral vascular disease, cardiovascular disease, chronic wounds, chronic kidney disease, dialysis dependence, intravenous drug use
- Preexisting skin lesions (burns, eczematous dermatitis, etc)
- Hereditary or iatrogenic neutrophil disorder

involving only the face, whereas for others it is used interchangeably with nonpurulent cellulitis of any body location. Impetigo has very distinct clinical characteristics and management. With respect to other SSTI, given confusion with nomenclature from region to region and practitioner to practitioner, we believe the 2 major categories of skin infection should be (i) nonpurulent skin infection (ie, cellulitis), and (ii) purulent skin infection, either abscess or purulent cellulitis.

Impetigo

Impetigo, which is limited to the dermal layer, can generally be managed with local wound care and topical antimicrobial therapy in an immunocompetent host.[28] Mupirocin and fusidic acid are most commonly used, although increasing antibiotic resistance has been noted.[29] Severe cases of impetigo (bullous lesions or widespread distribution) may warrant systemic antimicrobial therapy.[30]

Nonpurulent Skin Infection

Nonpurulent skin infections (ie, cellulitis) are caused primarily by *Streptococcus pyogenes*, with a minor contribution from *S aureus*. The predominance of streptococcal species is largely based on circumstantial data. In systematic review of 607 patients with nonpurulent skin infection, only 4.6% had positive blood cultures, of which 75% were streptococci and 14% were *S aureus*.[31] An investigation using acute and convalescent phase serologic testing for *S pyogenes* (anti–streptolysin-O and anti–DNase-B) or blood cultures in hospitalized patients attributed 73% of cases of nonpurulent skin infection to beta-hemolytic streptococci.[19] In outpatient clinical trials of mild to moderate nonpurulent SSTI, the addition of an anti-MRSA agent to an antistaphylococcal beta-lactam regimen did not improve outcome, suggesting that MRSA does not play a significant role in nonpurulent skin infection.[32–34] These trials support the general impression that streptococcal species are the most common etiology of nonpurulent cellulitis. However, given the potentially disastrous consequences of inappropriate empiric coverage, we recommend inclusion of anti-MRSA therapy in severely ill patients with nonpurulent skin infection.

Purulent Skin Infection with or Without Cellulitis

Furuncles (or "boils") are localized inflammatory nodules of the hair follicle. A coalescence of adjacent furuncles is termed a carbuncle. Clinically, carbuncles are considered to be abscesses. Given the difficulty in clearly distinguishing these entities, we prefer the term purulent skin infection for any skin infection with pus. It should be noted that some patients presenting with "purulent cellulitis" may have self-lanced the abscess before care or the abscess may have spontaneously opened and the pus is present only by patient history. Incision and drainage is the cornerstone of therapy. *S aureus* is the most common cultured pathogen from purulent skin infections.[12,16]

Deep Tissue S aureus Infections

Deep soft tissue infections are commonly caused by *S aureus* either as a single or contributing pathogen. We provide a brief overview of deeper skin and soft tissues infections in which *S aureus* commonly plays a role.

Necrotizing soft tissue infections

Necrotizing soft tissue infections (NSTI) historically have not involved *S aureus*. The emergence of *S aureus* as a cause of NSTI was first described in a case series in association with the CA-MRSA USA300 clone and has since been frequently reported.[35,36] *S aureus* NSTI is more commonly described as purulent at presentation, typically monomicrobial, and may be of milder severity than polymicrobial NSTI given its apparent lower mortality.[35] NSTIs are further addressed elsewhere in this issue.

Surgical site infection

Surgical site infections accounts for 20% of SSTIs in hospitalized patients[13] of which approximately 30% are due to S aureus.[37] Diagnosis and management of surgical site infection is beyond the scope of this article and we refer the reader to current guidelines.[27]

Diabetic foot infections

S aureus is a very common pathogen in diabetic foot infections. These infections are discussed elsewhere in this issue.

DIAGNOSIS OF SKIN AND SOFT TISSUE INFECTIONS

The diagnostic workup of SSTI is predominantly clinical and augmented by results of microbiologic and imaging studies and surgical interventions. The initial evaluation of cellulitis is to determine whether is it purulent or nonpurulent, the latter suggesting a non–S aureus infection. Noninfectious alternative diagnoses, termed pseudocellulitis, such as venous stasis dermatitis or deep vein thrombosis, are typically nonpurulent and should be considered if there are bilateral or atypical features.[38,39]

C-reactive protein and total white blood cell count are often elevated in SSTI, but have limited positive or negative predictive value.[40] In mild-to-moderate cellulitis, blood cultures are rarely positive (approximately 2%) and not recommended.[27,41] In severe cellulitis requiring hospitalization, the rate of bacteremia ranges from 2% to 18%, arguing for the use of blood cultures.[17,27,42]

Imaging may be of benefit. In a prospective emergency department study of 216 patients, ultrasound examination changed management in 71 patients (56%) in regard to the need for drainage of an underlying abscess.[43] Alternative imaging modalities, such as MRI, are less effective at delineating cellulitis from edema, but do provide useful information regarding depth and extent of tissue involvement (such as fascial involvement or bone).[44] Thermal imaging, an emerging modality, compares temperature of the affected limb with the contralateral unaffected limb, may improve diagnostic accuracy to differentiate cellulitis versus pseudocellulitis.[45]

APPROACH TO THERAPY

SSTI treatment guidelines were published by the Infectious Diseases Society of America in 2014, but predated several pivotal SSTI clinical trials and FDA approval of several newer antibiotics.

We believe antibiotic choice for S aureus treatment primarily should be predicated on illness severity and then further refined according to local susceptibility patterns, drug-related costs, toxicity or contraindications, and availability (eg, formulary restrictions). Decision-making processes for admitting patients to the hospital for SSTI is complex, often subjective, and beyond the scope of this article, although in general infections that are rapidly spreading, have evidence of systemic inflammatory response, and have failed oral therapy and worsening should be treated with intravenous antibiotics (see **Fig. 2**). In purulent SSTI, empiric coverage for MRSA is recommended both for oral and for intravenous antimicrobial therapy with pathogen-based targeting of therapy if, or when, culture data are available.

Numerous antimicrobial agents are available for treatment of S aureus SSTI with little consensus and fewer data as to which is best.[27,46–49] A network meta-analysis of randomized control trials from 1966 to 2017 for SSTI (not specific to *S aureus*) found that each antibiotic class had similar cure rates and there was no signal of overwhelming superiority of any drug class (Go-Wheeler MG, Mann SC, Hean S, et al. A network meta-analysis of antibiotic efficacy for the treatment of skin and soft tissue infections. [Submitted for publication]). Therefore, empiric management of SA-SSTI requires an understanding of pharmacokinetic and pharmacodynamics of the different antimicrobial classes, tolerability, side effects, and knowledge of local rates of antimicrobial resistance to inform the choice of empiric coverage to minimize treatment failures.[50]

Antibiotic duration for nonpurulent and purulent skin infections clinical trials has ranged from 6 to 14 days. Antibiotic stewardship advocates argue that "shorter is better," providing that clinical outcomes are similar.[51] Two SSTI clinical trials have addressed SSTI treatment duration. Five days of therapy was noninferior to 10 days for outpatient therapy of uncomplicated, nonpurulent cellulitis in 1 study.[52] Similarly, in complicated SSTI, 6 days of tedizolid was noninferior to 10 days linezolid.[53] Pushing for very short antibiotic durations may be problematic. In a randomized trial of 3 versus 10 days of trimethoprim–sulfamethoxazole (TMP-SMX) after incision and drainage for MRSA SSTI in children, failure and relapse were more common in the 3-day treatment group.[54] In severe, complicated infection, we suggest selecting the antibiotic duration based on individual clinical response and limiting it to 5 to 7 days in patients who have a good initial response, including those with diabetes.

For those treated with intravenous antibiotics, we recommend early switch to oral therapy after initial clinical improvement. Delaying the switch to oral treatment adds unnecessary risks associated with intravenous access and prolonged hospitalization.[55]

Occasionally, patients may not require hospitalization or are requesting to leave the hospital, yet oral therapy may be inappropriate because of the severity of infection, poor adherence to the treatment regimen, concern for poor oral drug absorption, drug resistance, or toxicity. Treatment with a single dose of a long-acting glycopeptide, oritavancin or dalbavancin, could be considered, as discussed elsewhere in this article.

The benefit of the addition of antibiotics after incision and drainage for uncomplicated abscesses has been an object of debate.[56] Although the 2014 Infectious Diseases Society of America guidelines recommended against the use of antibiotics for uncomplicated abscesses after drainage,[27] after publication of these guidelines, 2 large placebo-controlled clinical trials demonstrated higher cure rates with active antibiotics compared with placebo.[57,58] One trial of 786 outpatient adults and children with a single skin abscess less than 5 cm diameter that underwent incision and drainage found significantly lower cure rates with placebo (69%) compared with clindamycin or TMP-SMX (83% and 82%).[58] Another trial of 1247 patients with abscesses of any size that underwent incision and drainage found cure rates were significantly higher with TMP-SMX compared with placebo (80% vs 73%).[57] Additionally, TMP-SMX decreased requirements for subsequent drainage and skin infection during the subsequent 1 to 2 weeks.[57] In both studies, even abscesses of small size (eg, 1 cm) benefited from antibiotic therapy compared with placebo.[59,60] These high-quality, well-powered trials support the universal use of adjunctive antibiotic therapy to incision and drainage for uncomplicated abscesses.

For simple abscesses that cannot undergo incision and drainage (patient refusal, medical care access issues, or early phlegmatous stage), we recommend the use of warm compress and antimicrobial coverage that includes MRSA.

ORAL ANTIBIOTICS WITH BOTH METHICILLIN-SUSCEPTIBLE *S AUREUS* AND METHICILLIN-RESISTANT *S AUREUS* COVERAGE

A summary of antibiotics used to treat S aureus skin infections is found in **Table 1**. Following that, we explore the data on efficacy and safety of these antibiotics.

Trimethoprim–Sulfamethoxazole

Several studies have evaluated the efficacy and safety of TMP-SMX in uncomplicated SSTI. A large randomized trial of uncomplicated SSTI compared TMP-SMX with clindamycin and found similar cure rates.[61] A notable benefit of TMP-SMX compared with clindamycin was less diarrhea, 22% versus 11% ($P = .001$). MRSA susceptibility to TMP-SMX in the United States is typically greater than 90%, permitting its empiric use for mild to moderate infections.[62] This low resistance prevalence despite decades of use highlights a relatively high barrier to the emergence of resistance among S aureus. TMP-SMX has been combined with beta-lactams owing to concerns of poor streptococcal coverage with TMP-SMX alone. However, a large randomized trial of 524 patients with cellulitis (purulent or nonpurulent) comparing TMP-SMX with clindamycin found no difference in clinical cure in the subset of nonpurulent cellulitis.[61] Initial concerns for lack of TMP-SMX efficacy for streptococcal infections were based on inaccurate in vitro methodology that has since been modified.[63] Thus, for the treatment of cellulitis with or without abscess, TMP-SMX can be prescribed as monotherapy and additional antimicrobial therapy is unnecessary.

There are limited trials for TMP-SMX in severe SSTI. Vancomycin was superior to TMP-SMX in a randomized trial of 101 patients with severe S aureus infections associated with intravenous drug use, including 31% SSTI. Cure rate overall was 86% and 98% ($P = .01$) for TMP-SMX and vancomycin, respectively. However, only 2 of 7 failures occurred outside of the context of infective endocarditis.[64] In areas with limited antibiotic availability, TMP-SMX could be considered if other agents are not viable options owing to drug resistance, allergies, or other considerations. Rash, hyperkalemia, gastrointestinal discomfort, and pseudoelevation of the creatinine are all commonly reported with TMP-SMX use. Importantly, TMP-SMX use in patients with chronic kidney disease receiving angiotensin-converting enzyme inhibitors, angiotensin receptor blockers, and spironolactone has been associated with increased mortality in observational studies, suggesting that coadministration might have risks.[65] Additionally, coadministration with sulfonylureas is associated with clinically relevant hypoglycemia.[65]

Clindamycin

Clindamycin, a lincosamide protein synthesis inhibitor available in both oral and intravenous formulations, has been widely used for SSTI. It maintains coverage of S aureus (including MRSA), streptococcal species, and anaerobic bacteria. Overall, clindamycin is fairly well-tolerated, with gastrointestinal intolerance as the most common mild side effect. *Clostridium difficile*-associated diarrhea is a concern, but in 2 large published trials of outpatient SSTI treatment, no cases occurred among the 464 participants randomized to clindamycin.[58,61] This low incidence underscores the low risk for C difficile–associated diarrhea in outpatients with SSTI, likely owing to younger age, fewer comorbidities, and lower exposure to C difficile in the outpatient compared with hospitalized setting. Satisfactory cure rates for uncomplicated cellulitis have been found in a large clinical trial and, compared with TMP-SMX, recurrence of infection was lower in the clindamycin arm.[61] Reasons for higher rates of recurrence with TMP-SMX are unclear but may be due to clindamycin's ability to decolonize S aureus

Table 1
Antibiotics for _S aureus_ skin infection

IV Therapy for Purulent SA-SSTI	Standard Dosing[a]	_S Aureus_ Resistance[b]	Cost[c] (7-d Course)	Additional Comments
Cefazolin	IV: 1–2 g q8h	No MRSA activity	$105	Penicillin allergic patients <5% cross-reactivity Dosing with dialysis favorable
Ceftaroline	IV: 600 mg IV q12h	<1%	$731	Well-tolerated Penicillin allergic patients <5% cross-reactivity Broad gram-negative spectrum of activity AE: rash, headache, GI intolerance
Cephalexin	PO: 500 mg q6h	No MRSA activity	$35	Penicillin-allergic patients <5% cross-reactivity
Clindamycin	IV/PO: 300–600 mg q8h	30%	$78	AE: diarrhea
Dalbavancin	IV: 1000 mg over 30 min d 1, 500 mg over 30 min d 8 IV: 1500 mg over 30 min single dose	Rare	$5364	Long-acting antimicrobial, single dose Limitations: up-front cost
Daptomycin	IV: 4–6 mg/kg q24h	Rare	$3404	8–10 mg/kg if concomitant bacteremia Do not use if treating concomitant pneumonia Dosing with dialysis favorable AE: myopathy, eosinophilic pneumonia
Delafloxacin	IV: 300 mg q12h PO: 450 mg q12h	Rare	$1190	Broad gram-negative spectrum of activity AE: presumed similar to fluoroquinolone class MRSA resistance up to 75% to other fluoroquinolones (ciprofloxacin and levofloxacin)

(continued on next page)

Table 1 (continued)				
IV Therapy for Purulent SA-SSTI	**Standard Dosing[a]**	***S Aureus* Resistance[b]**	**Cost[c] (7-d Course)**	**Additional Comments**
Dicloxacillin	PO: 500 mg q6h	No MRSA activity	$34	Avoid if known moderate to severe penicillin allergy
Doxycycline[d]	IV/PO: 200 mg load then 100 mg q12h	6%	$16	Reduced bioavailability with food Administer in a fasting state AE: Photosensitivity
Fusidic acid	IV/PO: 500 mg q8–12h	10%[e]	–	Not available in the United States AE: GI intolerance (nausea, vomiting, abdominal pain), hyperbilirubinemia (more common with IV formulation) Less favorable for *S pyogenes* infections
Linezolid	IV/PO: 600 mg q12h	Rare	Varies[f]	AE: serotonergic drug interactions, thrombocytopenia
Oritavancin	IV: 1200 mg over 3 h single dose	Rare	$1160	Long-acting antimicrobial, single dose Limitations: up-front cost
Oxacillin/nafcillin	IV: 2 g q4h	NA	$744	Avoid if known moderate to severe penicillin allergy
Tedizolid	IV/PO: 200 mg q24h	Rare	$2602	–
Telavancin	IV: 10 mg/kg over 60 min q24h	Rare	$2996	AE: nephrotoxicity, QTc prolongation
Trimethoprim–sulfamethoxazole	IV: 160–320 mg (TMP component) q12h PO: 160/800 mg tab q12h	4%	$16	AE: rash, pseudoelevation creatinine, hyperkalemia, GI-related diarrhea Caution use in patients with chronic kidney disease

(continued on next page)

Table 1 (continued)				
IV Therapy for Purulent SA-SSTI	Standard Dosing[a]	S Aureus Resistance[b]	Cost[c] (7-d Course)	Additional Comments
Vancomycin	IV: 15 mg/kg q12h	Rare	$109	Inexpensive, widely available Dosing with dialysis favorable AE: nephrotoxicity. Monitor serum levels in patients with CKD or AKI

Abbreviations: AE, adverse effects; AKI, acute kidney injury; CKD, chronic kidney disease; GI, gastrointestinal; IV, intravenous; MRSA; methicillin-resistant *S aureus;* MSSA, methicillin-sensitive *S aureus;* PO, per oral; q##h, every ## hours.
   [a] Reference: Stevens et al. 2014. Dosage and frequency are based on patients with normal renal function.
   [b] Reference: Diekema et a. 2019. Resistance data from 2016. Includes all *S aureus* infections, not limited to SSTI.
   [c] Prices are representative of the average wholesale price (Johns Hopkins POC-IT ABX guide, Editor John G. Bartlett; 2020).
   [d] Minocycline as an alternative dosed IV/PO 100 mg q12h with similar efficacy and susceptibility to MRSA.
   [e] Reference: Castanheira et al. 2008.
   [f] Although, listed as $2571, the average wholesale price in Johns Hopkins POC-IT ABX guide (editor John G. Bartlett, 2020), of linezolid is available as a generic formulation and prices are substantially lower in some health care systems (eg, goodRx.com lists cost in September 2020 as $49.56 for 10-d oral course).

colonized persons.[66] We do not recommend empiric clindamycin for severe infections given a paucity of data as well as increasing population-level resistance rates among MRSA that exceed 25%.[62] Additionally, caution is warranted to recognize isolates reported as erythromycin resistant and clindamycin susceptible. Approximately 50% of these isolates harbor an erythromycin-inducible ribosomal methylase. Spontaneous clindamycin-resistant mutants constitutively expressing this enzyme can be selected out by clindamycin, leading to treatment failure.[58,67] Clinicians should be aware of whether their local laboratory tests for this inducible resistance mechanism.

Doxycycline and Minocycline

Doxycycline and minocycline are second-generation tetracycline protein synthesis inhibitors and are well-tolerated with good bioavailability and tissue concentrations. CA-MRSA and hospital-acquired MRSA isolates are typically (>90%) susceptible.[62] However, clinical microbiology laboratories in the United States do not routinely test for susceptibility to these agents and instead test for tetracycline susceptibility. All tetracycline-susceptible isolates will be susceptible to doxycycline and minocycline. Tetracycline-resistant isolates in which resistance is due to a tetracycline efflux pump (approximately 60%–80%) are susceptible to doxycycline and minocycline.[62,68] In general, we favor doxycycline over minocycline given fewer side effects, including dizziness and hypersensitivity reactions.[69] Clinical data on doxycycline or minocycline for SSTI are limited; however, observational studies have cure rates of 85% or more for a wide spectrum of clinical infections with *S aureus*, including a cure rate of CA-MRSA SSTI of 94% (15/16).[70] A small randomized controlled trial of 34 patients with purulent uncomplicated SSTI comparing doxycycline with TMP-SMX found similar efficacy in each treatment group.[71] A larger randomized, controlled trial comparing doxycycline with TMP-SMX in uncomplicated SSTI and abscess is currently enrolling (clinicaltrials.gov NCT03637400). Historically, doxycycline has not been recommended for treatment of nonpurulent cellulitis, owing to limited activity against *S pyogenes*.[27]

Rifampin

Rifampin is a protein synthesis inhibitor routinely active against *S aureus*, including MRSA. Owing to rapid acquisition of resistance, monotherapy is not recommended.[27] In *S aureus* bacteremia, the addition of rifampin to therapy did not improve clinical outcomes, but increased drug-related side effects.[72] Systematic reviews of *S aureus* treatment have found no clinical data to support its use for skin infections.[73] Given the lack of data supporting improved efficacy for SSTI and concerns for side effects and drug–drug interactions, the authors do not recommend rifampin use for SA-SSTI.

Fusidic Acid

Fusidic acid, a protein synthesis inhibitor introduced in the 1960s, is active against *S aureus* and has been used in topical, oral, and intravenous preparations. It is not available in the United States. Resistance is a concern with overuse of topical formulations and gusidic acid's low barrier to resistance.[74,75] In a phase II randomized controlled trial (n = 155), oral fusidic acid dosed 600 mg every 12 hours (after a loading dose of 1500 mg every 12 hours on day 1) was found to have similar efficacy to linezolid.[76] Gastrointestinal intolerance is most commonly reported side effect. Hyperbilirubinemia, especially with intravenous formulations, is another notable side effect.[74]

Oxazolidinones

Linezolid

Linezolid, the first oxazolidinone, has substantial clinical trial data supporting its use in complicated SSTI. Its mechanism of action is inhibition of protein synthesis, including toxin production. It is available both for oral and for intravenous administration. The oral formation has 100% bioavailability. Linezolid has excellent penetration into skin structures and bullae fluid.[55] *S aureus* resistance to linezolid is very rare.[62] In 1 study, hospital length of stay was shorter with use of linezolid compared with vancomycin.[77]

In a trial of 1200 patients with complicated SSTI comparing linezolid (oral or intravenous) with vancomycin (1 g every 12 hours), efficacy was similar (92% vs 89%; *P* = .06).[46] Cost and antibiotic stewardship priorities have limited the clinical use of linezolid for SSTI, although generic preparations are now available at a lower cost. Drug–drug interactions occur with serotonergic drugs, which should not be coadministered.[78] Toxicity of linezolid when given for short durations is uncommon. Thrombocytopenia, peripheral neuropathy, and optic neuritis are known side effects, but described typically with durations of therapy longer than necessary to treat SSTI.[79] Linezolid offers a safe oral option for the treatment of moderate to severe infections, pending or lacking microbiologic susceptibility data owing to low rates of resistance. As with any antibiotic class, we worry that widespread use will drive the emergence of oxazolidinone-resistant *S aureus* strains.

Tedizolid

Tedizolid, a newer oxazolidinone with oral and intravenous preparations, is highly bioavailable, dosed daily, and has less overall reported toxicity (neuropathy, thrombocytopenia) than linezolid.[78] Like linezolid, robust data support its efficacy and safety in

SSTI.[53,80] Gastrointestinal symptoms were the most common side effects and, unlike linezolid, there are no drug–drug interactions with serotonergic drugs.[53]

Fluoroquinolones

The fluoroquinolone class, including levofloxacin, ciprofloxacin, and moxifloxacin, are no longer recommended by the Infectious Diseases Society of America for the treatment of *S aureus* infections.[27] Despite efficacy in large clinical trials of fluoroquinolones for SSTI, including those caused by *S aureus*, these were generally conducted before 2000 and secular decreases in MRSA susceptibility to fluoroquinolones as well as increasing recognition of adverse events limit their benefits.[27]

A newer generation, nonzwitterionic fluroquinolone, delafloxacin, was approved for ABSSSI in 2017. Delafloxacin has improved gram-positive activity compared with levofloxacin, including reliable activity against *S aureus* and MSRA, as well as many gram-negative organisms, including *Pseudomonas aeruginosa*. Delafloxacin compared with vancomycin plus aztreonam for complicated ABSSSI has a similar efficacy, safety, and tolerability profile.[81] In the MRSA subset, cure rates with delafloxacin was greater than 98%. The FDA issued warnings on fluoroquinolone use because of rare but serious adverse events (eg, tendinopathy, peripheral neuropathy, mental health side effects, and aortic aneurysm) and are likely to pertain to delafloxacin as well (fda.gov/drugs/information-drug-class). An overly broad spectrum of activity, cost, and stewardship concerns limit upfront use of delafloxacin. However, practical benefits for monotherapy in selected situations may make a clinician consider this drug as an option.

Omadacycline

Omadacycline, approved in 2018, is a once daily tetracycline antibiotic available in both oral and intravenous formulations. It has broad gram-positive activity, including MRSA, as well as some limited gram-negative and anaerobic activity.[82] It is unaffected by common tetracycline resistance mechanisms and some doxycycline-resistant strains remain omandacycline susceptible.[83] Two large clinical trials (n = 655 and n = 735) found its efficacy and safety similar to that of linezolid.[84,85]

Omadacycline has poor oral bioavailability, especially when taken within 4 hours of food containing fat or divalent cations.[82] Gastrointestinal intolerance is common (>25%) and there are limited long-term safety data regarding adverse effects associated with the tetracycline class.[82,84] An overly broad spectrum of activity, cost, and stewardship concerns limit practicality of omadacycline use in most SSTI situations.

Guide to selection of empiric oral therapy

The authors prefer the use of doxycycline or TMP-SMX in uncomplicated purulent SSTI. In the absence of concerns for toxicity (eg, kidney disease) or drug–drug interactions with TMP-SMX (as discussed elsewhere in this article), either agent is a reasonable choice, assuming good local antimicrobial susceptibility profiles. We believe clindamycin is not first line in many areas of the United States given the increasing prevalence of resistance among *S aureus*; the side effect of diarrhea, albeit mild in severity, is another limitation. Antibiotic stewardship considerations and cost (less of a consideration now that linezolid is available as a generic) limit the generalized use of oxazolidinones, although these are an excellent choice in situations such as multiple drug allergies and for treatment highly antibiotic-resistant *S aureus* SSTI. Similarly, the authors' perspective of the other oral agents is that none are first line and their use is principally that of a "back pocket" regimen when other options are problematic. Stewardship and cost issues preclude their widespread use.

PARENTERAL ANTIBIOTICS WITH BOTH METHICILLIN-SUSCEPTIBLE *S AUREUS* AND METHICILLIN-RESISTANT *S AUREUS* COVERAGE

Linezolid, tedizolid, delafloxacin, and omadacycline are available in intravenous formulation for treatment of severe infections, as discussed in the oral regimens.

Glycopeptides

Vancomycin

Vancomycin, a bactericidal glycopeptide, had been a traditional first-line agent for complicated SSTI, and is the reference of standard of care for treatment of complicated MRSA SSTI infections owing to its proven efficacy, reliable activity, and lack of resistance among common gram-positive pathogens causing skin infections. Resistant *S aureus* isolates remain very rare despite many decades of vancomycin use, highlighting its high barrier to emergence of resistance among *S aureus*.[62]

Shortfalls with vancomycin therapy are multiple. It must be administered intravenously to achieve therapeutic concentrations in skin. Nephrotoxicity is the most common and serious adverse event, and risk is increased if coadministered with other nephrotoxic agents (piperacillin–tazobactam) or at higher serum troughs (>15 mg/L).[86] The 2020 vancomycin treatment guidelines recommend pharmacist-based dosing targeting a serum area under the concentration curve over 24 hours to minimum inhibitory concentration ratio of 400 to 600 μg/mL × hour rather than trough levels, which will incur ancillary labor and testing costs.[86] Of note, these guidelines for vancomycin dosing are based on considerations for bacteremia and there are no data to suggest that the target area under the concentration curve over 24 hours to minimum inhibitory concentration ratio is relevant for the treatment of SSTI. Skin and soft tissue concentrations seem to be generally adequate, although variable with the standard vancomycin dosing of 30 mg/kg/d.[87] No randomized controlled trial has demonstrated superiority of any other agent over vancomycin for the treatment of complicated SSTI. Vancomycin is widely available and inexpensive and thus remains a drug of choice, despite the availability of alternative intravenous agents with more favorable toxicity profiles and dosing. Interestingly, in an observational study, vancomycin plus clindamycin therapy was associated with a decreased length of hospital stay and readmission compared with vancomycin monotherapy.[88] Further evaluation with a randomized controlled trial should be done confirm the association before this combination is introduced into routine clinical practice.

Telavancin

Telavancin is a lipoglycopeptide that in a clinical trial of 579 evaluable patients was noninferior to vancomycin (88% vs 87% cure).[89] Nephrotoxicity is a complication with telavancin with similar or greater rates compared with vancomycin and it has a black box warning.[90] Telavancin's advantages over vancomycin include once daily dosing and a lack of drug monitoring requirements.

Dalbavancin and oritavancin

Dalbavancin and oritavancin are lipoglyopeptides with the unique pharmacokinetic property of long half-lives, permitting for single or weekly intravenous dosing, allowing outpatient intravenous delivery. Dalbavancin, dosed 1000 mg on day 1 and 500 mg day 8, was compared with in either vancomycin with oral linezolid step down or to intravenous linezolid with oral linezolid step down for complicated SSTI.[91,92] Cure rates were similar to comparators. Safety and tolerability were likewise similar. Nausea, diarrhea, and pruritus were the most common side effects of dalbavancin. No allergic reactions to dalbavancin were reported. A subsequent study of dalbavancin as a single 1500 mg dose was similarly noninferior to comparators.[93]

Oritavancin as a single 1200-mg infusion has been compared with vancomycin with oral stepdown therapy.[94] Cure rates and safety profiles were similar with nausea, headache and vomiting most commonly reported side effects of oritavancin.

Although the high cost of drug acquisition is a limiting factor for their use, dalbavancin or oritavancin may have a role for treatment of patients with severe infections who are seen in the emergency department, permitting them to be sent home; to facilitate early discharge from the hospital; or for patient who may not be a candidate for oral therapy, such as medication adherence concerns (**Fig. 3**). A lack of robust data in bacteremia or bone infections warrants caution when patients have these concomitant conditions.

Daptomycin

Daptomycin is a cyclic lipopeptide, dosed intravenously once daily, with excellent MRSA activity. In a clinical trial of 534 patients with complicated SSTI, it had similar efficacy and safety to a comparator arm of vancomycin or antistaphylococcal beta-lactam.[48] Culture-confirmed MRSA infections were limited (n = 64) and cure rates were similar between groups. A meta-analysis of 6 randomized trials evaluating daptomycin for complicated SSTI demonstrated similar efficacy versus comparators, including 120 patients who had infections with MRSA.[95] Toxicity is relatively low, yet prescribers should be prudent to monitor for (reversible) myopathy by checking creatinine kinase routinely. Coadministration of statins should be avoided to prevent increased myopathy risk.[96] The absence of nephrotoxicity makes daptomycin a favorable alternative to vancomycin in patients with kidney injury. Drug costs and perhaps

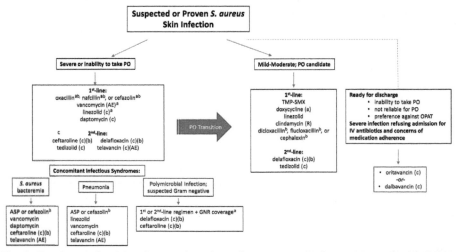

Fig. 3. Treatment algorithm for purulent skin infection suspected or proven to be caused by *S aureus*. [a]Author's preference for first-line therapy. [b]Proven MSSA only. [c]Higher cost considerations. a, alternative includes minocycline; AE, adverse effects considerations; IV, intravenous; OPAT, outpatient parenteral antibiotic treatment; PO, per oral; R, antimicrobial resistance considerations for empiric therapy; TMP-SMX, trimethoprim–sulfamethoxazole.

stewardship concerns remain barriers to recommending daptomycin as a first-line therapy. The recommended dose is 4 to 6 mg/kg/d for complicated SSTI, but a higher dose of 8 to 10 mg/kg/d is recommended for severe infection with bacteremia.[97]

Ceftaroline

Ceftaroline is the first FDA-approved cephalosporin with activity against MRSA. It has gram-negative and gram-positive activity similar to that of ceftriaxone. When compared with vancomycin and aztreonam in hospitalized patients with complicated SSTI, clinical cure rates were similar (85% vs 86%).[49] Similar to other cephalosporins, ceftaroline seems to be safe and well-tolerated for the short courses that are used for SSTI. Nausea, headache, and diarrhea are the most common side effects. Limited to intravenous therapy only, benefits over vancomycin include its lower toxicity profile and ease of dosing without monitoring levels. Higher cost limits its attractiveness as a first-line therapy.

Tigecycline

Tigecycline, a glycylcycline, is essentially is a broad spectrum intravenous tetracycline analogue with broad gram-positive activity, including MRSA, and efficacy against many gram-negative pathogens.[98] The broad antimicrobial spectrum and high rate of gastrointestinal disturbances (approximately 25%) are limitations that severely limit its use.

BETA-LACTAM ANTIBIOTICS FOR THE TREATMENT OF METHICILLIN-SUSCEPTIBLE *S AUREUS* SKIN AND SOFT TISSUE INFECTIONS

MSSA infection will respond to all the drugs listed for MRSA. However, MSSA is rarely diagnosed at point of care and distinguishing MRSA from MSSA by clinical features is not possible.[99] Once diagnosed, beta-lactam therapy is first line for severe infections, in which case an antistaphylococcal penicillin (oxacillin or nafcillin) or a first-generation cephalosporin (cefazolin) is preferred over vancomycin with better outcomes, including lower mortality, demonstrated in severe infections complicated by bacteremia,[97] although such benefits have not been demonstrated with SSTI. With more prolonged therapy, cefazolin demonstrates nearly 30% fewer side effects and discontinuations than oxacillin; however, this problem is less likely to occur given the short courses required for treatment of SSTI.[100] Ongoing debate between the use of antistaphylococcal penicillins versus cefazolin continues.[100,101] Concerns for inducible beta-lactamase–mediated resistance to cefazolin in high inoculum infections (in which NSTI or abscesses would be included) and the potential for treatment failure, although infrequent, lead many providers to choose an antistaphylococcal penicillin upfront. For complicated SSTI with MSSA, the authors' preference is for cefazolin with its fewer side effects, unless there is concomitant bacteremia or undrained foci of infection, in which case an antistaphylococcal penicillin is preferred until bacteremia is controlled and/or source control is achieved.

Oral beta-lactam options for mild to moderate infections include flucloxacillin, dicloxacillin, and cephalexin, which have demonstrated equivalent efficacy in management of cellulitis compared with clindamycin or TMP-SMX, respectively.[33,34] Although well-tolerated with minimal side effects, dosing requirements every 6 hours make adherence challenging outside of clinical trials. The frequent dosing required gives us concern about the efficacy of oral beta-lactams owing to the risk of medication nonadherence, which is common in patients with SSTI treatment and is associated with worse clinical outcomes.[102] Therefore, we believe there is no compelling reason to prefer oral beta-lactams over non–beta-lactams for proven MSSA cases and we typically prefer non–beta-lactam options owing to their ease of dosing and equivalent efficacy.

Amoxicillin–clavulanic acid, which has activity against MSSA, also has had clinically success in treating SSTI, primarily associated with animal bites or trauma.[27] Benefits include every 12-hour dosing but its overly broad spectrum that includes activity against community acquired gram-negative pathogens and anaerobic pathogens, should limit its routine use outside of consensus indications, for example, animal bites.

NEWER AGENTS

Iclaprim is a broad-spectrum diaminopyrimidine antibiotic inhibiting dihydrofolate reductase with broad gram-positive activity. It has increased potency against gram-positive organisms similar to TMP-SMX. The absence of a companion sulfonamide makes it more appealing with the potential for fewer side effects.[103] Two phase III studies have demonstrated similar efficacy in complicated SSTI compared with vancomycin.[104,105] Iclaprim was declined approval by the FDA in 2019 owing to need for additional data concerning the risk of liver toxicity. Its fate remains uncertain.

Lefamulin, a member of a novel drug class, pleuromutilins, inhibits protein synthesis by binding to the 50S ribosomal subunit. It is available in both intravenous and oral formulations. Microbiological activity is primarily against gram-positive organisms, including MRSA and MSSA, with some anaerobic and atypical gram-negative coverage.[106] In a phase II clinical trial (n = 207) of complicated SSTI, lefamulin dosed at 100 mg and 150 mg had similar cure rates compared with vancomycin.[106] The most common side effects included headache, nausea, and diarrhea.

SUMMARY

S aureus SSTI present an ongoing challenge in patient care and burden to the medical system. The primary treatment is source control with incision and drainage and a relatively short course of antibiotic therapy. Wound cultures are important for establishing local antimicrobial susceptibility patterns. In the future, changes in antibiotic susceptibility and transition of newer drugs to generic therapies may change treatment considerations to favor less expensive, safer, and better tolerated medications with high barriers to the emergence of resistance.

CLINICAL CARE POINTS

- *S aureus* is the most common cause of SSTIs.
- The most common types of skin infections can be categorized into nonpurulent skin infection, and purulent skin infection with or without cellulitis, the latter of which is typically caused by *S aureus*.
- After incision and drainage, antibiotic treatment for an uncomplicated abscess is generally recommended, regardless of abscess size.
- Antibiotic choice should be based on disease severity, infection location, host comorbidities, and a regimens' safety and tolerability, local formulary and availability, and cost.

DISCLOSURE

Dr L.G. Miller has received grants from Merck. Dr T.J. Hatlen has nothing to disclose.

REFERENCES

1. Moran GJ, Krishnadasan A, Gorwitz RJ, et al. Methicillin-resistant S. aureus infections among patients in the emergency department. N Engl J Med 2006; 355(7):666–74.
2. Food and Drug Administration Center for Drug Evaluation and Research. Guidance for industry acute bacterial skin and skin structure infections: developing drugs for treatment. Available at: http://https://www.fda.gov/files/drugs/published/Acute-Bacterial-Skin-and-Skin-Structure-Infections—Developing-Drugs-for-Treatment. pdf. Published Oct 2013. Accessed November 11, 2020.
3. DeLeo FR, Diep BA, Otto M. Host defense and pathogenesis in Staphylococcus aureus infections. Infect Dis Clin North Am 2009;23(1):17–34.
4. Kobayashi SD, Malachowa N, DeLeo FR. Pathogenesis of Staphylococcus aureus abscesses. Am J Pathol 2015;185(6):1518–27.
5. Abad CL, Pulia MS, Safdar N. Does the nose know? An update on MRSA decolonization strategies. Curr Infect Dis Rep 2013;15(6):455–64.
6. Safdar N, Bradley EA. The risk of infection after nasal colonization with Staphylococcus aureus. Am J Med 2008;121(4):310–5.
7. Miller LG, Eells SJ, Taylor AR, et al. Staphylococcus aureus colonization among household contacts of patients with skin infections: risk factors, strain discordance, and complex ecology. Clin Infect Dis 2012;54(11):1523–35.
8. Williams RE. Healthy carriage of Staphylococcus aureus: its prevalence and importance. Bacteriol Rev 1963;27:56–71.
9. McKinnell JA, Huang SS, Eells SJ, et al. Quantifying the impact of extranasal testing of body sites for methicillin-resistant Staphylococcus aureus colonization at the time of hospital or intensive care unit admission. Infect Control Hosp Epidemiol 2013;34(2):161–70.
10. Tong SYC, Davis JS, Eichenberger E, et al. Staphylococcus aureus infections: epidemiology, pathophysiology, clinical manifestations, and management. Clin Microbiol Rev 2015;28(3):603–61.
11. Suaya JA, Mera RM, Cassidy A, et al. Incidence and cost of hospitalizations associated with Staphylococcus aureus skin and soft tissue infections in the United States from 2001 through 2009. BMC Infect Dis 2014;14:296.
12. Talan DA, Krishnadasan A, Gorwitz RJ, et al. Comparison of Staphylococcus aureus from skin and soft-tissue infections in US emergency department patients, 2004 and 2008. Clin Infect Dis 2011;53(2):144–9.
13. Miller LG, Eisenberg DF, Liu H, et al. Incidence of skin and soft tissue infections in ambulatory and inpatient settings, 2005-2010. BMC Infect Dis 2015;15:362.
14. Shallcross LJ, Fragaszy E, Johnson AM, et al. The role of the Panton-Valentine leucocidin toxin in staphylococcal disease: a systematic review and meta-analysis. Lancet Infect Dis 2013;13(1):43–54.
15. Hamilton SM, Bryant AE, Carroll KC, et al. In vitro production of panton-valentine leukocidin among strains of methicillin-resistant Staphylococcus aureus causing diverse infections. Clin Infect Dis 2007;45(12):1550–8.
16. Ray GT, Suaya JA, Baxter R. Microbiology of skin and soft tissue infections in the age of community-acquired methicillin-resistant Staphylococcus aureus. Diagn Microbiol Infect Dis 2013;76(1):24–30.
17. Lipsky BA, Kollef MH, Miller LG, et al. Predicting bacteremia among patients hospitalized for skin and skin-structure infections: derivation and validation of a risk score. Infect Control Hosp Epidemiol 2010;31(8):828–37.

18. Chira S, Miller LG. Staphylococcus aureus is the most common identified cause of cellulitis: a systematic review. Epidemiol Infect 2010;138(3):313–7.

19. Jeng A, Beheshti M, Li J, et al. The role of beta-hemolytic streptococci in causing diffuse, nonculturable cellulitis: a prospective investigation. Medicine (Baltimore) 2010;89(4):217–26.

20. Eells SJ, McKinnell JA, Wang AA, et al. A comparison of clinical outcomes between healthcare-associated infections due to community-associated methicillin-resistant Staphylococcus aureus strains and healthcare-associated methicillin-resistant S. aureus strains. Epidemiol Infect 2013;141(10):2140–8.

21. Choo EJ. Community-associated methicillin-resistant Staphylococcus aureus in nosocomial infections. Infect Chemother 2017;49(2):158–9.

22. Kim S-H, Kim K-H, Kim H-B, et al. Outcome of vancomycin treatment in patients with methicillin-susceptible Staphylococcus aureus bacteremia. Antimicrobial Agents Chemother 2008;52(1):192–7.

23. Huang SS, Singh R, McKinnell JA, et al. Decolonization to reduce postdischarge infection risk among MRSA carriers. N Engl J Med 2019;380(7):638–50.

24. Ray GT, Suaya JA, Baxter R. Trends and characteristics of culture-confirmed Staphylococcus aureus infections in a large U.S. integrated health care organization. J Clin Microbiol 2012;50(6):1950–7.

25. Russo A, Concia E, Cristini F, et al. Current and future trends in antibiotic therapy of acute bacterial skin and skin-structure infections. Clin Microbiol Infect 2016; 22(Suppl 2):S27–36.

26. Daum RS. Clinical practice. Skin and soft-tissue infections caused by methicillin-resistant Staphylococcus aureus. N Engl J Med 2007;357(4):380–90.

27. Stevens DL, Bisno AL, Chambers HF, et al. Practice guidelines for the diagnosis and management of skin and soft tissue infections: 2014 update by the infectious diseases society of America. Clin Infect Dis 2014;59(2):e10–52.

28. Koning S, van der Sande R, Verhagen AP, et al. Interventions for impetigo. Cochrane Database Syst Rev 2012;1:CD003261.

29. Edge R, Argáez C. Topical antibiotics for impetigo: a review of the clinical effectiveness and guidelines. Canadian Agency for Drugs and Technologies in Health. 2017. Available at: http://www.ncbi.nlm.nih.gov/books/NBK447580/. Accessed June 17, 2020.

30. Bowen AC, Tong SYC, Andrews RM, et al. Short-course oral co-trimoxazole versus intramuscular benzathine benzylpenicillin for impetigo in a highly endemic region: an open-label, randomised, controlled, non-inferiority trial. Lancet 2014;384(9960):2132–40.

31. Gunderson CG, Martinello RA. A systematic review of bacteremias in cellulitis and erysipelas. J Infect 2012;64(2):148–55.

32. Pallin DJ, Binder WD, Allen MB, et al. Clinical trial: comparative effectiveness of cephalexin plus trimethoprim-sulfamethoxazole versus cephalexin alone for treatment of uncomplicated cellulitis: a randomized controlled trial. Clin Infect Dis 2013;56(12):1754–62.

33. Moran GJ, Krishnadasan A, Mower WR, et al. Effect of cephalexin plus trimethoprim-sulfamethoxazole vs cephalexin alone on clinical cure of uncomplicated cellulitis: a randomized clinical trial. JAMA 2017;317(20):2088–96.

34. Brindle R, Williams OM, Davies P, et al. Adjunctive clindamycin for cellulitis: a clinical trial comparing flucloxacillin with or without clindamycin for the treatment of limb cellulitis. BMJ Open 2017;7(3):e013260.

35. Miller LG, Perdreau-Remington F, Rieg G, et al. Necrotizing fasciitis caused by community-associated methicillin-resistant Staphylococcus aureus in Los Angeles. N Engl J Med 2005;352(14):1445–53.
36. Lee Y-T, Lin J-C, Wang N-C, et al. Necrotizing fasciitis in a medical center in northern Taiwan: emergence of methicillin-resistant Staphylococcus aureus in the community. J Microbiol Immunol Infect 2007;40(4):335–41.
37. Sievert DM, Ricks P, Edwards JR, et al. Antimicrobial-resistant pathogens associated with healthcare-associated infections: summary of data reported to the National healthcare safety network at the centers for disease control and prevention, 2009-2010. Infect Control Hosp Epidemiol 2013;34(1):1–14.
38. Rabuka CE, Azoulay LY, Kahn SR. Predictors of a positive duplex scan in patients with a clinical presentation compatible with deep vein thrombosis or cellulitis. Can J Infect Dis 2003;14(4):210–4.
39. David CV, Chira S, Eells SJ, et al. Diagnostic accuracy in patients admitted to hospitals with cellulitis. Dermatol Online J 2011;17(3):1.
40. Chan Y-L, Liao H-C, Tsay P-K, et al. C-reactive protein as an indicator of bacterial infection of adult patients in the emergency department. Chang Gung Med J 2002;25(7):437–45.
41. Peralta G, Padrón E, Roiz MP, et al. Risk factors for bacteremia in patients with limb cellulitis. Eur J Clin Microbiol Infect Dis 2006;25(10):619–26.
42. Perl B, Gottehrer NP, Raveh D, et al. Cost-effectiveness of blood cultures for adult patients with cellulitis. Clin Infect Dis 1999;29(6):1483–8.
43. Tayal VS, Hasan N, Norton HJ, et al. The effect of soft-tissue ultrasound on the management of cellulitis in the emergency department. Acad Emerg Med 2006; 13(4):384–8.
44. Rahmouni A, Chosidow O, Mathieu D, et al. MR imaging in acute infectious cellulitis. Radiology 1994;192(2):493–6.
45. Ko LN, Raff AB, Garza-Mayers AC, et al. Skin surface temperatures measured by thermal imaging aid in the diagnosis of cellulitis. J Invest Dermatol 2018; 138(3):520–6.
46. Weigelt J, Itani K, Stevens D, et al. Linezolid versus vancomycin in treatment of complicated skin and soft tissue infections. Antimicrobial Agents Chemother 2005;49(6):2260–6.
47. Agarwal R, Bartsch SM, Kelly BJ, et al. Newer glycopeptide antibiotics for treatment of complicated skin and soft tissue infections: systematic review, network meta-analysis and cost analysis. Clin Microbiol Infect 2018;24(4):361–8.
48. Arbeit RD, Maki D, Tally FP, et al. Daptomycin 98-01 and 99-01 Investigators. The safety and efficacy of daptomycin for the treatment of complicated skin and skin-structure infections. Clin Infect Dis 2004;38(12):1673–81.
49. Wilcox MH, Corey GR, Talbot GH, et al. CANVAS 2: the second Phase III, randomized, double-blind study evaluating ceftaroline fosamil for the treatment of patients with complicated skin and skin structure infections. J Antimicrob Chemother 2010;65(Suppl 4):iv53–65.
50. Ruhe JJ, Smith N, Bradsher RW, et al. Community-onset methicillin-resistant Staphylococcus aureus skin and soft-tissue infections: impact of antimicrobial therapy on outcome. Clin Infect Dis 2007;44(6):777–84.
51. Spellberg B. The new antibiotic mantra-"shorter is better". JAMA Intern Med 2016;176(9):1254–5.
52. Hepburn MJ, Dooley DP, Skidmore PJ, et al. Comparison of short-course (5 days) and standard (10 days) treatment for uncomplicated cellulitis. Arch Intern Med 2004;164(15):1669–74.

53. Moran GJ, Fang E, Corey GR, et al. Tedizolid for 6 days versus linezolid for 10 days for acute bacterial skin and skin-structure infections (ESTABLISH-2): a randomised, double-blind, phase 3, non-inferiority trial. Lancet Infect Dis 2014;14(8):696–705.

54. Holmes L, Ma C, Qiao H, et al. Trimethoprim-sulfamethoxazole therapy reduces failure and recurrence in methicillin-resistant Staphylococcus aureus skin abscesses after surgical drainage. J Pediatr 2016;169:128–34.e1.

55. Eckmann C, Nathwani D, Lawson W, et al. Comparison of vancomycin and linezolid in patients with peripheral vascular disease and/or diabetes in an observational European study of complicated skin and soft-tissue infections due to methicillin-resistant Staphylococcus aureus. Clin Microbiol Infect 2015; 21(Suppl 2):S33–9.

56. Fahimi J, Singh A, Frazee BW. The role of adjunctive antibiotics in the treatment of skin and soft tissue abscesses: a systematic review and meta-analysis. CJEM 2015;17(4):420–32.

57. Talan DA, Mower WR, Krishnadasan A, et al. Trimethoprim-sulfamethoxazole versus placebo for uncomplicated skin abscess. N Engl J Med 2016;374(9): 823–32.

58. Daum RS, Miller LG, Immergluck L, et al. A placebo-controlled trial of antibiotics for smaller skin abscesses. N Engl J Med 2017;376(26):2545–55.

59. Talan DA, Moran GJ, Krishnadasan A, et al. Subgroup analysis of antibiotic treatment for skin abscesses. Ann Emerg Med 2018;71(1):21–30.

60. Lake JG, Miller LG, Fritz SA. Antibiotic duration, but not abscess size, impacts clinical cure of limited skin and soft tissue infection after incision and drainage. Clin Infect Dis 2019. https://doi.org/10.1093/cid/ciz1129. Published online.

61. Miller LG, Daum RS, Creech CB, et al. Clindamycin versus trimethoprim-sulfamethoxazole for uncomplicated skin infections. N Engl J Med 2015; 372(12):1093–103.

62. Diekema DJ, Pfaller MA, Shortridge D, et al. Twenty-year trends in antimicrobial susceptibilities among Staphylococcus aureus from the SENTRY antimicrobial surveillance program. Open Forum Infect Dis 2019;6(Suppl 1):S47–53.

63. Bowen AC, Lilliebridge RA, Tong SYC, et al. Is Streptococcus pyogenes resistant or susceptible to trimethoprim-sulfamethoxazole? J Clin Microbiol 2012; 50(12):4067–72.

64. Markowitz N, Quinn EL, Saravolatz LD. Trimethoprim-sulfamethoxazole compared with vancomycin for the treatment of Staphylococcus aureus infection. Ann Intern Med 1992;117(5):390–8.

65. Ho JM-W, Juurlink DN. Considerations when prescribing trimethoprim-sulfamethoxazole. CMAJ 2011;183(16):1851–8.

66. Hogan PG, Rodriguez M, Spenner AM, et al. Impact of systemic antibiotics on Staphylococcus aureus colonization and recurrent skin infection. Clin Infect Dis 2018;66(2):191–7.

67. Siberry GK, Tekle T, Carroll K, et al. Failure of clindamycin treatment of methicillin-resistant Staphylococcus aureus expressing inducible clindamycin resistance in vitro. Clin Infect Dis 2003;37(9):1257–60.

68. Schwartz BS, Graber CJ, Diep BA, et al. Doxycycline, not minocycline, induces its own resistance in multidrug-resistant, community-associated methicillin-resistant Staphylococcus aureus clone USA300. Clin Infect Dis 2009;48(10): 1483–4.

69. Shapiro LE, Knowles SR, Shear NH. Comparative safety of tetracycline, minocycline, and doxycycline. Arch Dermatol 1997;133(10):1224–30.

70. Ruhe JJ, Monson T, Bradsher RW, et al. Use of long-acting tetracyclines for methicillin-resistant Staphylococcus aureus infections: case series and review of the literature. Clin Infect Dis 2005;40(10):1429–34.
71. Cenizal MJ, Skiest D, Luber S, et al. Prospective randomized trial of empiric therapy with trimethoprim-sulfamethoxazole or doxycycline for outpatient skin and soft tissue infections in an area of high prevalence of methicillin-resistant Staphylococcus aureus. Antimicrobial Agents Chemother 2007;51(7):2628–30.
72. Thwaites GE, Scarborough M, Szubert A, et al. Adjunctive rifampicin for Staphylococcus aureus bacteraemia (ARREST): a multicentre, randomised, double-blind, placebo-controlled trial. Lancet 2018;391(10121):668–78.
73. Perlroth J, Kuo M, Tan J, et al. Adjunctive use of rifampin for the treatment of Staphylococcus aureus infections: a systematic review of the literature. Arch Intern Med 2008;168(8):805–19.
74. Whitby M. Fusidic acid in the treatment of methicillin-resistant Staphylococcus aureus. Int J Antimicrob Agents 1999;12(Suppl 2):S67–71.
75. Castanheira M, Watters AA, Mendes RE, et al. Occurrence and molecular characterization of fusidic acid resistance mechanisms among Staphylococcus spp. from European countries (2008). J Antimicrob Chemother 2010;65(7):1353–8.
76. Craft JC, Moriarty SR, Clark K, et al. A randomized, double-blind phase 2 study comparing the efficacy and safety of an oral fusidic acid loading-dose regimen to oral linezolid for the treatment of acute bacterial skin and skin structure infections. Clin Infect Dis 2011;52(Suppl 7):S520–6.
77. Itani KMF, Weigelt J, Li JZ, et al. Linezolid reduces length of stay and duration of intravenous treatment compared with vancomycin for complicated skin and soft tissue infections due to suspected or proven methicillin-resistant Staphylococcus aureus (MRSA). Int J Antimicrob Agents 2005;26(6):442–8.
78. Durkin MJ, Corey GR. New developments in the management of severe skin and deep skin structure infections - focus on tedizolid. Ther Clin Risk Manag 2015; 11:857–62.
79. Gerson SL, Kaplan SL, Bruss JB, et al. Hematologic effects of linezolid: summary of clinical experience. Antimicrobial Agents Chemother 2002;46(8): 2723–6.
80. Prokocimer P, De Anda C, Fang E, et al. Tedizolid phosphate vs linezolid for treatment of acute bacterial skin and skin structure infections: the ESTABLISH-1 randomized trial. JAMA 2013;309(6):559–69.
81. O'Riordan W, McManus A, Teras J, et al. A Comparison of the efficacy and safety of intravenous followed by oral delafloxacin with vancomycin plus aztreonam for the treatment of acute bacterial skin and skin structure infections: a phase 3, multinational, double-blind, randomized study. Clin Infect Dis 2018; 67(5):657–66.
82. Zhanel GG, Esquivel J, Zelenitsky S, et al. Omadacycline: a novel oral and intravenous aminomethylcycline antibiotic agent. Drugs 2020;80(3):285–313.
83. Draper MP, Weir S, Macone A, et al. Mechanism of action of the novel aminomethylcycline antibiotic omadacycline. Antimicrobial Agents Chemother 2014; 58(3):1279–83.
84. O'Riordan W, Green S, Overcash JS, et al. Omadacycline for acute bacterial skin and skin-structure infections. N Engl J Med 2019;380(6):528–38.
85. O'Riordan W, Cardenas C, Shin E, et al. Once-daily oral omadacycline versus twice-daily oral linezolid for acute bacterial skin and skin structure infections (OASIS-2): a phase 3, double-blind, multicentre, randomised, controlled, non-inferiority trial. Lancet Infect Dis 2019;19(10):1080–90.

86. Rybak MJ, Le J, Lodise TP, et al. Executive summary: therapeutic monitoring of vancomycin for serious methicillin-resistant Staphylococcus aureus infections: a revised consensus guideline and review of the American Society of Health-System Pharmacists, the Infectious Diseases Society of America, the Pediatric Infectious Diseases Society, and the Society of Infectious Diseases Pharmacists. Pharmacotherapy 2020;40(4):363–7.

87. Stein GE, Wells EM. The importance of tissue penetration in achieving successful antimicrobial treatment of nosocomial pneumonia and complicated skin and soft-tissue infections caused by methicillin-resistant Staphylococcus aureus: vancomycin and linezolid. Curr Med Res Opin 2010;26(3):571–88.

88. Wargo KA, McCreary EK, English TM. Vancomycin combined with clindamycin for the treatment of acute bacterial skin and skin-structure infections. Clin Infect Dis 2015;61(7):1148–54.

89. Stryjewski ME, Graham DR, Wilson SE, et al. Telavancin versus vancomycin for the treatment of complicated skin and skin-structure infections caused by gram-positive organisms. Clin Infect Dis 2008;46(11):1683–93.

90. Polyzos KA, Mavros MN, Vardakas KZ, et al. Efficacy and safety of telavancin in clinical trials: a systematic review and meta-analysis. PLoS ONE 2012;7(8): e41870.

91. Boucher HW, Wilcox M, Talbot GH, et al. Once-weekly dalbavancin versus daily conventional therapy for skin infection. N Engl J Med 2014;370(23):2169–79.

92. Jauregui LE, Babazadeh S, Seltzer E, et al. Randomized, double-blind comparison of once-weekly dalbavancin versus twice-daily linezolid therapy for the treatment of complicated skin and skin structure infections. Clin Infect Dis 2005;41(10):1407–15.

93. Dunne MW, Puttagunta S, Giordano P, et al. A randomized clinical trial of single-dose versus weekly dalbavancin for treatment of acute bacterial skin and skin structure infection. Clin Infect Dis 2016;62(5):545–51.

94. Corey GR, Good S, Jiang H, et al. Single-dose oritavancin versus 7-10 days of vancomycin in the treatment of gram-positive acute bacterial skin and skin structure infections: the SOLO II noninferiority study. Clin Infect Dis 2015; 60(2):254–62.

95. Wang SZ, Hu JT, Zhang C, et al. The safety and efficacy of daptomycin versus other antibiotics for skin and soft-tissue infections: a meta-analysis of randomised controlled trials. BMJ Open 2014;4(6):e004744.

96. Dare RK, Tewell C, Harris B, et al. Effect of statin coadministration on the risk of daptomycin-associated myopathy. Clin Infect Dis 2018;67(9):1356–63.

97. Liu C, Bayer A, Cosgrove SE, et al. Clinical practice guidelines by the Infectious Diseases Society of America for the treatment of methicillin-resistant Staphylococcus aureus infections in adults and children. Clin Infect Dis 2011;52(3): e18–55.

98. Sacchidanand S, Penn RL, Embil JM, et al. Efficacy and safety of tigecycline monotherapy compared with vancomycin plus aztreonam in patients with complicated skin and skin structure infections: results from a phase 3, randomized, double-blind trial. Int J Infect Dis 2005;9(5):251–61.

99. Miller LG, Perdreau-Remington F, Bayer AS, et al. Clinical and epidemiologic characteristics cannot distinguish community-associated methicillin-resistant Staphylococcus aureus infection from methicillin-susceptible S. aureus infection: a prospective investigation. Clin Infect Dis 2007;44(4):471–82.

100. Youngster I, Shenoy ES, Hooper DC, et al. Comparative evaluation of the tolerability of cefazolin and nafcillin for treatment of methicillin-susceptible

Staphylococcus aureus infections in the outpatient setting. Clin Infect Dis 2014; 59(3):369–75.

101. Miller WR, Seas C, Carvajal LP, et al. The cefazolin inoculum effect is associated with increased mortality in methicillin-susceptible Staphylococcus aureus bacteremia. Open Forum Infect Dis 2018;5(6):ofy123.

102. Eells SJ, Nguyen M, Jung J, et al. Relationship between adherence to oral antibiotics and postdischarge clinical outcomes among patients hospitalized with Staphylococcus aureus skin infections. Antimicrobial Agents Chemother 2016; 60(5):2941–8.

103. Noviello S, Magnet S, Hawser S, et al. In vitro activity of iclaprim against isolates in two phase 3 clinical trials (REVIVE-1 and -2) for acute bacterial skin and skin structure infections. Antimicrobial Agents Chemother 2019;63(4). https://doi. org/10.1128/AAC.02239-18.

104. Holland TL, O'Riordan W, McManus A, et al. A Phase 3, randomized, double-blind, multicenter study to evaluate the safety and efficacy of intravenous iclaprim versus vancomycin for treatment of acute bacterial skin and skin structure infections suspected or confirmed to be due to gram-positive pathogens (REVIVE-2 Study). Antimicrobial Agents Chemother 2018;62(5). https://doi.org/ 10.1128/AAC.02580-17.

105. Huang DB, O'Riordan W, Overcash JS, et al. A Phase 3, randomized, double-blind, multicenter study to evaluate the safety and efficacy of intravenous iclaprim vs vancomycin for the treatment of acute bacterial skin and skin structure infections suspected or confirmed to be due to gram-positive pathogens: REVIVE-1. Clin Infect Dis 2018;66(8):1222–9.

106. Prince WT, Ivezic-Schoenfeld Z, Lell C, et al. Phase II clinical study of BC-3781, a pleuromutilin antibiotic, in treatment of patients with acute bacterial skin and skin structure infections. Antimicrobial Agents Chemother 2013;57(5):2087–94.

Decolonization of *Staphylococcus aureus*

Sima L. Sharara, MD, Lisa L. Maragakis, MD, MPH, Sara E. Cosgrove, MD, MS*

KEYWORDS

- Decolonization • Staphylococcus aureus colonization • Chlorhexidine bathing
- Nasal mupirocin

KEY POINTS

- Strategies for decolonization of *Staphylococcus aureus* include topical nasal antibiotics and antiseptic body washes and have been found to reduce the risk of invasive and noninvasive infections in some populations.
- Current evidence suggests that *S aureus* decolonization with nasal mupirocin and chlorhexidine gluconate bathing for 5 days reduces the risk of *S aureus* surgical site infections, particularly in patients undergoing joint replacements or cardiac surgery.
- Both targeted and universal decolonization of *S aureus* have been studied in the intensive care unit setting and reduce the risk of hospital-acquired infections in these studies.
- Decolonization has also been studied in persons with recurrent skin and soft tissue infections, critically ill neonatal patients and their families, non–critically ill hospitalized patients, nursing home residents, and after hospital discharge with mixed results.
- The risks of decolonization include toxicity from the agents and selection for more resistant organisms, and guidelines should recommend surveillance of *S aureus* susceptibility to decolonization agents and the development of alternative agents for decolonization.

BACKGROUND

Staphylococcus aureus infections are associated with increased morbidity, mortality, hospital length of stay, and health-care costs.[1–4] *S aureus*, including both methicillin-susceptible and resistant strains, is the second most common causative pathogen of all health care–associated infections, and the most common cause of surgical site infections (SSI) and ventilator-associated pneumonia.[5] *S aureus* colonization has been shown to increase risk for invasive and noninvasive infections.[6–10] More than 80% of *S aureus* strains causing infections are endogenous and are genetically similar to strains isolated from the nares of corresponding colonized patients.[11–14]

Division of Infectious Diseases, Department of Medicine, Johns Hopkins University School of Medicine, 600 North Wolfe Street, Baltimore, MD 21287, USA
* Corresponding author.
E-mail address: scosgro1@jhmi.edu

Infect Dis Clin N Am 35 (2021) 107–133
https://doi.org/10.1016/j.idc.2020.10.010
0891-5520/21/© 2020 Elsevier Inc. All rights reserved.

Given the role of colonization in the pathogenesis of S aureus infection, prevention strategies have included decolonization with the use of antimicrobial or antiseptic agents to suppress or eliminate S aureus carriage as a means of preventing auto-infection or transmission.[7] In this article, we summarize the recent literature on decolonization of S aureus, highlighting important clinical studies, to guide current practice.

Although there has been a focus on methicillin-resistant S aureus (MRSA) decolonization strategies, studies suggest that morbidity and mortality of invasive MRSA and methicillin-susceptible S aureus (MSSA) infection in hospitalized patients are similar.[15] Further, there is a decreasing incidence of MRSA skin and soft tissue infection (SSTI) in children and adults, and an increase in MSSA SSTI.[16] Thus, we address decolonization of both MSSA and MRSA and also highlight important studies exclusively examining MRSA decolonization.

PREVALENCE

Between 15% and 32% of the population is thought to be nasally colonized with MSSA, and 1% to 3% is colonized with MRSA.[7,17–19] Identification of S aureus carriage is usually performed using nasal swabs, and results can be available within 2 hours using real-time polymerase chain reaction.[20] S aureus can also colonize the oropharynx, skin folds (groin, axilla), and rectum. S aureus screening from additional sites in addition to the nares at the time of hospital or intensive care unit (ICU) admission has been shown to increase detection of MRSA compared with nasal screening alone.[21] Although the nose is often the only site swabbed during surveillance, the risk of developing infection is higher when more sites are colonized with MRSA.[22]

Nasal S aureus carriage patterns in humans include noncarriers who never have positive cultures, intermittent carriers, and persistent carriers. Intermittent carriers have less than 80% of cultures positive for S aureus, and persistent carriers have more than 80% of cultures positive with genotypically identical S aureus isolates.[10,23] Persistent carriers seem to have the highest risk of infection.[24–27] However, decolonization interventions target both intermittent and persistent carriers to decrease the risk of invasive disease.

S AUREUS DECOLONIZATION STRATEGIES

Strategies for decolonization of S aureus include topical nasal agents (eg, mupirocin, retapamulin, and povidone-iodine [PI]) and antiseptic body washes (eg, chlorhexidine gluconate [CHG] or sodium hypochlorite [dilute bleach]). Oral antimicrobial therapy is recommended only for active treatment of infection, and is not routinely recommended for S aureus decolonization.[28] These strategies have been evaluated either alone or in combination, and there are varying approaches. Twice daily mupirocin for 5 days is used for nasal decolonization for both MSSA and MRSA.[29] Retapamulin also is applied twice daily to the nares for 5 days, but has not been robustly studied. PI mainly has been studied in the setting of SSI prevention, and applied once or twice within 24 hours before the operation. CHG or dilute beach baths are used daily or every other day for 5 to 14 days.[28]

Decolonization of carriers has proven effective in decreasing staphylococcal infections in certain patient settings. However, because screening for S aureus largely depends on detection of nasal carriage, this strategy may lead to misclassification of patients with other sites of colonization that might stand to benefit from decolonization. Further, recolonization following decolonization is frequent, with between 30% and 60% of patients found to be recolonized after 7 to 18 months.[30–32]

Two main decolonization strategies, targeted and universal decolonization, are applied to large populations in the studies discussed elsewhere in this article. Targeted decolonization relies on the detection of carriers through surveillance swabs, whereas universal decolonization is applied to an entire population of people, regardless of their colonization status and without screening.

USEFULNESS OF *S AUREUS* DECOLONIZATION BY PATIENT POPULATION

A summary of select larger and more recent studies discussed in this article can be found in **Table 1**.

Surgical Patients

S aureus is the most common pathogen associated with SSI overall, as well as the most common pathogen in orthopedic, obstetrics and gynecology, and cardiac SSIs.[5] *S aureus* colonization has been shown to increase the risk of *S aureus* SSIs. In response, several studies have been conducted implementing decolonization interventions in an effort to reduce the risk of postoperative *S aureus* SSI. Herein, we summarize the randomized controlled trials (RCTs) and multicenter studies that examine the usefulness of *S aureus* decolonization in surgical patients.

A large, RCT in the United States that included general, gynecologic, cardiac, and neurologic surgery patients regardless of baseline *S aureus* nasal carriage status (n = 3864) who were treated with nasal mupirocin before the procedure did not show an overall decrease in the rate of *S aureus* SSIs.[14] However, in the subgroup of patients with preoperative nasal carriage (23% of patients in each arm), fewer postoperative *S aureus* health care–associated infections occurred in patients treated with mupirocin (4.0% vs 7.7%; $P = .02$). The odds of SSI in *S aureus* carriers was 4.5 times higher compared with noncarriers in the placebo group ($P<.001$). This study suggests that mupirocin decolonization of nasal carriers may be an effective strategy to prevent *S aureus* infections after surgery.

A randomized, double-blind, placebo-controlled multicenter trial conducted in the Netherlands found that rapid detection of *S aureus* nasal carriage through real-time polymerase chain reaction followed by immediate decolonization of nasal and extranasal sites with nasal mupirocin and CHG soap significantly decrease the risk of hospital-acquired *S aureus* infections[6] (see **Table 1**). Decolonization therapy was begun at the time of admission for 5 days, regardless of surgery performed during the course of treatment, and was repeated at 3 and 6 weeks for patients who were still hospitalized. The eradication of *S aureus* was found to decrease the rate of *S aureus* health care–associated infections by 58%, and this effect was more pronounced for *S aureus* deep SSIs (79% reduction). In the cohort, more than 88% of patients underwent a surgical procedure and no patients had MRSA; thus, inferences regarding the usefulness of this approach in nonsurgical patients or those with MRSA cannot be drawn.

A meta-analysis including 39 studies found that implementing a bundle of screening for *S aureus* nasal carriage, decolonizing carriers with nasal mupirocin and CHG bathing, and using vancomycin for perioperative prophylaxis among MRSA carriers was associated with lower rates of *S aureus* SSI in patients undergoing cardiac or orthopedic surgeries.[33] This evidence-based prevention bundle with targeted decolonization and prophylaxis based on nasal *S aureus* carrier status was tested in the STOP-SSI trial, a multicenter, pragmatic intervention among patients undergoing cardiac, hip, or knee surgery[34] (see **Table 1**). The study included 20 hospitals in the United States, with 42,534 operations among 38,409 patients and found that the prevention bundle

Table 1
Select large recent clinical studies evaluating decolonization strategies in different populations

Author/Year	Sample Size/Patient Population	Study Design	Setting	Number of Sites	Intervention	Control/Placebo	Outcomes	Resistance to Decolonizing Medications	Conclusions	Limitations
Bode et al,[6] 2010	917 adults	Patient-level randomized, double-blind, placebo-controlled trial	General medicine and surgery	5 hospitals	Patients were screened for SA on admission by means of a real-time PCR assay SA nasal carriers received IN mupirocin 2% twice daily and CHG soap (40 mg/mL) daily both for 5 d, starting on admission	SA nasal carriers received IN placebo ointment	Primary: cumulative incidence of SA health care–associated infections in the 6 week-period after discharge Secondary: all-cause in-hospital mortality; LOS; time to onset of SA health care–associated infection	No SA resistance to mupirocin found on screenings	Decrease in SA SSIs (RR of infection, 0.42; 95% CI, 0.23–0.75) and LOS (crude estimate, 12.2 vs 14.0 d; P = .04)	Low proportion of nonsurgical patients (12%); no MRSA; intervention did not substantially reduce exogenous infections
Schweizer et al,[34] 2015	42,534 cardiac/orthopedic operations	Pre-post quality improvement study	Surgery	20 hospitals	MRSA nasal carriers received IN mupirocin twice daily for 5 d, CHG baths twice preop and then daily for up to 5 d and vancomycin perioperative prophylaxis in addition to a cephalosporin	Routine care during the preintervention period	Primary: complex (deep incisional or organ space) SA SSIs Secondary: postoperative LOS; 90-d readmissions for SSIs	1 isolate with high-level mupirocin resistance; 1 isolate with CHG MIC of 4 μ g/mL	Reduction in complex SA SSIs compared with historical data (rate ratio, 0.58; 95% CI, 0.37–0.92)	Patients and facilities were not randomized; SSI surveillance methods differed among sites

Huang et al,[61] 2013	74,256 adults	Cluster-randomized trial	ICU	43 hospitals	Targeted decolonization (screening, isolation, and decolonization of MRSA carriers) or universal decolonization (decolonization of all patients): Decolonization with IN mupirocin twice daily for 5 d and CHG cloths daily for 5 d (targeted decolonization) or full ICU stay (universal decolonization).	MRSA screening and isolation without decolonization	Primary: ICU-attributable, MRSA-positive clinical cultures Secondary: ICU-attributable MRSA BSIs; any ICU-attributable BSIs	Not mentioned	Compared with baseline, for ICU-attributable MRSA positive clinical cultures HR = 0.92 for nondecolonization, HR = 0.75 for targeted decolonization and HR = 0.63 for universal decolonization (P = .01 for test of all groups being equal). Compared with baseline, for ICU-attributable all-cause BSI HR = 0.99 for nondecolonization, HR = 0.78 for targeted decolonization and HR = 0.56 for universal decolonization (P = .01 for test of all groups being equal). No significant difference for MRSA BSI	Baseline rates of ICU-attributable all-cause BSI were higher in the universal decolonization group
Kotloff et al,[80] 2019	155 infants	Patient-level RCT	NICU	8 NICUs	SA nasal carriers received IN, periumbilical, perianal mupirocin 2% if positive 3 times daily for 5 d	SA nasal carriers did not receive mupirocin	Primary: decolonization of the IN, periumbilical, and perianal areas after 8 and 22 d; solicited AEs; moderate and severe unsolicited AEs Secondary: SA infections through day 22; non-SA invasive infections; stage II to III NEC	No emergence of mupirocin resistance in treated infants; greater proportion of infants colonized with mupirocin-resistant strains at enrollment toward the end of the study period	In the treatment group, SA decolonization occurred more often after 8 d (P<.001) and after 22 (P<.001)	More rashes in the treatment group; many infants who remained in the hospital became recolonized with SA; the open-label design may have led to reporting bias

(continued on next page)

Table 1
(continued)

Author/Year	Sample Size/Patient Population	Study Design	Setting	Number of Sites	Intervention	Control/Placebo	Outcomes	Resistance to Decolonizing Medications	Conclusions	Limitations
Milstone et al,[79] 2020	236 neonates	Double-blinded randomized trial; neonate-parent groupings were randomized	NICU	2 NICUs	Parents received IN mupirocin 2% twice daily and 2% CHG cloths daily for 5 d	Placebo IN ointment and nonmedicated soap cloths for 5 d	Primary: concordant SA acquisition Secondary: any SA acquisition; SA infection; BSI by any organism	Not mentioned	SA decolonization of parents led to their newborns being less likely to be colonized by a strain concordant with their parents' strains after 90 d (HR, 0.43; 95.2% CI, 0.16–0.79)	The amount of parent-neonate interaction was not measured; the study was not powered to evaluate SA infections
Huang et al,[90] 2019	528,983 adults	Cluster-randomized trial	General medicine and surgery	53 hospitals	MRSA carriers received IN mupirocin twice daily for 5 d All patients showered/bathed with CHG daily	Routine care	Primary: combined MRSA or VRE clinical cultures attributable to a participating unit Secondary: clinical cultures of MDRGNRs attributable to a participating unit; all-pathogen BSI attributable to a participating unit	Not mentioned	In non-critical care patients, CHG bathing and mupirocin treatment of MRSA carriers did not reduce MRSA or VRE clinical isolates (P = .17), MDRGNR clinical isolates (P = .16), or all-pathogen BSIs (P = .43).	Quality of CHG application may have varied; low baseline rates of resistant organisms

| Huang et al,[111] 2019 | 2121 adults | Patient-level RCT | Hospital units and nursing homes | 17 hospitals and 7 nursing homes | MRSA carriers received postdischarge hygiene education They also received IN mupirocin and CHG mouthwash twice daily and bathed/showered with CHG daily, each for 5 d twice per month for 6 mo | Postdischarge hygiene education only | Primary: MRSA infection within 1 y Secondary: infection-related rehospitalization within 1 y; infection from any cause per CDC criteria | 9.4% and 3.1% of MRSA isolates with high-level and low-level mupirocin resistance, respectively, post intervention 1.5% of MRSA strains with emergent high-level mupirocin-resistant strains 2 MRSA isolates with CHG MIC of 8 μ g/mL | Postdischarge MRSA decolonization reduced the risks of postdischarge MRSA infections by 30% (HR, 0.70; 95% CI, 0.52–0.96; *P* = .03) and rehospitalization owing to infection (HR, 0.76; 95% CI, 0.62–0.93) | Unblinded; substantial attrition; mild infections may not have been detected; treatment effects for the secondary outcomes should be interpreted with caution |

Abbreviations: AE, adverse event; BSI, bloodstream infection; CDC, Centers for Disease Control and Prevention; CHG, chlorhexidine; CI, confidence interval; HR, hazard ratio; ICU, intensive care unit; IN, intranasal; LOS, length of stay; MDRGNR, multidrug-resistant gram-negative rod; MIC, minimum inhibitory concentration; MRSA, methicillin-resistant *Staphylococcus aureus*; MSSA, methicillin-sensitive *S aureus*; NEC, necrotizing enterocolitis; NICU, neonatal intensive care unit; PCR, polymerase chain reaction; RCT, randomized controlled trial; RR, relative risk; SA, *S aureus*; SSI, surgical-site infection; VRE, vancomycin-resistant enterococci.

was associated with reduced deep incisional or organ space S aureus SSIs. Subgroup analyses showed a significant decrease in S aureus SSI in hip and knee arthroplasties, but not in cardiac operations. The intervention was not associated with a significant decrease in postoperative length of stay or readmissions. Full bundle adherence was seen in only 39% of cases, suggesting the difficulty in achieving adherence to complicated bundled protocols, particularly in hospital settings without strong quality improvement infrastructures. The findings of these studies have been echoed in other studies and meta-analyses.[35,36]

PI solutions have also been used for decolonization of nasal S aureus in surgical patients. The benefits of PI include the large number of S aureus strains in the nares sensitive to PI, lower cost, rapid bactericidal activity, and effectiveness with a single application.[37] A randomized, nonblinded placebo-controlled trial found that a single nasal application of 10% PI significantly reduced MRSA at 1 and 6 hours after application, but suppression was not sustained at 12 and 24 hours.[38] This result suggests that PI applications may be effective for short-term suppression of S aureus during the perioperative period. An RCT investigating SSI after arthroplasty or spine fusion compared nasal mupirocin ointment for 5 days with 2 applications of 5% PI within 2 hours of surgical incision; all patients received CHG cloths for skin cleansing.[39] There was no significant difference in deep SSI or S aureus deep SSI within 3 months after the surgery between the 2 groups in the intent-to-treat analysis. In the per-protocol analysis, PI was more effective in reducing S aureus deep SSI ($P = .03$). In a prospective study, use of CHG cloths and oral rinse (0.12%) and nasal PI solution (5%) the night before and the morning of surgery in patients undergoing elective orthopedic surgery with hardware implantation was associated with a lower 30-day SSI rate compared with a preintervention control group (1.1% vs 3.8%; $P = .02$).[40]

The guidelines for preoperative antimicrobial prophylaxis developed by the American Society of Health-System Pharmacists, the Infectious Diseases Society of America, the Surgical Infection Society, and the Society for Healthcare Epidemiology of America (SHEA) recommend the use of decolonization with preoperative nasal mupirocin as an adjunctive measure to prevent S aureus SSI, with a particular focus on patients undergoing cardiac and orthopedic procedures, but the guidelines do not comment on CHG bathing.[41] The adoption of screening and decolonization interventions to decrease SSIs vary significantly, with between 40% and 60% of physicians not screening for S aureus preoperatively.[42,43] Further, decolonization of S aureus before surgery often only targets MRSA carriers, despite the greater frequency of MSSA infections and colonization in this population.[34,43]

Current evidence suggests that S aureus decolonization with nasal mupirocin and CHG bathing for 5 days decreases the risk of S aureus SSI, particularly in patients undergoing joint replacements or cardiac surgery. Although the optimal timing and duration of administration are not standardized, 70% of patients who are initially colonized with MSSA or MRSA remained decolonized at 156 days with 5 days of nasal mupirocin and a single CHG preoperative shower.[31] PI solutions may be a reasonable alternative if mupirocin resistance or allergy is a concern. If a program to decolonize surgical patients is desired, consideration should be given to how to ensure that it is successfully operationalized, including who orders and performs the testing, how the topical agents are provided to patients in the appropriate preoperative time frame, and whether there will be modification to perioperative systemic antibiotic prophylaxis based on the results. Universal preoperative decolonization is not supported by existing data; additional research is required to quantify its risks and benefits.

Patients with Recurrent Skin and Soft Tissue Infections

Patients with recurrent SSTIs are often reinfected with the same strain of *S aureus*.[44–46] Thus, decolonization of *S aureus* has been used as a method to interrupt the cycle of recurrent infection.

The data regarding the efficacy of *S aureus* decolonization in preventing recurrent SSTI are mixed. Although *S aureus* decolonization may be effective in decreasing carriage, it remains unclear whether that contributes to a decreased risk of SSTI recurrence. A 1-year trial of a monthly 5-day course of nasal mupirocin in patients with 3 or more staphylococcal skin infections who were carriers was found to reduce the prevalence of nasal colonization and the risk of recurrent skin infection compared with placebo (n = 34, 17 per arm).[47] An RCT of 987 children with probable community-acquired *S aureus* SSTIs or invasive infections found that dilute bleach baths plus hygiene education over a 3-month period was associated with a nonsignificant decrease in recurrent SSTI compared with hygiene education alone.[48] A retrospective review of 399 pediatric patients with culture-positive MRSA abscesses found that a decolonization prescription for 2 weeks of daily nasal mupirocin and dilute sodium hypochlorite baths or CHG cloth washes 2 to 3 times per week did not decrease rates of SSTI recurrence.[49] An RCT of 244 patients with community-onset SSTI and *S aureus* colonization in the nares, axilla, or inguinal fold who were randomized to personal and household education or education with 3 different decolonization strategies (nasal mupirocin, nasal mupirocin and CHG washes, or nasal mupirocin and dilute bleach baths, all for 5 days) found that participants in all study arms experienced a substantial rate of recurrent SSTIs.[50] Only the participants in the education, mupirocin, and CHG arms had a significantly lower rate of SSTI at 1 month compared with controls, but this effect was not seen at 4 and 6 months.[50]

The rates of recurrent *S aureus* SSTIs remain high, even after decolonization, indicating the need to understand and mitigate risk factors for recurrent infection. The Infectious Diseases Society of America clinical practice guidelines recommend decolonization in the setting of ongoing transmission from household members or close contacts,[28] because household members are thought to serve as reservoirs contributing to reinfection.[51] A randomized trial implementing decolonization in household members of children with community-acquired *S aureus* SSTI found that decolonization of all household members was more effective in preventing recurrent infection compared with decolonization of the index patient alone, with the effect lasting for up to 1 year.[52] A multicenter study of 223 households of adult or children with index community-onset MRSA SSTI found no significant difference in time to clearance of MRSA colonization between the hygiene education group and the decolonization group, but compliance with the intervention was only reported in 26% of the households.[53] An RCT comparing household versus personal decolonization with twice-daily nasal mupirocin and daily dilute bleach water baths for 5 days in children with MRSA SSTI found that the personal approach was noninferior in preventing SSTI compared with decolonization of all household members after 12 months.[54]

Although data are equivocal regarding the effectiveness of decolonization strategies to prevent recurrent SSTIs, for patients experiencing recurrent SSTI, or in households in which multiple members have experienced SSTI, decolonization can be considered. Decolonization of patients and households in the community setting should be based on the individual's (or household's) burden of disease and recurrence risk.[55] A recommended decolonization regimen includes the application of nasal mupirocin and antiseptic body washes with CHG or dilute bleach water baths. For patients who continue to experience recurrent SSTI, periodic decolonization should be considered.

However, the optimal regimen, frequency of application, and duration of decolonization for recurrent SSTIs remain unclear and require further study. In addition to decolonization, it is important to emphasize education regarding S aureus transmission, wound care, and personal and household hygiene measures.[51]

Hospitalized Patients

Patients in the intensive care unit

S aureus is the third most common cause of central line–associated bloodstream infections after coagulase-negative staphylococci and Candida albicans, and the most common cause of ventilator-associated pneumonia in the ICU setting.[5] Colonization with S aureus in the ICU significantly increases the risk of developing S aureus infections.[56] Hospitals commonly screen ICU patients for nasal carriage of MRSA and many implement contact isolation precautions for patients who are carriers. Two main strategies have been studied in the ICU setting: universal and targeted decolonization.

Several studies have examined the use of universal decolonization for all patients in the ICU and its association with a reduced risk of acquisition of multidrug-resistant organisms—including MRSA—and the development of health care–associated infection.[57–59] Further, universal decolonization in a large ICU was shown to contribute to a decrease in the spread and incidence of MRSA across an entire hospital[60] (see **Table 1**). The REDUCE-MRSA trial was a pragmatic, cluster randomized trial including 43 hospitals and 74 ICUs implementing 3 intervention strategies for MRSA prevention: (1) MRSA screening and isolation with contact precautions (also the baseline period strategy) without decolonization, (2) MRSA screening, contact isolation, and targeted decolonization of MRSA carriers with daily CHG bathing and twice-daily nasal mupirocin, and (3) universal decolonization of all patients with the same regimen.[61] Compared with the baseline period, hazard ratios for having a clinical culture growing MRSA (primary outcome) were 0.92 for the nondecolonization strategy, 0.75 for the targeted decolonization strategy, and 0.63 for the universal decolonization strategy ($P = .01$ for test of all groups being equal). Similar results were observed for the secondary outcome of ICU-attributable all-cause bloodstream infections, but a significant difference was not observed for the secondary outcome of ICU-attributable MRSA bloodstream infection. Universal decolonization in the ICU was significantly more effective than the nondecolonization strategy for decreasing all outcomes. Targeted decolonization in the ICU was significantly more effective than the nondecolonization strategy for reducing ICU-attributable all-cause bloodstream infection, but not ICU-attributable clinical cultures growing MRSA or MRSA bloodstream infections. Of note, the baseline rates of ICU-attributable all-cause bloodstream infection were higher in the universal decolonization group; thus, these units may have been engaged in other activities besides the study intervention to decrease bloodstream infections during the intervention period. Overall, this study suggests that population-level decolonization strategies seem to prevent health care–associated infections with a potential additive benefit of universal decolonization over targeted decolonization in this cohort. It is important to note that the study interventions were successfully implemented as a part of routine practice across various hospital settings.

Fewer studies examine targeted S aureus colonization alone, and most are single-center, observational, cohort studies, with a focus on MRSA. Targeted decolonization of MRSA-colonized patients with nasal mupirocin and daily CHG bathing in the ICU of a Veterans Affairs Medical Center was found to decrease incident cases of MRSA colonization or infection by 52%.[62] A 5-year study implementing routine treatment of MRSA nasal carriers in the ICU with CHG bathing and nasal mupirocin resulted in a significant decrease in MRSA health care–associated infections in Brazil.[63] A retrospective quasiexperimental study in *S aureus* nasal carriers in a medical ICU showed that active surveillance and decolonization with nasal mupirocin and CHG baths was associated with a significantly decreased incidence of both MSSA and MRSA colonization, and *S aureus* health care–associated infections and ventilator-associated pneumonia.[64] Of note, there was no significant difference in the incidence of *S aureus* bloodstream infections.

Both targeted and universal decolonization are recommended as potential strategies to prevent MRSA health care–associated infections in the compendium published by the SHEA, the Infectious Diseases Society of America, the American Hospital Association, the Association for Professionals in Infection Control and Epidemiology, and the Joint Commission.[65] A National Healthcare Safety Network survey found substantial variation in the adoption of MRSA screening and infection prevention measures.[66] The benefits of universal decolonization include the decrease of skin colonization with several potential pathogens and protecting patients from subsequent infection,[57,67,68] a decrease in the environmental microbial burden and the risk of patient-to-patient transmission, avoiding delays in decolonization pending screening test results,[61] and decreasing the costs associated with MRSA surveillance cultures and contact precautions.[69-71] The risk of universal decolonization is the potential emergence of resistance to mupirocin and CHG with widespread use that could contribute to decolonization failure.[72] A recent model found that universal decolonization could lead to a significantly higher prevalence of mupirocin resistance among MRSA strains when compared with targeted decolonization after 5 years (21% vs 9% estimated prevalence of mupirocin resistance, respectively).[73] There has not yet been a trial comparing CHG bathing alone with CHG bathing plus mupirocin for decolonization, an approach that could minimize mupirocin resistance. High rates of CHG resistance have been found in the ICU settings, with reports as high as 33% of *S aureus* isolates.[74,75] In 2017, the US Food and Drug Administration released a warning about the rare but serious allergic reactions with skin antisepsis with CHG, including anaphylaxis, which may also limit widespread use.[76] The impact of these risks would be expected to be minimized with targeted decolonization. Of note, a targeted strategy provides information on MRSA colonization status, which is helpful in understanding risk for MRSA infection and in antimicrobial stewardship decisions around MRSA treatment and vancomycin de-escalation in the ICU.[77]

Neonatal intensive care unit patients and families

S aureus is a leading cause of health care–associated infections in the neonatal ICU (NICU).[78] Neonates are particularly vulnerable to *S aureus* colonization owing to their immature microbiome at the time of NICU admission, and the high risk of exposure to people and objects in the environment.[79] The nares and umbilicus are the 2 most common site of initial neonatal colonization.[12] *S aureus* colonization of NICU infants is a strong predictor of subsequent invasive infections, which are often caused by the same *S aureus* strain.[12] Interventions to prevent *S aureus* infections in critically ill infants have the potential to decrease adverse outcomes, length of hospital stay, antibiotic use, and health care costs.[80] Although the majority of these interventions target MRSA, morbidity and mortality from MSSA in the NICU seems to be equivalent to MRSA.[81]

A 7-year study in Taiwan that included standard infection control measures to decrease MRSA spread in the NICU found that surveillance cultures and decolonization of MRSA with nasal and periumbilical mupirocin significantly reduced rates of MRSA colonization (8.6% vs 41%) and infection (1.1% vs 12%) compared with the period of surveillance cultures without decolonization.[82] A phase II multicenter, open-label, randomized trial of nasal, periumbilical, and perianal mupirocin in S aureus colonized critically ill infants less than 24 months of age (79% MSSA, 20% MRSA) found that primary decolonization occurred in up to 94% of treated infants, but that more than one-half of those who remained hospitalized were recolonized within 2 to 3 weeks and no statistically significant decrease in S aureus infections was noted.[80] The trial found that the application of mupirocin to S aureus-colonized infants in the NICU is generally well-tolerated and safe, but could result in rashes (usually mild and perianal).

As in the adult ICU, the use of universal decolonization has been studied in the NICU setting. A 5-year study applying twice daily mupirocin to all infants admitted to a NICU in Hawaii revealed a significant decrease in S aureus colonization and infections, and this was not found to contribute to mupirocin resistance.[83] However, a study in France found that the use of mupirocin in health care staff and NICU patients did not control an MRSA outbreak, and that other measures such as hand hygiene audits and training, as well as cohort isolation of neonates, were more effective.[84]

Targeted decolonization strategies in the NICU have showed minimal success. A retrospective cohort study found that using aggressive infection prevention measures, including routine surveillance cultures, contact precautions, decolonization of infants and health care workers, and increasing hand hygiene compliance did not prevent ongoing MRSA transmission and infection in the NICU.[85] Forty-two percent of infections developed before infants were identified as MRSA colonized. Further, 16% of infants decolonized with CHG cloths and nasal mupirocin developed MRSA infection. The study highlighted the limitation of MRSA decolonization as an infection prevention strategy in a setting with high-endemicity of community-acquired MRSA and the need to investigate other sources of potential to decrease the risk of S aureus transmission in this high-risk population.

Guidelines for S aureus decolonization in the NICU are lacking; thus, there is significant variation in approaches to S aureus colonization in the NICU.[86] A survey conducted by the SHEA on the identification and eradication of MRSA in the NICU found that, although 86% of respondents screened patients for MRSA colonization, approaches to the number of anatomic sites screened, use of admission cultures, empiric isolation, and MRSA decolonization greatly varied.[87] Only 37% of respondents attempted decolonization of MRSA carriers (21% decolonized all MRSA carriers, 12% decolonized select patients, and 4% decolonized MRSA-infected infants). All of the respondents reported using mupirocin, with 35% using a topical antiseptic bath.

The US Food and Drug Administration advises caution with the use of 2% CHG cloths in premature infants and infants under 2 months of age owing to the risk of irritation and chemical burns. However, the majority of NICUs use CHG, commonly for central venous catheter site preparation and maintenance.[88] Premature infants are especially vulnerable to adverse reactions to CHG exposure owing to their underdeveloped and highly permeable skin leading to local toxicity and systemic absorption, their decreased ability for metabolizing and clearing of drugs, and concern for potential neurotoxicity.[89]

Owing to the high rate of recolonization of NICU infants, studies have targeted parents as a source of potential S aureus colonization, predisposing neonates to invasive S aureus disease. A recent double-blind RCT in 2 tertiary care NICUs examined whether treating S aureus-colonized parents can decrease a key reservoir of transmission and prevent or delay neonatal acquisition of S aureus in neonates. S aureus–colonized parents of NICU patients were treated with nasal mupirocin and 2% CHG bathing cloths versus placebo for 5 days.[79] Neonates whose parents were treated had a reduced risk of both concordant and any S aureus colonization within

90 days of randomization as well as up to 8 weeks after randomization compared with placebo. However, there remained high rates of S aureus acquisition in both groups at 8 weeks (31.5% in the intervention group and 44.6% in the placebo group), which indicates the need for other strategies to decrease S aureus colonization and infection in this high-risk population. Further, this study was only conducted in 2 centers (which have a comprehensive S aureus surveillance and decolonization program), so the generalizability of these findings requires studies that replicate these findings and further research.

Non–critically ill hospitalized patients

Despite the high-risk nature of patients in the ICU, most health care–associated infections occur in non–critical care units, because of the larger patient population.[90] S aureus is the most frequently reported central line–associated bloodstream infections pathogen in hospital wards.[5] Universal decolonization strategies could be a way to prevent these infections; however, experimental evidence for this approach in the non–critical care setting is limited and shows mixed results. A survey of hospital practices of the SHEA Research Network regarding the use of CHG bathing for the prevention of health care–associated infection found that 38% of respondents reported CHG bathing in some non-ICU units and 17% reported hospital-wide use of CHG bathing for S aureus decolonization.[91]

A prospective crossover study of daily CHG bathing In 4 medical inpatient units in Canada over a 7-month period showed a significant decrease in MRSA (55%) and vancomycin-resistant enterococci (VRE) (36%) infection and colonization compared with controls.[92] However, compliance with CHG bathing was only 58%. A similar study of daily CHG bathing in 4 general medicine units over 14 months showed a 64% decreased risk of the composite incidence of MRSA and VRE health care–associated infections compared with historical controls.[93] Another study of hospital-wide CHG bathing for 19 months with a 4-month washout period reported a significant decrease in *Clostridioides difficile* infection, but no impact on the composite measure of colonization and infection rates of VRE and MRSA.[94] A randomized, double-blind placebo controlled trial comparing 2% mupirocin nasal treatment to placebo for 5 days in nonsurgical hospitalized patients found no statistical difference in the rate of nosocomial S aureus infections, mortality, or duration of hospitalization.[95]

The ABATE (Active Bathing To Eliminate infection) trial was a cluster-randomized trial of 53 hospitals (with 194 non–critical care units) that compared routine bathing with decolonization with universal CHG and targeted nasal mupirocin (for known MRSA carriers) in non–critical care units[90] (see **Table 1**). These interventions did not significantly decrease unit-attributable multidrug-resistant clinical cultures or all-cause bloodstream infection in non–critical care patients. Contrary to the benefit of universal decolonization in the ICU setting, the lack of apparent benefit in non–critically ill patients can be driven by multiple factors. General inpatients have fewer medical devices, are less likely to undergo invasive procedures, have shorter durations of hospital stay, and are better able to maintain self-care and personal hygiene compared with critically ill patients.[90]

Post hoc analyses of the ABATE trial revealed that patients with medical devices did benefit from the intervention, with a 32% greater decrease in all-cause bloodstream infection and a 37% greater decrease in MRSA or VRE clinical cultures compared with routine care group. Patients who had medical devices accounted for only 10% of the patients in the routine care group during the intervention period, but had 37% of MRSA or VRE cultures and 56% of the bloodstream infections. However, this benefit seen for patients with medical devices was in the context of universal CHG bathing, emphasizing the need for targeted studies examining bathing and nasal decolonization exclusively for patients with medical devices in general inpatient settings. Decolonization for S aureus in non–critically ill hospitalized patients should be selectively used in patients with medical devices and central lines. Consideration should be given to the operationalization of decolonization of these patients given that, in contrast with the ICU setting, patients on the hospital wards are more likely to be self-administering the treatment.

Dialysis patients

Patients on hemodialysis (HD) and peritoneal dialysis are a unique patient population with frequent health care contact. Dialysis patients have a rate of S aureus colonization between 20% to 50%, and are particularly vulnerable to subsequent S aureus infections.[10,32,96–98]

HD patients colonized with MRSA have an increased risk of subsequent S aureus infection, mortality, and increased health care costs.[99–103] There remain limited data on the clinical consequences and guidance for screening of MSSA in HD patients, although the majority of S aureus carrier isolates are methicillin susceptible.[32] A study of HD patients found that, after decolonization of S aureus (>90% MSSA), only 36% of patients were decolonized after 18 months.[32] The patients who failed to eradicate S aureus were more likely to have an episode of S aureus bacteremia within the study period compared with those who were successfully decolonized. A 2-year study of HD patients found that nasal mupirocin led to eradication of nasal S aureus carriage in 96.3% of surveillance cultures and led to a 4-fold decrease in incidence of S aureus bacteremia per patient-year.[104] A study in the Netherlands found that elimination of S aureus carriage with nasal mupirocin was effective in 98.5% of HD patients, persisted up to 6 months in 91% of patients, and was associated with a significantly lower risk of S aureus bacteremia compared with historic controls.[105] A Cochrane review on the use of nasal mupirocin in S aureus carriers found that mupirocin was associated with a reduction in S aureus (particularly MSSA) health care–associated infections, primarily among patients receiving dialysis.[106]

Similarly, continuous peritoneal dialysis patients with persistent S aureus carriage were found to have higher rates of continuous peritoneal dialysis-related infections compared with noncarriers and intermittent carriers, including exit site infections and peritonitis.[10] The Mupirocin Study group conducted a multicenter study of 267 continuous peritoneal dialysis patients that revealed that use of nasal mupirocin in nasal carriers of S aureus significantly reduced the rate of exit-site infections with the organism compared with placebo.[107] A Cochrane review of agents preventing peritonitis in peritoneal dialysis patients found that nasal S aureus decolonization had an uncertain effect on the risk of peritonitis owing to the low quality of existing studies.[108]

A meta-analysis of 10 studies and 2445 dialysis patients found that the use of mupirocin decreased the rate of S aureus infections by 68%, with a subgroup analysis revealing a risk reduction of 80% in HD patients and 63% in peritoneal dialysis patients.[109] Another systemic review and meta-analysis on the use of mupirocin decolonization to prevent S aureus infection in nonsurgical settings found that mupirocin decrease the risk of S aureus infections by 59% in dialysis patients and 40% in nondialysis settings.[110]

Dialysis patients are more frequently colonized with S aureus than the general population,[98] and it is recommended to routinely screen for S aureus and attempt to decolonize.[32] Although topical mupirocin has been mainly studied in this population, further clinical trials and investigation of alternative agents is needed to guide infection prevention in this population, particularly CHG bathing.

After Hospital Discharge

Rates of invasive MRSA infection are highest within 6 months after hospital discharge and do not normalize for at least 1 year.[111] Most infections in newly detected MRSA carriers occur after discharge, and the risk of MRSA infection among chronically ill carriers persists for up to 1 year after hospital discharge.[82] A study of patients who underwent *S aureus* screening and decolonization before elective orthopedic surgery found that 30% were not decolonized at repeat testing after a mean of 213 days.[31] Another study using CHG washes, nasal mupirocin, and oral rifampin and doxycycline for 7 days for eradication of MRSA colonization found that 25% of patients were recolonized after 3 months and 45% were recolonized at 8 months.[30] This persistent risk has led to the development of targeted prevention strategies at hospital discharge.

Project CLEAR was a multicenter, RCT examining whether decolonization plus hygiene education was superior to education alone after hospital discharge in decreasing the likelihood of postdischarge MRSA infection among MRSA carriers[111] (see **Table 1**). The study included 17 hospitals and 7 nursing homes with 2121 enrolled participants. The education group received and reviewed an educational binder about MRSA, how it spreads, and recommendations for personal hygiene, laundry, and household cleaning, whereas the decolonization group also underwent decolonization with CHG mouthwash, CHG baths, and nasal mupirocin for 5 days twice monthly for 6 months after hospital discharge in addition to the education. Postdischarge MRSA decolonization with CHG and mupirocin led to a 30% lower risk of MRSA infection compared with education alone at 1 year of follow-up. The decolonization group had a significantly lower hazard of MRSA and lower risks of hospitalization owing to MRSA infection, clinically judged infection from any cause, and infection-related hospitalization. However, the limitations of this study include the intense regimen with concerns for adherence in a nonstudy setting, the confounding factors related to adherence (adherent participants had fewer coexisting conditions and devices and required less bathing assistance), and the possible risk of emergence of resistance to CHG and mupirocin, although no difference was reported in resistance rates between the 2 groups. Further studies need to be conducted to evaluate the usefulness of *S aureus* decolonization after hospital discharge.

Nursing Homes

Elderly patients are particularly vulnerable to *S aureus* colonization and infection owing to comorbidities, frequent exposure to health care settings and antibiotics, and chronic skin ulcers.[112–114] Despite this situation, there is limited research examining infection prevention and control strategies for decolonization of *S aureus* in nursing home residents.[115] A cluster randomized study of 104 nursing homes in Switzerland screened residents for MRSA carriage at baseline and at 12 months, with all MRSA carriers undergoing topical decolonization including nasal mupirocin, CHG gargle and bathing, and environmental disinfection.[112] This study found that universal screening followed by decolonization of MRSA carriers did not significantly reduce prevalence of MRSA carriage at 1 year. Although the nursing homes did not subsequently adopt a decolonization approach, a follow-up study 4 years later found that the MRSA prevalence in the intervention group was significantly lower than at the start of the study; this difference was not seen in the control group, suggesting a possible long-term benefit of decolonization.

Another cluster randomized 2-year trial examined the impact of MRSA surveillance, education and targeted decolonization at 3 long-term care facilities.[116] In the first year, residents were randomly assigned to undergo targeted decolonization with nasal mupirocin, CHG bathing, and enhanced environmental cleaning with bleach every 4 months, with decolonization of newly admitted MRSA carriers. Residents of control units were screened but not decolonized. In the second year, all units followed the intervention protocol. The planned interventions of screening and decolonization were successful at lowering MRSA colonization; after the first year, the proportion colonized on intervention units was 11.6% and was significantly lower compared with baseline (16.6%); the proportion colonized on control units was unchanged from baseline (17.8%). In the second year, the proportion colonized was 10.5%, which was significantly lower compared with baseline.

A randomized, double-blind, placebo-controlled trial of residents in 2 long-term care facilities found that twice daily mupirocin for 2 weeks in persistent *S aureus* carriers was highly effective in decolonization compared with placebo, and persistent for 45 days after therapy, with a decrease in decolonization efficacy by 90 days. The intervention also resulted in a trend toward reduction in infections with mupirocin treatment ($P = .1$). Four patients (7%) in the mupirocin group failed to be decolonized with mupirocin and 3 of these had mupirocin-resistant strains (only 1 developed resistance during the study).

There are currently no recommendations for routine *S aureus* carriage screening on nursing home admission and decolonization of carriers is not routinely recommended but is often used on a case-by-case basis.[117] A national survey of nursing homes in the United States found that a majority (75%) do not decolonize MRSA carriers.[117] Further guidance is required to decrease the risk of *S aureus* colonization, transmission, and infection in this population.

RESISTANCE TO DECOLONIZATION AGENTS

The main concern highlighted with decolonization strategies is the selection for more resistant organisms.[28] Low-level resistance to decolonization agents is associated with an increased rate of failure of decolonization, and possible hospital outbreaks with resistant strains.[118,119] Reported rates of mupirocin and CHG resistance vary widely in existing literature.

Mupirocin can exhibit both low-level resistance with a minimum inhibitory concentration (MIC) of 8 or greater to 256 μg/mL caused by point mutations in the native isoleucyl-tRNA synthase gene and high-level resistance with a MIC of 512 μg/mL or greater owing to mechanisms that include a plasmid-mediated gene (*mupA*) coding for an isoleucyl-tRNA synthase with less affinity to mupirocin.[72,120] High-level resistance has been associated with decolonization failure.[30] The clinical significance of low-level resistance is not known, but is hypothesized to temporarily suppress the growth of isolates, although it does not result in sustained decolonization.[72,121] The increased and prolonged use of mupirocin is associated with the development of mupirocin resistance, as shown in a study where widespread mupirocin use in Canada led to a rapid increase in the rate of mupirocin resistance in MRSA isolates from 2.7% in 1990 to 65% in 1993.[122] Several studies have reported increased mupirocin resistance in association with mupirocin use both in the hospital and community setting.[30,122–125] Resistance to mupirocin varies between hospitals and countries, with a reported prevalence of high-level mupirocin resistance reaching as high as 31% to 79% and low-level mupirocin resistance of up to 28%.[126]

However, some recent studies have shown that the development of mupirocin resistance may be less common. A 7-year study of targeted MRSA decolonization with mupirocin in neonates did not lead to the emergence of mupirocin resistance in unit-acquired MRSA isolates.[127] Similarly, universal mupirocin prophylaxis in the

NICU setting was not associated with development of resistance in *S aureus* isolates.[83] Another study found that the median mupirocin MIC slightly increased from 0.25 to 0.75 µg/mL after 1 month of universal mupirocin prophylaxis in the NICU.[128] A study of 1089 patients with community-onset SSTI who were followed for 12 months with repeat colonization cultures found that 2.1% carried mupirocin-resistant *S aureus* strain and 0.9% had a CHG-resistant strain.[129] Several studies of decolonization report a low level of mupirocin or CHG resistance in both MRSA and MSSA isolates.[14,106]

CHG resistance is most commonly defined as a MIC of 4 µg/mL or greater by broth dilution, although this definition is not standardized and may not be relevant clinically.[130,131] Resistance to CHG is conferred by 2 gene families, *qac* (*qac A/B, qacC*) and *smr*. The *qac* are plasmid-mediated genes that encode proton-dependent multidrug efflux pumps, which can result in high-level resistance to antiseptics, whereas the *smr* gene confers low-level resistance.[126,132] The reported prevalence of *qac* and *smr* genes in staphylococci varies according to geographic location, ranging from 1% in the Eastern United States to 80% in Brazil.[131] ICU patients carrying *qacA/B*-positive MRSA were found to be more likely have a clinical isolate (rather than just a surveillance MRSA isolate) and longer hospital stays compared with patients carrying *qacA/B*-negative MRSA.[74,130] The *qacA/B*-carrying *S aureus* isolates have been associated with invasive bloodstream infections and reduced susceptibility to other systemic antimicrobials in children.[133]

A concern with the widespread use of CHG antisepsis is the selection of resistant strains. An interrupted time-series study in the ICU setting found that CHG-based antisepsis was associated with a significant decrease in MRSA transmission, but an increase in the acquisition and spread of strains carrying *qac A/B* genes, with a 3-fold increase in the minimum bacterial concentrations to CHG in vitro.[134] In the REDUCE-MRSA trial, a follow-up study of 3173 isolates found that only 2 were not susceptible to CHG (both of which occurred during periods without CHG/mupirocin decolonization), and 0.6% carried *qacA* or *qacB*.[135] Given the growing number of indications for its use, the potential for emergence of reduced susceptibility to mupirocin and CHG remains a concern,[136] and guidelines should recommend surveillance of *S aureus* susceptibility to decolonization agents.[41,137] A challenge to clinicians remains the paucity of commercially available resistance testing for mupirocin and CHG, because there are currently no interpretive breakpoints established by the US Food and Drug Administration.[138]

FUTURE DIRECTIONS

The foundational principles of hand hygiene and standard precautions, SSI and device-associated prevention bundles, and environmental disinfection are critical interventions to decrease the risk of infection in the health care setting and at home. Some, but not all, studies evaluating the decolonization of *S aureus* have shown a decreased risk of subsequent *S aureus* infection, with the greatest impact seen in patients undergoing cardiac and orthopedic surgery, with indwelling vascular devices, residing in adult ICUs, or undergoing HD or continuous peritoneal dialysis. However, there are conflicting data on the usefulness of hospital-wide universal and targeted decolonization strategies and uncertainty regarding the optimal decolonization treatment modalities (eg, CHG alone or in combination with nasal decolonization). Additional data are needed on the potential adverse consequences of widespread decolonization, including skin toxicity and resistance, and the development of alternative agents for decolonization should be pursued.

CLINICS CARE POINTS

- Strategies for decolonization of S aureus include topical nasal antibiotics (mupirocin, retapamulin, and PI) and antiseptic body washes (CHG or dilute bleach), either alone or in combination.

- S aureus decolonization can decrease the risk of SSIs, particularly in the setting of orthopedic or cardiac surgery.

- Decolonization should be considered for patients with recurrent SSTIs, possibly including household members, based on individual burden of disease and recurrence risk.

- Targeted and universal decolonization of S aureus have been studied in the ICU and can significantly reduce the risk of hospital-acquired infections and acquisition of multidrug-resistant organisms, including MRSA.

- Optimal strategies for S aureus decolonization in the neonatal intensive care remain to be determined.

- Decolonization of S aureus in non–critically ill hospitalized patients should be used selectively in patients with medical devices and central lines.

- Dialysis patients are more frequently colonized with S aureus than the general population, and it is recommended to routinely screen for S aureus and attempt to decolonize in this setting.

- S aureus decolonization after hospital discharge may contribute to a reduced risk of S aureus infection and hospitalization.

DISCLOSURE

The authors have no financial conflicts of interest to report. No funding was received for this article.

REFERENCES

1. Schmidt A, Bénard S, Cyr S. Hospital cost of staphylococcal infection after cardiothoracic or orthopedic operations in France: a retrospective database analysis. Surg Infect 2015;16(4):428–35.
2. Anderson DJ, Kaye KS, Chen LF, et al. Clinical and financial outcomes due to methicillin resistant Staphylococcus aureus surgical site infection: a multi-center matched outcomes study. PLoS One 2009;4(12):e8305.
3. McGarry SA, Engemann JJ, Schmader K, et al. Surgical-site infection due to Staphylococcus aureus among elderly patients: mortality, duration of hospitalization, and cost. Infect Control Hosp Epidemiol 2004;25(6):461–7.
4. Campbell RS, Emons MF, Mardekian J, et al. Adverse Clinical Outcomes and Resource Utilization Associated with Methicillin-Resistant and Methicillin-Sensitive Staphylococcus aureus Infections after Elective Surgery. Surg Infect 2015;16(5):543–52.
5. Weiner-Lastinger LM, Abner S, Edwards JR, et al. Antimicrobial-resistant pathogens associated with adult healthcare-associated infections: summary of data reported to the National Healthcare Safety Network, 2015–2017. Infect Control Hosp Epidemiol 2020;41(1):1–18.
6. Bode LGM, Bogaers D, Troelstra A, et al. Preventing Surgical-Site Infections in Nasal Carriers of Staphylococcus aureus. N Engl J Med 2010;362:9–17.

7. Septimus EJ, Schweizer ML. Decolonization in Prevention of Health Care-Associated Infections. Clin Microbiol Rev 2016;29(2):201–22.
8. Davis KA, Stewart JJ, Crouch HK, et al. Methicillin-resistant Staphylococcus aureus (MRSA) nares colonization at hospital admission and its effect on subsequent MRSA infection. Clin Infect Dis 2004;39(6):776–82.
9. Kalmeijer MD, van Nieuwland-Bollen E, Bogaers-Hofman D, et al. Nasal carriage of Staphylococcus aureus is a major risk factor for surgical-site infections in orthopedic surgery. Infect Control Hosp Epidemiol 2000;21(5):319–23.
10. Nouwen J, Schouten J, Schneebergen P, et al. Staphylococcus aureus Carriage Patterns and the Risk of Infections Associated with Continuous Peritoneal Dialysis. J Clin Microbiol 2006;44(6):2233–6.
11. von Eiff C, Becker K, Machka K, et al. Nasal carriage as a source of Staphylococcus aureus bacteremia. Study Group. N Engl J Med 2001;344(1):11–6.
12. Huang Y-C, Chou Y-H, Su L-H, et al. Methicillin-resistant Staphylococcus aureus colonization and its association with infection among infants hospitalized in neonatal intensive care units. Pediatrics 2006;118(2):469–74.
13. Wertheim HF, Melles DC, Vos MC, et al. The role of nasal carriage in Staphylococcus aureus infections. Lancet Infect Dis 2005;5(12):751–62.
14. Perl TM, Cullen JJ, Wenzel RP, et al. Intranasal mupirocin to prevent postoperative Staphylococcus aureus infections. N Engl J Med 2002;346(24):1871–7.
15. Wang J-L, Chen S-Y, Wang J-T, et al. Comparison of both clinical features and mortality risk associated with bacteremia due to community-acquired methicillin-resistant Staphylococcus aureus and methicillin-susceptible S. aureus. Clin Infect Dis 2008;46(6):799–806.
16. Acree ME, Morgan E, David MZ. S. aureus infections in Chicago, 2006-2014: increase in CA MSSA and decrease in MRSA incidence. Infect Control Hosp Epidemiol 2017;38(10):1226–34.
17. Mendy A, Vieira ER, Albatineh AN, et al. Staphylococcus aureus colonization and long-term risk for death, United States. Emerg Infect Dis 2016;22(11). https://doi.org/10.3201/eid2211.160220.
18. Graham PL, Lin SX, Larson EL. A U.S. population-based survey of Staphylococcus aureus colonization. Ann Intern Med 2006;144(5):318–25.
19. Charlebois ED, Bangsberg DR, Moss NJ, et al. Population-based community prevalence of methicillin-resistant Staphylococcus aureus in the urban poor of San Francisco. Clin Infect Dis 2002;34(4):425–33.
20. Botelho-Nevers E, Gagnaire J, Verhoeven PO, et al. Decolonization of Staphylococcus aureus carriage. Med Mal Infect 2017;47(5):305–10.
21. McKinnell JA, Huang SS, Eells SJ, et al. Quantifying the impact of extranasal testing of body sites for methicillin-resistant Staphylococcus aureus colonization at the time of hospital or intensive care unit admission. Infect Control Hosp Epidemiol 2013;34(2):161–70.
22. Heng Sim BL, McBryde E, Street AC, et al. Multiple site surveillance cultures as a predictor of methicillin-resistant Staphylococcus aureus infections. Infect Control Hosp Epidemiol 2013;34(8):818–24.
23. VandenBergh MF, Yzerman EP, van Belkum A, et al. Follow-up of Staphylococcus aureus nasal carriage after 8 years: redefining the persistent carrier state. J Clin Microbiol 1999;37(10):3133–40.
24. Nouwen JL, Fieren MWJA, Snijders S, et al. Persistent (not intermittent) nasal carriage of Staphylococcus aureus is the determinant of CPD-related infections. Kidney Int 2005;67(3):1084–92.

25. Walsh AL, Fields AC, Dieterich JD, et al. Risk factors for Staphylococcus aureus nasal colonization in joint arthroplasty patients. J Arthroplasty 2018;33(5): 1530–3.

26. Hidron AI, Kourbatova EV, Halvosa JS, et al. Risk factors for colonization with methicillin-resistant Staphylococcus aureus (MRSA) in patients admitted to an urban hospital: emergence of community-associated MRSA nasal carriage. Clin Infect Dis 2005;41(2):159–66.

27. Verhoeven PO, Gagnaire J, Botelho-Nevers E, et al. Detection and clinical relevance of Staphylococcus aureus nasal carriage: an update. Expert Rev Anti Infect Ther 2014;12(1):75–89.

28. Liu C, Bayer A, Cosgrove SE, et al. Clinical practice guidelines by the Infectious Diseases Society of America for the treatment of methicillin-resistant Staphylococcus aureus infections in adults and children. Clin Infect Dis 2011;52(3): e18–55.

29. McConeghy KW, Mikolich DJ, LaPlante KL. Agents for the decolonization of methicillin-resistant Staphylococcus aureus. Pharmacotherapy 2009;29(3): 263–80.

30. Simor AE, Phillips E, McGeer A, et al. Randomized controlled trial of chlorhexidine gluconate for washing, intranasal mupirocin, and rifampin and doxycycline versus no treatment for the eradication of methicillin-resistant Staphylococcus aureus colonization. Clin Infect Dis 2007;44(2):178–85.

31. Immerman I, Ramos NL, Katz GM, et al. The persistence of Staphylococcus aureus decolonization after mupirocin and topical chlorhexidine: implications for patients requiring multiple or delayed procedures. J Arthroplasty 2012; 27(6):870–6.

32. Price A, Sarween N, Gupta I, et al. Methicillin-resistant Staphylococcus aureus and methicillin-susceptible Staphylococcus aureus screening in a cohort of haemodialysis patients: carriage, demographics and outcomes. J Hosp Infect 2015;90(1):22–7.

33. Schweizer M, Perencevich E, McDanel J, et al. Effectiveness of a bundled intervention of decolonization and prophylaxis to decrease Gram positive surgical site infections after cardiac or orthopedic surgery: systematic review and meta-analysis. BMJ 2013;346:f2743.

34. Schweizer ML, Chiang H-Y, Septimus E, et al. Association of a Bundled Intervention With Surgical Site Infections Among Patients Undergoing Cardiac, Hip, or Knee Surgery. JAMA 2015;313(21):2162–71.

35. Sporer SM, Rogers T, Abella L. Methicillin-resistant and methicillin-sensitive Staphylococcus aureus screening and decolonization to reduce surgical site infection in elective total joint arthroplasty. J Arthroplasty 2016;31(9 Suppl): 144–7.

36. Saraswat MK, Magruder JT, Crawford TC, et al. Preoperative Staphylococcus aureus screening and targeted decolonization in cardiac surgery. Ann Thorac Surg 2017;104(4):1349–56.

37. Rezapoor M, Nicholson T, Tabatabaee RM, et al. Povidone-iodine–based solutions for decolonization of nasal Staphylococcus aureus: a randomized, prospective, placebo-controlled study. J Arthroplasty 2017;32(9):2815–9.

38. Ghaddara HA, Kumar JA, Cadnum JL, et al. Efficacy of a povidone iodine preparation in reducing nasal methicillin-resistant Staphylococcus aureus in colonized patients. Am J Infect Control 2020;48(4):456–9.

39. Phillips M, Rosenberg A, Shopsin B, et al. Preventing surgical site infections: a randomized, open-label trial of nasal mupirocin ointment and nasal povidone-iodine solution. Infect Control Hosp Epidemiol 2014;35(7):826–32.
40. Bebko SP, Green DM, Awad SS. Effect of a preoperative decontamination protocol on surgical site infections in patients undergoing elective orthopedic surgery with hardware implantation. JAMA Surg 2015;150(5):390–5.
41. Bratzler DW, Dellinger EP, Olsen KM, et al. Clinical practice guidelines for antimicrobial prophylaxis in surgery. Am J Health Syst Pharm 2013;70(3):195–283.
42. Kline S, Highness M, Herwaldt LA, et al. Variable screening and decolonization protocols for Staphylococcus aureus carriage prior to surgical procedures. Infect Control Hosp Epidemiol 2014;35(7):880–2.
43. Diekema D, Johannsson B, Herwaldt L, et al. Current practice in Staphylococcus aureus screening and decolonization. Infect Control Hosp Epidemiol 2011;32(10):1042–4.
44. Al-Zubeidi D, Burnham C-AD, Hogan PG, et al. Molecular epidemiology of recurrent cutaneous methicillin-resistant Staphylococcus aureus infections in children. J Pediatr Infect Dis Soc 2014;3(3):261–4.
45. Rodriguez M, Hogan PG, Burnham C-AD, et al. Molecular epidemiology of Staphylococcus aureus in households of children with community-associated S aureus skin and soft tissue infections. J Pediatr 2014;164(1):105–11.
46. Chen C-J, Su L-H, Lin T-Y, et al. Molecular analysis of repeated methicillin-resistant Staphylococcus aureus infections in children. PLoS One 2010;5(12): e14431.
47. Raz R, Miron D, Colodner R, et al. A 1-year trial of nasal mupirocin in the prevention of recurrent staphylococcal nasal colonization and skin infection. Arch Intern Med 1996;156(10):1109–12.
48. Kaplan SL, Forbes A, Hammerman WA, et al. Randomized Trial of "Bleach Baths" Plus Routine Hygienic Measures vs Routine Hygienic Measures Alone for Prevention of Recurrent Infections. Clin Infect Dis 2014;58(5):679–82.
49. Papastefan ST, Buonpane C, Ares G, et al. Impact of Decolonization Protocols and Recurrence in Pediatric MRSA Skin and Soft-Tissue Infections. J Surg Res 2019;242:70–7.
50. Fritz SA, Camins BC, Eisenstein KA, et al. Effectiveness of measures to eradicate Staphylococcus aureus carriage in patients with community-associated skin and soft tissue infections: a randomized trial. Infect Control Hosp Epidemiol 2011;32(9):872–80.
51. McNeil JC, Fritz SA. Prevention strategies for recurrent community-associated Staphylococcus aureus skin and soft tissue infections. Curr Infect Dis Rep 2019;21(4):12.
52. Fritz SA, Hogan PG, Hayek G, et al. Household versus individual approaches to eradication of community-associated Staphylococcus aureus in children: a randomized trial. Clin Infect Dis 2012;54(6):743–51.
53. Cluzet VC, Gerber JS, Metlay JP, et al. The effect of total household decolonization on clearance of colonization with methicillin-resistant Staphylococcus aureus. Infect Control Hosp Epidemiol 2016;37(10):1226–33.
54. Hogan PG, Parrish KL, Mork RL, et al. HOME2: household vs. personalized decolonization in households of children with methicillin-resistant Staphylococcus aureus skin and soft tissue infection - a randomized clinical trial. Clin Infect Dis 2020. https://doi.org/10.1093/cid/ciaa752.

55. Kaur I, Souder E. Developing guidelines for S. aureus decolonization a difficult task. AAP News 2020. Available at: https://www.aappublications.org/news/2017/05/01/Decolonization050117. Accessed June 5, 2020.

56. Honda H, Krauss MJ, Coopersmith CM, et al. Staphylococcus aureus nasal colonization and subsequent infection in intensive care unit patients: does methicillin resistance matter? Infect Control Hosp Epidemiol 2010;31(6):584–91.

57. Climo MW, Yokoe DS, Warren DK, et al. Effect of Daily Chlorhexidine Bathing on Hospital-Acquired Infection. N Engl J Med 2013. https://doi.org/10.1056/NEJMoa1113849.

58. Derde LPG, Cooper BS, Goossens H, et al. Interventions to reduce colonisation and transmission of antimicrobial-resistant bacteria in intensive care units: an interrupted time series study and cluster randomised trial. Lancet Infect Dis 2014; 14(1):31–9.

59. Swan JT, Ashton CM, Bui LN, et al. Effect of chlorhexidine bathing every other day on prevention of hospital-acquired infections in the surgical ICU: a single-center, randomized controlled trial. Crit Care Med 2016;44(10):1822–32.

60. Bradley CW, Wilkinson MAC, Garvey MI. The effect of universal decolonization with screening in critical care to reduce MRSA across an entire hospital. Infect Control Hosp Epidemiol 2017;38(4):430–5.

61. Huang SS, Septimus E, Kleinman K, et al. Targeted versus universal decolonization to prevent ICU infection. N Engl J Med 2013;368(24):2255–65.

62. Ridenour G, Lampen R, Federspiel J, et al. Selective use of intranasal mupirocin and chlorhexidine bathing and the incidence of methicillin-resistant Staphylococcus aureus colonization and infection among intensive care unit patients. Infect Control Hosp Epidemiol 2007;28(10):1155–61.

63. Sandri AM, Dalarosa MG, Ruschel de Alcantara L, et al. Reduction in incidence of nosocomial methicillin-resistant Staphylococcus aureus (MRSA) infection in an intensive care unit: role of treatment with mupirocin ointment and chlorhexidine baths for nasal carriers of MRSA. Infect Control Hosp Epidemiol 2006; 27(2):185–7.

64. Fraser TG, Fatica C, Scarpelli M, et al. Decrease in Staphylococcus aureus colonization and hospital-acquired infection in a medical intensive care unit after institution of an active surveillance and decolonization program. Infect Control Hosp Epidemiol 2010;31(8):779–83.

65. Calfee DP, Salgado CD, Milstone AM, et al. Strategies to prevent methicillin-resistant Staphylococcus aureus transmission and infection in acute care hospitals: 2014 update. Infect Control Hosp Epidemiol 2014;35(7):772–96.

66. Pogorzelska M, Stone PW, Larson EL. Wide variation in adoption of screening and infection control interventions for multidrug-resistant organisms: a national study. Am J Infect Control 2012;40(8):696–700.

67. Climo MW, Sepkowitz KA, Zuccotti G, et al. The effect of daily bathing with chlorhexidine on the acquisition of methicillin-resistant Staphylococcus aureus, vancomycin-resistant Enterococcus, and healthcare-associated bloodstream infections: results of a quasi-experimental multicenter trial. Crit Care Med 2009;37(6):1858–65.

68. Popovich KJ, Hota B, Hayes R, et al. Effectiveness of routine patient cleansing with chlorhexidine gluconate for infection prevention in the medical intensive care unit. Infect Control Hosp Epidemiol 2009;30(10):959–63.

69. Lee Y-J, Chen J-Z, Lin H-C, et al. Impact of active screening for methicillin-resistant Staphylococcus aureus (MRSA) and decolonization on MRSA

infections, mortality and medical cost: a quasi-experimental study in surgical intensive care unit. Crit Care 2015;19:143.

70. Whittington MD, Atherly AJ, Curtis DJ, et al. Recommendations for methicillin-resistant Staphylococcus aureus prevention in adult ICUs: a cost-effectiveness analysis*. Crit Care Med 2017;45(8):1304–10.

71. Huang SS, Septimus E, Avery TR, et al. Cost savings of universal decolonization to prevent intensive care unit infection: implications of the REDUCE MRSA trial. Infect Control Hosp Epidemiol 2014;35(Suppl 3):S23–31.

72. Patel JB, Gorwitz RJ, Jernigan JA. Mupirocin Resistance. Clin Infect Dis 2009; 49(6):935–41.

73. Deeny SR, Worby CJ, Tosas Auguet O, et al. Impact of mupirocin resistance on the transmission and control of healthcare-associated MRSA. J Antimicrob Chemother 2015;70(12):3366–78.

74. Cho O-H, Park K-H, Song JY, et al. Prevalence and microbiological characteristics of qacA/B-positive methicillin-resistant Staphylococcus aureus isolates in a surgical intensive care unit. Microb Drug Resist 2017;24(3):283–9.

75. Lu Z, Chen Y, Chen W, et al. Characteristics of qacA/B-positive Staphylococcus aureus isolated from patients and a hospital environment in China. J Antimicrob Chemother 2015;70(3):653–7.

76. FDA. FDA warns about rare but serious allergic reactions with the skin antiseptic chlorhexidine gluconate. 2017. Available at: https://www.fda.gov/media/102986/download. Accessed June 21, 2020.

77. Chotiprasitsakul D, Tamma PD, Gadala A, et al. The role of negative methicillin-resistant Staphylococcus aureus nasal surveillance swabs in predicting the need for empiric vancomycin therapy in intensive care unit patients. Infect Control Hosp Epidemiol 2018;39(3):290–6.

78. Lake JG, Weiner LM, Milstone AM, et al. See I. Pathogen distribution and anti-microbial resistance among pediatric healthcare-associated infections reported to the National Healthcare Safety Network, 2011–2014. Infect Control Hosp Epidemiol 2018;39(1):1–11.

79. Milstone AM, Voskertchian A, Koontz DW, et al. Effect of treating parents colonized with Staphylococcus aureus on transmission to neonates in the intensive care unit: a randomized clinical trial. JAMA 2020;323(4):319–28.

80. Kotloff KL, Shirley D-AT, Creech CB, et al. Mupirocin for Staphylococcus aureus decolonization of infants in neonatal intensive care units. Pediatrics 2019;143(1). https://doi.org/10.1542/peds.2018-1565.

81. Shane AL, Hansen NI, Stoll BJ, et al. Methicillin-resistant and susceptible Staphylococcus aureus bacteremia and meningitis in preterm infants. Pediatrics 2012;129(4):e914–22.

82. Huang SS, Hinrichsen VL, Datta R, et al. Methicillin-resistant Staphylococcus aureus infection and hospitalization in high-risk patients in the year following detection. PLoS One 2011;6(9):e24340.

83. Delaney HM, Wang E, Melish M. Comprehensive strategy including prophylactic mupirocin to reduce Staphylococcus aureus colonization and infection in high-risk neonates. J Perinatol 2013;33(4):313–8.

84. Lepelletier D, Corvec S, Caillon J, et al. Eradication of methicillin-resistant Staphylococcus aureus in a neonatal intensive care unit: which measures for which success? Am J Infect Control 2009;37(3):195–200.

85. Popoola VO, Budd A, Wittig SM, et al. Methicillin-resistant Staphylococcus aureus transmission and infections in a neonatal intensive care unit despite

active surveillance cultures and decolonization: challenges for infection prevention. Infect Control Hosp Epidemiol 2014;35(4):412–8.

86. Nelson MU, Bizzarro MJ, Dembry LM, et al. One size does not fit all: why universal decolonizaiton strategies to prevent methicillin-resistant Staphylococcus aureus colonization and infection in adult intensive care units may be inappropriate for neonatal intensive care units. J Perinatol 2014;34(9):653–5.

87. Milstone AM, Song X, Coffin S, et al. Identification and eradication of methicillin-resistant Staphylococcus aureus colonization in the neonatal intensive care unit: results of a national survey. Infect Control Hosp Epidemiol 2010;31(7):766–8.

88. Tamma PD, Aucott SW, Milstone AM. Chlorhexidine use in the neonatal intensive care unit: results from a national survey. Infect Control Hosp Epidemiol 2010; 31(8):846–9.

89. Chapman AK, Aucott SW, Milstone AM. Safety of chlorhexidine gluconate used for skin antisepsis in the preterm infant. J Perinatol 2012;32(1):4–9.

90. Huang SS, Septimus E, Kleinman K, et al. Chlorhexidine versus routine bathing to prevent multidrug-resistant organisms and all-cause bloodstream infections in general medical and surgical units (ABATE Infection trial): a cluster-randomised trial. Lancet 2019;393(10177):1205–15.

91. Shuman E, Harpe J, Calfee DP. 1383 Survey of hospital practices regarding use of chlorhexidine gluconate bathing for prevention of healthcare-associated infections. Open Forum Infect Dis 2014;1(suppl_1):S363–4.

92. Lowe CF, Lloyd-Smith E, Sidhu B, et al. Reduction in hospital-associated methicillin-resistant Staphylococcus aureus and vancomycin-resistant Enterococcus with daily chlorhexidine gluconate bathing for medical inpatients. Am J Infect Control 2017;45(3):255–9.

93. Kassakian SZ, Mermel LA, Jefferson JA, et al. Impact of chlorhexidine bathing on hospital-acquired infections among general medical patients. Infect Control Hosp Epidemiol 2011;32(3):238–43.

94. Rupp ME, Cavalieri RJ, Lyden E, et al. Effect of hospital-wide chlorhexidine patient bathing on healthcare-associated infections. Infect Control Hosp Epidemiol 2012;33(11):1094–100.

95. Wertheim HFL, Vos MC, Ott A, et al. Mupirocin prophylaxis against nosocomial Staphylococcus aureus infections in nonsurgical patients: a randomized study. Ann Intern Med 2004;140(6):419–25.

96. Lu P-L, Tsai J-C, Chiu Y-W, et al. Methicillin-resistant Staphylococcus aureus carriage, infection and transmission in dialysis patients, healthcare workers and their family members. Nephrol Dial Transplant 2008;23(5):1659–65.

97. Ghavghani FR, Rahbarnia L, Naghili B, et al. Nasal and extra nasal MRSA colonization in hemodialysis patients of north-west of Iran. BMC Res Notes 2019; 12(1):260.

98. Scheuch M, Freiin von Rheinbaben S, Kabisch A, et al. Staphylococcus aureus colonization in hemodialysis patients: a prospective 25 months observational study. BMC Nephrol 2019;20(1):153.

99. Lai C-F, Liao C-H, Pai M-F, et al. Nasal carriage of methicillin-resistant Staphylococcus aureus is associated with higher all-cause mortality in hemodialysis patients. Clin J Am Soc Nephrol 2011;6(1):167–74.

100. Schmid H, Romanos A, Schiffl H, et al. Persistent nasal methicillin-resistant staphylococcus aureus carriage in hemodialysis outpatients: a predictor of worse outcome. BMC Nephrol 2013;14:93.

101. Zacharioudakis IM, Zervou FN, Ziakas PD, et al. Meta-analysis of methicillin-resistant Staphylococcus aureus colonization and risk of infection in dialysis patients. J Am Soc Nephrol 2014;25(9):2131–41.

102. Yeoh LY, Tan FLG, Willis GC, et al. Methicillin-resistant Staphylococcus aureus carriage in hospitalized chronic hemodialysis patients and its predisposing factors. Hemodial Int 2014;18(1):142–7.

103. Lee BY, Song Y, McGlone SM, et al. The economic value of screening haemodialysis patients for methicillin-resistant Staphylococcus aureus in the USA. Clin Microbiol Infect 2011;17(11):1717–26.

104. Boelaert JR, Van Landuyt HW, Godard CA, et al. Nasal mupirocin ointment decreases the incidence of Staphylococcus aureus bacteraemias in haemodialysis patients. Nephrol Dial Transplant 1993;8(3):235–9.

105. Kluytmans JA, Manders MJ, van Bommel E, et al. Elimination of nasal carriage of Staphylococcus aureus in hemodialysis patients. Infect Control Hosp Epidemiol 1996;17(12):793–7.

106. van Rijen M, Bonten M, Wenzel R, et al. Mupirocin ointment for preventing Staphylococcus aureus infections in nasal carriers. Cochrane Database Syst Rev 2008;(4):CD006216.

107. Nephrology AS of. Nasal mupirocin prevents Staphylococcus aureus exit-site infection during peritoneal dialysis. Mupirocin Study Group. J Am Soc Nephrol 1996;7(11):2403–8.

108. Campbell D, Mudge DW, Craig JC, et al. Antimicrobial agents for preventing peritonitis in peritoneal dialysis patients. Cochrane Database Syst Rev 2017;(4):CD004679.

109. Tacconelli E, Carmeli Y, Aizer A, et al. Mupirocin prophylaxis to prevent Staphylococcus aureus infection in patients undergoing dialysis: a meta-analysis. Clin Infect Dis 2003;37(12):1629–38.

110. Nair R, Perencevich EN, Blevins AE, et al. Clinical effectiveness of mupirocin for preventing Staphylococcus aureus infections in nonsurgical settings: a meta-analysis. Clin Infect Dis 2016;62(5):618–30.

111. Huang SS, Singh R, McKinnell JA, et al. Decolonization to reduce postdischarge infection risk among MRSA carriers. N Engl J Med 2019;380(7):638–50.

112. Bellini C, Petignat C, Masserey E, et al. Universal screening and decolonization for control of MRSA in nursing homes: a cluster randomized controlled study. Infect Control Hosp Epidemiol 2015;36(4):401–8.

113. Trick WE, Weinstein RA, DeMarais PL, et al. Colonization of skilled-care facility residents with antimicrobial-resistant pathogens. J Am Geriatr Soc 2001;49(3):270–6.

114. Mendelson G, Yearmack Y, Granot E, et al. Staphylococcus aureus carrier state among elderly residents of a long-term care facility. J Am Med Dir Assoc 2003;4(3):125–7.

115. Hughes C, Smith M, Tunney M, et al. Infection control strategies for preventing the transmission of methicillin-resistant Staphylococcus aureus (MRSA) in nursing homes for older people. Cochrane Database Syst Rev 2011;(12):CD006354.

116. Schora DM, Boehm S, Das S, et al. Impact of Detection, Education, Research and Decolonization without Isolation in Long-term care (DERAIL) on methicillin-resistant Staphylococcus aureus colonization and transmission at 3 long-term care facilities. Am J Infect Control 2014;42(10 Suppl):S269–73.

117. Ye Z, Mukamel DB, Huang SS, et al. Healthcare-associated pathogens and nursing home policies and practices: results from a national survey. Infect Control Hosp Epidemiol 2015;36(7):759–66.

118. Harbarth S, Dharan S, Liassine N, et al. Randomized, placebo-controlled, double-blind trial to evaluate the efficacy of mupirocin for eradicating carriage of methicillin-resistant Staphylococcus aureus. Antimicrob Agents Chemother 1999;43(6):1412–6.

119. Lee AS, Macedo-Vinas M, François P, et al. Impact of combined low-level mupirocin and genotypic chlorhexidine resistance on persistent methicillin-resistant Staphylococcus aureus carriage after decolonization therapy: a case-control study. Clin Infect Dis 2011;52(12):1422–30.

120. Sakr A, Brégeon F, Rolain J-M, et al. Staphylococcus aureus nasal decolonization strategies: a review. Expert Rev Anti Infect Ther 2019;17(5):327–40.

121. Walker ES, Vasquez JE, Dula R, et al. Mupirocin-resistant, methicillin-resistant Staphylococcus aureus: does mupirocin remain effective? Infect Control Hosp Epidemiol 2003;24(5):342–6.

122. Miller MA, Dascal A, Portnoy J, et al. Development of mupirocin resistance among methicillin-resistant Staphylococcus aureus after widespread use of nasal mupirocin ointment. Infect Control Hosp Epidemiol 1996;17(12):811–3.

123. Perumal N, Murugesan S, Ramanathan V, et al. High occurrence of high-level mupirocin & chlorhexidine resistant genes in methicillin resistant staphylococcal isolates from dialysis unit of a tertiary care hospital. Indian J Med Res 2016; 143(6):824.

124. Upton A, Lang S, Heffernan H. Mupirocin and Staphylococcus aureus: a recent paradigm of emerging antibiotic resistance. J Antimicrob Chemother 2003; 51(3):613–7.

125. Jones JC, Rogers TJ, Brookmeyer P, et al. Mupirocin resistance in patients colonized with methicillin-resistant Staphylococcus aureus in a surgical intensive care unit. Clin Infect Dis 2007;45(5):541–7.

126. Poovelikunnel T, Gethin G, Humphreys H. Mupirocin resistance: clinical implications and potential alternatives for the eradication of MRSA. J Antimicrob Chemother 2015;70(10):2681–92.

127. Suwantarat N, Carroll KC, Tekle T, et al. Low prevalence of mupirocin resistance among hospital-acquired methicillin-resistant Staphylococcus aureus isolates in a neonatal intensive care unit with an active surveillance cultures and decolonization program. Infect Control Hosp Epidemiol 2015;36(2):232–4.

128. Hitomi S, Kubota M, Mori N, et al. Control of a methicillin-resistant Staphylococcus aureus outbreak in a neonatal intensive care unit by unselective use of nasal mupirocin ointment. J Hosp Infect 2000;46(2):123–9.

129. Fritz SA, Hogan PG, Camins BC, et al. Mupirocin and chlorhexidine resistance in Staphylococcus aureus in patients with community-onset skin and soft tissue infections. Antimicrob Agents Chemother 2013;57(1):559–68.

130. Madden GR, Sifri CD. Antimicrobial resistance to agents used for Staphylococcus aureus decolonization: is there a reason for concern? Curr Infect Dis Rep 2018;20(8):26.

131. Horner C, Mawer D, Wilcox M. Reduced susceptibility to chlorhexidine in staphylococci: is it increasing and does it matter? J Antimicrob Chemother 2012; 67(11):2547–59.

132. Longtin J, Seah C, Siebert K, et al. Distribution of antiseptic resistance genes qacA, qacB, and smr in methicillin-resistant Staphylococcus aureus isolated

in Toronto, Canada, from 2005 to 2009. Antimicrob Agents Chemother 2011; 55(6):2999–3001.

133. McNeil JC, Kok EY, Vallejo JG, et al. Clinical and molecular features of decreased chlorhexidine susceptibility among nosocomial Staphylococcus aureus isolates at Texas Children's Hospital. Antimicrob Agents Chemother 2016;60(2):1121–8.

134. Batra R, Cooper BS, Whiteley C, et al. Efficacy and limitation of a chlorhexidine-based decolonization strategy in preventing transmission of methicillin-resistant Staphylococcus aureus in an intensive care unit. Clin Infect Dis 2010;50(2): 210–7.

135. Hayden MK, Lolans K, Haffenreffer K, et al. Chlorhexidine and mupirocin susceptibility of methicillin-resistant Staphylococcus aureus Isolates in the REDUCE-MRSA trial. J Clin Microbiol 2016;54(11):2735–42.

136. Harbarth S, Tuan Soh S, Horner C, et al. Is reduced susceptibility to disinfectants and antiseptics a risk in healthcare settings? A point/counterpoint review. J Hosp Infect 2014;87(4):194–202.

137. Muto CA, Jernigan JA, Ostrowsky BE, et al. SHEA guideline for preventing nosocomial transmission of multidrug-resistant strains of Staphylococcus aureus and enterococcus. Infect Control Hosp Epidemiol 2003;24(5):362–86.

138. Creech CB, Al-Zubeidi DN, Fritz SA. Prevention of recurrent staphylococcal skin infections. Infect Dis Clin North Am 2015;29(3):429–64.

Necrotizing Soft Tissue Infections

Dennis L. Stevens, PhD, MD[a], Amy E. Bryant, PhD[b],*, Ellie JC. Goldstein, MD[c,d]

KEYWORDS

- Necrotizing soft tissue infection • Necrotizing fasciitis • Myonecrosis
- Gas gangrene • Group A streptococcus • Clostridium • Polymicrobial infection

KEY POINTS

- Necrotizing soft tissue infections are severe, life-threatening conditions characterized by widespread tissue destruction, systemic signs of toxicity, hemodynamic collapse, organ failure and high mortality.
- Necrotizing soft tissue infection require prompt diagnosis and urgent medical treatment, including surgical intervention and intensive care measures.
- Risk factors include breaches in cutaneous or mucosal integrity, traumatic wounds, diabetes, or other immunosuppressing conditions. Disruption of barrier function provides microbial access to deeper soft tissues.
- Necrotizing soft tissue infection should be suspected with evidence of soft tissue infection plus signs of systemic involvement. Definitive diagnosis requires surgical exploration and Gram stain and culture.
- Treatment includes early and aggressive debridement of devitalized tissue, appropriate antibiotic therapy, and hemodynamic support.

NECROTIZING FASCIITIS

Necrotizing fasciitis (NF) is a deep-seated infection, the diagnosis of which is made by surgical inspection where the hallmarks include friability of the superficial fascia (ie, the so-called "gloved finger" sign) and dishwater gray appearance of inflammatory fluid with a notable absence of pus. The current incidence of NF is 4.0 to 15.5 cases per 100,000 population.[1,2] NF and other necrotizing skin and soft tissue infections have multiple etiologies, risk factors, anatomic locations, and different pathogenic

[a] Infectious Diseases Center of Biomedical Research Excellence, Veterans Affairs Medical Center, 500 West Fort Street (Mail Stop 151), Boise, ID 83702, USA; [b] Department of Biomedical and Pharmaceutical Sciences, College of Pharmacy, Idaho State University, 1311 East Central Drive, Meridian, ID 83642, USA; [c] David Geffen School of Medicine at UCLA, Los Angeles, CA 90074, USA; [d] R M Alden Research Laboratory, 2021 Santa Monica Boulevard, Suite #740 East, Santa Monica, CA 90404, USA
* Corresponding author.
E-mail address: bryaamy2@isu.edu

Infect Dis Clin N Am 35 (2021) 135–155
https://doi.org/10.1016/j.idc.2020.10.004
0891-5520/21/© 2020 Elsevier Inc. All rights reserved.

id.theclinics.com

mechanisms, but all are characterized by widespread destruction of tissue that may extend from the epidermis to the deep musculature. Other common features include blood vessel thrombosis, abundant bacteria spreading along fascial planes, and a marked absence of acute inflammatory cells in the tissues. Late cutaneous findings, including ecchymoses, bullae, and skin sloughing, portend a fatal outcome.

Necrotizing Fasciitis Type I

NF type I is a polymicrobial infection involving aerobic and anaerobic organisms and is usually associated with a breach of mucosal or cutaneous integrity. Predisposing factors include diabetic or decubitus ulcers, hemorrhoids, rectal fissures, episiotomies, colonic or urologic surgery, and gynecologic procedures. It is often associated with gas in the tissue and thus is difficult to distinguish from clostridial gangrene. Nonclostridial anaerobic cellulitis and synergistic necrotizing cellulitis are variants of NF type I. Both occur in diabetic patients and typically involve the feet with rapid extension into the leg. Although cellulitis also occurs commonly in diabetic patients, NF should be considered in those with systemic manifestations such as tachycardia, leukocytosis, acidosis, or marked hyperglycemia.

NF type I may also develop after surgery or instrumentation. In the head and neck region, dental surgery or extraction with bacterial penetration into the fascial compartments may result in Ludwig's angina or Lemierre's syndrome caused by *Fusobacterium necrophorum*, with or without concomitant NF and severe sepsis.[3,4] Breach of the gastrointestinal or urethral mucosa, as can occur even with simple procedures such as catheterization, may result in Fournier's gangrene. This infection begins abruptly with severe pain and may spread rapidly onto the anterior abdominal wall, into the gluteal muscles and, in males, the scrotum and penis. Last, an indolent polymicrobial infection known variably as "progressive bacterial synergistic gangrene," "postoperative progressive gangrene," or "large phagedenic ulcer of the abdomen"[5] usually follows surgery involving colostomy sites or wire sutures. Although large ulcerations often develop, the process does not involve the fascia. *Staphylococcus aureus* and microaerophilic streptococci injected together, but neither alone, produced similar lesions in a dog model.[6]

Necrotizing Fasciitis Type II

NF type II is monomicrobial in etiology and group A streptococcus (GAS) remains the most common pathogen.[1,2,7] Others include several clostridial species as well as *Aeromonas hydrophila*, *Vibrio vulnificus*, and *S aureus*.[8] Unlike NF type I, type II may occur in any age group and among those without underlying or complicated medical illnesses (reviewed in[9]).

NECROTIZING SOFT TISSUE INFECTIONS CAUSED BY GROUP A STREPTOCOCCUS
Incidence

The incidence of severe invasive *Streptococcus pyogenes* infections, including NF, remains steady at 3 to 5 cases per 100,000 population per year,[10] with an average mortality of 29%.[10] Mortality is higher in patients who develop streptococcal toxic shock syndrome (38%) or septic shock (45%).[10] Postpartum group A streptococcal infections also remain prevalent worldwide.[11]

Clinical Presentations

Two distinct clinical presentations are described: those with a defined portal of bacterial entry and those without.

Defined portal of entry

S pyogenes may reach the deep fascia from superficial cutaneous lesions (chicken pox, insect bites, lacerations), after breaches of skin or mucosal integrity (drug injections, surgical incisions, childbirth) or penetrating trauma. The initial lesion may seem to be only mildly erythematous, yet over the next 24 to 72 hours, inflammation becomes extensive, the skin becomes dusky and then purplish, and bullae appear. Bacteremia is frequently present, and metastatic infections may occur. Very rapidly, the skin becomes frankly gangrenous and undergoes extensive sloughing. The patient is now perilously ill, with a high fever and extreme prostration. Mortality rates are high, even with appropriate treatment.[10,12]

"No portal" infections

Forty percent to 80% of patients who develop group A streptococcal NF/myonecrosis have no obvious portal of bacterial entry. Instead, infection develops deep in the soft tissues, often at sites of nonpenetrating trauma such as a minor muscle strain, sprain, or bruise.[13–15] Initially, only fever and/or crescendo pain (sufficiently severe as to require ketorolac or narcotics) may be present and such pain is the main reason patients seek medical care. Mild fever, malaise, myalgias, diarrhea, and anorexia may also be present early (first 24 hours), but cutaneous manifestations are notably absent. Without these clinical clues, the correct diagnosis of these "cryptogenic" infections is initially missed or delayed, causing the mortality to exceed 70% (reviewed in[16]). By the time erythema, ecchymoses, and bullae develop, tissue destruction is extensive and patients usually exhibit fever, systemic toxicity, and evidence of organ failure. Emergent surgery, including extensive surgical debridement or amputation, is often required to ensure survival and necessitates a prolonged hospitalization.[14,17,18] Erroneous diagnoses include severe muscle strain or deep vein thrombophlebitis; food poisoning may also be included to explain the associated nausea, vomiting, and diarrhea. Although seeding of the deep tissues likely occurs via transient bacteremia from the nasopharynx, rarely do patients have a symptomatic pharyngitis.

Irrespective of whether a defined portal of bacterial entry exists, necrotizing group A streptococcal infections are severe and deep muscle involvement is common. Even with modern antibiotic regimens and intensive care measures, mortality rates remain between 30% and 80% and morbidity among survivors is extensive and life altering.

Nonsteroidal Anti-inflammatory Drugs and Group A Streptococcal Infection

Prior nonpenetrating soft tissue injury is an accepted risk factor for invasive GAS soft tissue infections. Epidemiologic factors that increase the risk of death from these infections have also been defined (eg, advanced age, diabetes, obesity)[19]; however, a large percentage of such infections occur in individuals with no identified risk factors or underlying illness.[19] In these settings, nonsteroidal anti-inflammatory drug (NSAID) use has been suggested to predispose to infection onset and/or worse outcomes, although controversy remains. Proponents recognize that NSAIDs suppress critical neutrophil functions and augment production of tumor necrosis factor-α, a key mediator of septic shock. Other investigators argue that NSAIDs merely mask the signs and symptoms of developing infection, such that diagnosis and treatment are delayed. Numerous clinical and epidemiologic studies have investigated, but not resolved, this issue (reviewed in[20]). In 2003, Aronoff and Bloch[21] reviewed this issue, analyzing studies published from 1966 to 2002. Because most studies lacked appropriate control groups or had other limitations, they could not confirm a causal role for NSAIDs in the establishment or worsening of GAS NF. Subsequently, additional clinical reports emerged, including prospective and case-matched active surveillance studies that demonstrated NSAID use was independently associated with increased risk of severe bacterial complications, including GAS infections (reviewed in[20]). Since 2015, 3 additional clinical studies have associated NSAID use with increased risk of peritonsillar abscess after GAS pharyngitis.[22–24]

Experimental studies in animals strongly suggest NSAIDs directly affect GAS disease pathogenesis. Specifically, 2 studies clearly showed that different nonselective NSAIDs (ketorolac, ibuprofen, and indomethacin) accelerated the course of established myonecrosis and worsened outcomes.[25,26] Further, addition of NSAIDs to therapeutic antibiotic regimens significantly decreased antibiotic efficacy.[25] Recently, a third laboratory reported another nonselective NSAID (diclofenac) increased the incidence of sepsis in mice challenged intramuscularly with GAS.[27] In addition, in our murine model of cryptogenic GAS infection, ketorolac significantly increased trafficking of circulating GAS to strain-injured muscles.[28] Thus, mounting clinical and experimental evidence support a direct causal relationship between NSAID use and the risk and severity of GAS infection.

NECROTIZING CLOSTRIDIAL INFECTIONS

Clostridial gas gangrene is an acute invasion of healthy living muscle and occurs in 2 different settings: traumatic and spontaneous. Rarely, recurrent gas gangrene has also been described, occurring several decades after primary infection.[29]

Traumatic Clostridial Infections: Contamination Versus Infection

Deeply penetrating injuries that compromise the blood supply create an anaerobic environment ideal for spore germination and bacterial proliferation (reviewed in[30]). Such trauma accounts for approximately 70% of cases of gas gangrene. Other predisposing conditions are bowel and biliary tract surgery, intramuscular injection of epinephrine, criminal abortion, retained placenta, prolonged rupture of the membranes, or intrauterine fetal demise in postpartum patients. *Clostridium perfringens* causes approximately 80% of such infections; other pathogens include *Clostridium septicum*, *C novyi*, *C histolyticum*, and others.

Data regarding contamination versus active infection of traumatic wounds comes from studies during World Wars I and II. In 1915, Fleming[31] documented that 60.4% of war wounds were contaminated with clostridia. MacLennan[32] later showed that active infection occurred in only 4.8 to 9.0 cases per thousand wounded, and resulted in either gas gangrene (myonecrosis) or "anaerobic cellulitis."[33] In 1941, Qvist[34] suggested that anaerobic cellulitis required only debridement of tissue damaged by trauma itself, whereas in gas gangrene, amputation was necessary to ensure survival—a premise that guides clinical practice today.

Spontaneous Gas Gangrene

Spontaneous (nontraumatic) gas gangrene is commonly caused by *C perfringens* or the more aerotolerant *C septicum*.[35] Most infections occur in patients with gastrointestinal portals of entry, such as adenocarcinoma,[35] or in those with congenital or cyclic neutropenia.[36]

Clostridium sordellii Infection

C sordellii infections affect women after natural childbirth, abortion, or other gynecologic manipulations, and men, women, and children after a variety of traumatic injuries and surgical procedures (reviewed in[37]). Infection has also been reported following intracutaneous injection ("skin popping") of black tar heroin. *C sordellii* infection is characterized by an absence of fever, profound hypotension, diffuse capillary leak, hemoconcentration (hematocrit of 50%–80%), and a marked leukemoid reaction (white blood cell count of 50,000–150,000/μL whole blood). In most cases, mortality is extreme (70%–100%) and occurs within 2 to 4 days of hospital admission. Survival is higher (≥50%) in patients who inject black tar heroin, likely caused by earlier recognition of infection at the injection site.

PATHOGENESIS
Pain and Rapid Tissue Destruction

The classical clinical and histologic features of necrotizing GAS infections, and those caused by clostridial species, are mediated by potent bacterial exotoxins (for a detailed review, see[16]). In high concentrations, some factors are cytotoxic—contributing directly to tissue destruction and organ dysfunction, whereas lower concentrations can hyperaugment cellular responses, including cytokine production, cell–cell interactions, and leukocyte degranulation. For instance, acute onset of severe pain and rapid destruction of healthy tissues have been attributed to vascular occlusion (**Fig. 1**) and tissue hypoxia mediated by toxin-induced formation of platelet–leukocyte complexes (reviewed in[38]). It is likely that this mechanism also accounts for the classic observations that dead and dying tissues in these infections do not bleed and that the tissue inflammatory response is markedly attenuated.[39]

Shock and Organ Failure

Cytokines clearly mediate shock and organ failure in bacterial infections. Multiple *S pyogenes* exotoxins are superantigens,[40] causing hyperproduction of both monocyte- and lymphocyte-derived cytokines.[40–46] In experimental streptococcal myonecrosis in baboons, neutralizing anti-tumor necrosis factor-α antibody restored normal blood pressure and decreased mortality by 50%.[47] Diffuse capillary leak is likely attributable

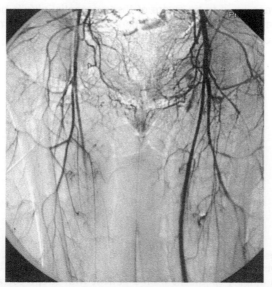

Fig. 1. Perfusion deficits in necrotizing infections. Arteriogram of patient with group A streptococcal NF/myonecrosis of the leg showing a marked vascular occlusion and reduced blood flow in the affected tissue.

to cytokines and other host mediators, as well as circulating exotoxins and M protein–fibrinogen complexes.[48]

Cardiomyopathy

Streptolysin O causes direct cardiomyocyte contractile dysfunction[49] by allowing an influx of calcium through streptolysin O–induced membrane pores.[49] Removal of streptolysin O restored normal function, suggesting membrane integrity and calcium homeostasis were reestablished. These observations are consistent with the clinical observation that cardiomyopathy is reversible among survivors of streptococcal toxic shock syndrome.[50] In addition, cardiomyocyte-derived cytokines ("cardiokines") are produced after direct S pyogenes stimulation and after exposure to S pyogenes-activated inflammatory cells.[51] Further, an uncharacterized S pyogenes-induced cardiomyocyte-derived stimulator/s boosted macrophage production of proinflammatory cytokines and cardiodepressant factors.[52]

Cryptogenic S pyogenes Infections

Using a murine muscle strain model, we have shown that circulating GAS specifically traffics to sites of injury.[28] Trafficking correlated with expression of vimentin[28]—a key group A streptococcal ligand[53] (**Fig. 2**). Because vimentin is highly expressed on activated muscle precursors (myoblasts) but not on mature myofibers,[54] our findings provide a molecular mechanism to explain the development of cryptogenic group A streptococcal infections at sites of nonpenetrating muscle trauma.

DIAGNOSIS OF NECROTIZING SOFT TISSUE INFECTIONS
Diagnostic Pitfalls

Early diagnosis of necrotizing infections may be confounded by the absence of fever or early cutaneous manifestations; nonspecific radiographic tests; a recent history of nonpenetrating trauma, surgery, or childbirth; and chronic underlying diseases (**Table 1**). Physicians need to be aware of these potential pitfalls because delays in diagnosis and treatment have dire consequences. A basic algorithm for diagnosis of necrotizing infections is shown in **Fig. 3**.

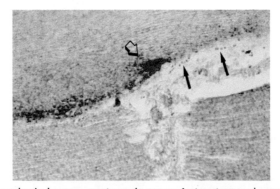

Fig. 2. Necrotic muscles in human cryptogenic group A streptococcal necrotizing soft tissue infection express vimentin. Immunohistochemistry for the GAS ligand, vimentin, was performed on human autopsy specimens from a patient with streptococcal toxic shock syndrome and myonecrosis. Vimentin was readily visible (*open arrowhead*; brown stain) in areas of muscle destruction and was frequently associated with adjacent GAS (*closed arrows*; blue stain).

Table 1	
Pitfalls in the diagnosis of necrotizing soft tissue infection	
Absence of fever	Fever is often absent in patients with necrotizing soft tissue infections because of NSAIDS that are self-administered or prescribed in the emergency department or in postsurgical settings. It is also absent in patients with necrotizing infection caused by *C sordellii*.
Absence of cutaneous manifestations	Spontaneous or cryptogenic necrotizing infections that begin in the deep soft tissues without an obvious bacterial portal of entry often lack cutaneous signs of infection until late in the course of disease.
Attributing severe pain to injury or procedures	Severe pain is a key finding in patients with necrotizing infections. However, when such infections develop after surgery or parturition, pain may be erroneously attributed to the procedure itself. Similarly, perineal pain may be attributed to hemorrhoids, epididymitis, or vaginal or rectal trauma. Severe pain associated with spontaneous or cryptogenic infections is often wrongly attributed to muscle strain or venous thrombosis. If the pain is out of proportion to clinical findings and/or requires opioids or ketorolac (Toradol) for management, a developing necrotizing infection should be considered. Pain may be absent caused by use of narcotics or NSAIDS or to neuropathy in diabetic patients.
Nonspecific imaging tests	In patients with necrotizing infections, radiographs may only show edema and an absence of gas in the deep tissue. Because such findings are consistent with noninfectious etiologies (eg, soft tissue injury, postsurgery and postpartum conditions), they may confound diagnosis.
Attributing systemic manifestations to other causes	Nausea, vomiting, and diarrhea may be early manifestations of toxemia from group A streptococcal infection though they are often wrongly attributed to food poisoning or viral illness.

Clinical Findings

Classical findings in NF include soft tissue edema (75%), erythema (72%), severe pain (72%), tenderness (68%), fever (60%), and skin blebs, bullae, or necrosis (38%).[55] In Ludwig's angina, patients exhibit slight inflammation, a "woody" hardness of the sublingual area, and swelling of the oral floor. In a recent case-controlled study, the significant factors that differentiated cellulitis from NF were recent surgery, pain out of proportion to clinical findings, hypotension, skin necrosis, and hemorrhagic bullae.[56]

In the approximately 50% of patients who develop cryptogenic (ie, no portal) group A streptococcal infection, the process begins deep in the tissues. In this setting, crescendo pain is the most important clinical clue and its onset typically occurs well

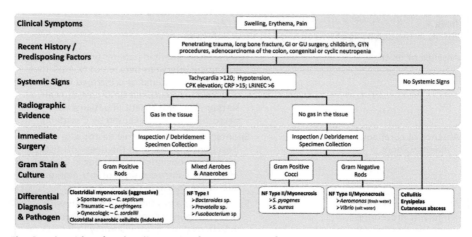

Fig. 3. Algorithm for the diagnosis of necrotizing infections.

before shock, renal impairment, or acute respiratory distress syndrome are manifest. Such pain, however, may be absent or attenuated in surgical, trauma, or postpartum patients receiving analgesics including NSAIDs. Alternatively, pain may be incorrectly attributed to normal postoperative discomfort rather than acute infection. Pain may also be absent in those with altered mental status or those with diabetes-related neuropathy. In these instances a strong clinical clue is lost, delaying the correct diagnosis and appropriate treatments, often with dire consequences. Thus, all patients presenting with sudden onset of severe pain in an extremity, with or without an obvious portal of bacterial entry or the presence of fever, should be evaluated for severe soft tissue infection on an emergent basis.

Imaging Tests

Radiographs, computed tomography scans, or MRI techniques will show soft tissue swelling in group A streptococcal infection, and gas in the tissues of patients with clostridial gas gangrene or NF type I. Imaging evidence of gas in the tissues, or the presence of crepitus, should prompt immediate surgical consultation. Findings of swelling alone may not be useful in patients with prior trauma, surgery, childbirth, and so on, because swelling does not distinguish between infection, trauma, and inflammation. Comparison by enhanced computed tomography scan of patients with documented NF versus those having other musculoskeletal infections suggested that a lack of fascial enhancement was specific for NF.[57]

Additional Testing

Gram stain of surgically obtained material is crucial to determine the infectious etiology and to guide empiric treatment. Percutaneous biopsy with frozen section has been proposed to aid in the diagnosis of necrotizing infection.[58,59] However, this technique suffers from sampling error and is not a good substitute for open surgical inspection and biopsy. Group A streptococcal necrotizing infection is characterized histologically by the destruction of muscle tissue, the paucity of infiltrating phagocytes, and large numbers of gram-positive bacteria adjacent to muscle cells. Similar histologic findings accompany clostridial myonecrosis, although with more evidence of edema and/or or gas formation.

Surrogate Markers for Early Diagnosis

Objective criteria to distinguish mild versus necrotizing infections in lieu of surgical diagnosis have been sought. A C-reactive protein of greater than 200,[60] a modestly increased white blood cell count with marked left shift,[61] or elevated serum creatinine in the absence of hypotension are suggestive of severe group A streptococcal infection. Marked leukemoid reactions (50,000–150,000 cells/μL) and profound hemoconcentration are characteristic of *C sordellii* infection. The combination of a white blood cell count of greater than 15,400 plus a serum sodium of less than 135 has been associated with NF, but failed to distinguish between NF in general and non-necrotizing soft tissue infections (positive predictive value, 26%) in a low prevalence setting.[61] Elevated serum creatine phosphokinase or serum glutamic-oxaloacetic transaminase may suggest deep infection involving muscle or fascia (as opposed to cellulitis).

In 2004, the Laboratory Risk Indicator for Necrotizing Fasciitis (LRINEC) scoring system was reported.[62] This system used total white blood cell count, hemoglobin, sodium, glucose, creatinine, and C-reactive protein to distinguish between mild soft tissue infections and NF.[62] For patients with LRINEC scores of 5.8 or greater, the positive predictive value ranged from 57% to 92%[1,62,63]; negative predictive values were 86% to 96%.[62,64] Yet, in children with NF, the median LRINEC score was only 3.7.[65] The disparity in scores and predictive values may be attributable, in part, to the fact that LRINEC's specificity is greatest for advanced disease. This notion is supported by a recent study in which 70% of patients admitted to the intensive care unit with NF had an LRINEC score of greater than 6 and the mortality was 29.3%[66]; patients with less severe disease were excluded. Subsequent studies have demonstrated the tool's limited sensitivity when scores are less than 6 and therefore it should not be used to rule out a necrotizing soft tissue infection.[64,67,68]

In summary, for suspected necrotizing infections, no single clinical laboratory test or group of tests adequately replaces timely surgical inspection.

THERAPEUTIC OPTIONS
Surgical Intervention

For patients with aggressive soft tissue infection or those with mild infection plus evidence of systemic toxicity, prompt surgical exploration is of extreme importance to (a) determine the extent of infection, (b) assess the need for debridement or amputation, and (c) obtain specimens for Gram stain and culture. When infection is near the vital structures of the neck, surgical intervention may be necessary to prevent airway obstruction.

There is universal agreement that early surgical debridement is crucial in managing these complex patients. Yet, using published reports to pinpoint the critical time for surgical intervention is problematic because many studies, particularly retrospective analyses, variably define the delays to surgical intervention relative to either (1) time from diagnosis, (2) time from recognition or (3) time from hospital admission. Studies from tertiary hospitals typically report shorter times to surgery, likely because the diagnosis was made elsewhere. Nevertheless, initial studies demonstrated a significant increase in survival among patients taken to surgery within 24 hours after admission versus those in whom surgery was delayed.[55,69] More recent studies document that survival is further improved with even earlier surgical intervention (eg, <6 hours),[70,71] supporting the notion that the earlier surgery occurs, the better the outcome.

Antimicrobial Treatment

Polymicrobial necrotizing infections

An array of organisms (often ≥5 pathogens per wound) can be cultured from involved tissues. As such, empiric antibiotic therapy must broadly cover both aerobes and anaerobes until microbes are identified and antibiotic susceptibilities determined. Empirical choices could include a beta-lactam–beta-lactamase inhibitor combination such as piperacillin–tazobactam or a carbapenem such as meropenem, imipenem, and perhaps some of the newer combinations if local resistance patterns warrant use, with or without vancomycin if methicillin-resistant S aureus risk factors exist (eg, prior colonization, diabetes, injectable drug use). The role of clindamycin to inhibit the ribosome and synthesis of exotoxins should also be considered, although not for its activity against anaerobes. It is recommended that susceptibility testing should be performed on those anaerobic isolates that grow in pure culture, including clostridia (especially those of the C ramosum, innocuum and clostridioforme group), those that are virulent and clinically important, and those from difficult to treat infections.[72]

Unfortunately, fewer clinicians are ordering, and fewer laboratories are performing, anaerobic cultures for susceptibility testing.[73] Consequently, clinicians must rely on a few published multicenter surveys[74–78] and Clinical and Laboratory Standards Institute reviews[72] to choose empirical therapy. Many anaerobic bacteria produce penicillinases (eg, Prevotella and Porphyromonas spp), mediating resistance to penicillin and ampicillin, and many anaerobes produce cephalosporinases.[78] Most Clostridium spp, including C perfringens and excluding C ramosum, C clostridioforme, and C innocuum, and gram-positive anaerobic cocci (eg, Finegoldia magna) are penicillin and ampicillin susceptible. Bacteroides fragilis is composed of at least 20 species (coupled with Parabacteroides spp.) with variable susceptibility patterns and with B fragilis generally the most susceptible member of the group species. Metronidazole resistance is rare in all Bacteroides spp. Comparative anaerobic susceptibility testing information is summarized in **Table 2**.

For mixed aerobic/anaerobic infections of the head and neck, either beta-lactams (ampicillin–sulbactam, cefoxitin, cephalosporins plus metronidazole, or carbapenem) or clindamycin can be effective treatments[78,79] covering aerobic (streptococci) and anaerobic (Prevotella, Porphyromonas, and gram-positive cocci) oral flora. B fragilis is rarely isolated from oral anaerobic cultures. Penicillin resistance is seen in approximately 10% of F necrophorum isolates as well as 30% of Prevotella spp and 7% of Veillonella spp. Treatment of mixed infections of the abdomen, perineum or gynecologic organs should empirically cover aerobic gram-negative rods as well as fecal anaerobes such as B fragilis group spp., Prevotella and Clostridia spp., plus gram-positive cocci such as F magna and Parvimonas micra. Gram stain, anaerobic culture, and susceptibility information, should be obtained. Empirical treatment should be based on updated Clinical and Laboratory Standards Institute data.[72] Broader aerobic gram-negative coverage may be necessary if the patient has been recently hospitalized or prescribed antibiotics, or when the prevalence of extended spectrum beta lactamase E coli and other resistant gram-negative aerobes is locally increased. Clindamycin and fluoroquinolone empirical therapy should be avoided.[79] If wound cultures are obtained, then therapy should be guided by those specific individual results. If empirical therapy is used, then the targeted therapy should be guided by local antibiograms because resistance varies geographically and may be specific to a particular locale such as a hospital or geographic region. Additional information on specific and alternative treatments can be found in the current Infectious Diseases Society of

Table 2
Antimicrobial resistance (% of isolates) among clinically important anaerobes associated with necrotizing soft tissue infection

Organism	Drug	Ampicillin-sulbactam	Piperacillin-tazobactam	Cefoxitin	Carbapenems	Clindamycin	Moxifloxacin	Metronidazole	Tedizolid	Tigecycline
						Percent Resistant				
B fragilis		4	1	6	1–2	24–28	19–38	0	1	2–3
B thetaiotaomicron		3	1–2	8–13	1–2	49–56	30–34	0	2	2
B fragilis group (general)		3–4	1–2	6–12	1	33–42	28–40	0	2	2

America guidelines for treatment of skin and soft tissue infections[80] and for treatment of diabetic foot infections.[81]

Monomicrobial necrotizing infections

a. *Group A Streptococcal Infections*: For the treatment of severe GAS infections, the Infectious Diseases Society of America guidelines recommend a combination of penicillin plus clindamycin for 10 to 14 days[79] and is based on the following: (a) clindamycin alone has proved efficacious in human studies[82–84]; (b) clindamycin is more efficacious than penicillin in experimental models of NF and myonecrosis[85] because of its ability to inhibit bacterial protein toxin production, its insensitivity to bacterial inoculum or physiologic state, and its ability to modulate the host's immune response; and (c) no in vitro antagonistic effects have been found for combinations of penicillin and clindamycin at clinically relevant concentrations.

b. *Emerging Antibiotic Resistance*: Macrolide/lincosamide resistance among GAS has increased worldwide. An early report of such resistance was from Japan in 1979 where 70% of strains causing pharyngitis were erythromycin-resistant.[86] In a European study of *S pyogenes* strains from 10 countries, the prevalence of erythromycin resistance had increased from 29.3% in 2002 to 2003 to 45.7% in 2004 to 2005 and this increase was highly associated with erythromycin consumption in individual countries.[87] In France, 16% of erythromycin resistant strains were also found to be resistant to clindamycin.[88] A 2014 report from China showed that 98.4% of strains isolated from children with tonsillitis or scarlet fever were resistant to both clindamycin and erythromycin,[89] and 90.4% of these displayed the cMLSB phenotype.[89] In a 2017 report from Wisconsin, 15% of pediatric pharyngeal isolates were resistant to both clindamycin and erythromycin.[90]In these reports, most resistance occurred in pharyngeal isolates, however this too is changing. For instance, in 1999 in San Francisco County, 32% of the isolates from invasive-disease-related specimens were resistant to erythromycin.[91] Two of the 39 erythromycin-resistant strains were also resistant to clindamycin and an additional 34 strains demonstrated inducible clindamycin resistance. A retrospective review of invasive GAS disease in Hawaii (2005–2007) identified 12 erythromycin- and clindamycin-resistant *emm90* GAS isolates that had identical pulse gel electrophoretic patterns, suggesting a clonal spread.[92] Lastly, from 2013 to 2017, 20% to 35% of invasive GAS isolates at Harborview Medical Center in Seattle, Washington displayed constitutive resistance to both erythromycin and clindamycin (F. Fang, Harborview Medical Center, Seattle, WA, personal communication, 2018).The emergence of such resistance poses a significant therapeutic dilemma for the treatment of necrotizing soft tissue infection caused by GAS. Recent studies in mice have demonstrated significant efficacy of oxazolidinones (linezolid, tedizolid) against fulminant myonecrosis caused by constitutive erythromycin/clindamycin GAS,[93] suggesting these agents may be useful in severe human GAS infections. Thus, the next iteration of Infectious Diseases Society of America treatment guidelines for severe *S pyogenes* infections will likely address the emerging worldwide problem of macrolide/lincosamide resistance.

c. *Clostridial Gas Gangrene*: For traumatic or spontaneous clostridial myonecrosis, treatment with penicillin together with clindamycin for 10 to 14 days is recommended.[79] Penicillin is recommended based on in vitro sensitivity data; clindamycin is recommended based on superior efficacy over penicillin in animal models of *C perfringens* gas gangrene.[94,95] Clinical trials in humans have not been performed.

d. *Emerging Antibiotic Resistance*: Although *C perfringens* remains largely susceptible to first-line antibiotics, antibiotic resistance has been reported, highlighting the importance of good anaerobic microbiology and susceptibility testing to guide optimal clinical management decisions for clostridial infections. Reports from the United Kingdom, Spain, Canada, and Taiwan isolated clindamycin-resistant *C perfringens* from various sites.[96–100] In a 2-year prospective study from Canada, 14.2% of clostridium species other than *C perfringens* were penicillin resistant and 21.6% clindamycin resistant.[100]

e. *Other Necrotizing Monomicrobial Infections.* Current guidelines recommend that *Aeromonas hydrophilia* infections be treated with doxycycline plus either ciprofloxacin or ceftriaxone.[80] A combination of doxycycline plus either ceftriaxone or cefotaxime is recommended for *V vulnificus* infections.[80] Treatment options for necrotizing infections caused by *S aureus* are discussed elsewhere in this publication (Timothy J. Hatlen and Loren G. Miller's article, "Staphylococcal Skin and Soft Tissue Infections," in this issue).

Intensive Care Unit Management

Management guidelines for critically ill patients have been recently published elsewhere.[101] Still, unique problems associated with necrotizing infections are of concern.

Capillary leak syndrome
Circulating streptococcal and clostridial toxins and host mediators cause diffuse endothelial damage. Intravenous fluid requirements may be extremely high (10–12 L of normal saline/day); however, profound hypoalbuminemia (0.5–1.0 g/dL) is also common and thus replacement with colloid (albumin) may be necessary to maintain oncostatic pressure.

Intravascular hemolysis
Streptococcal and clostridial hemolysins cause impressive and rapid reductions in hematocrit in the absence of disseminated intravascular hemolysis. Monitoring the hematocrit rather than hemoglobin may be a better indicator for the need for transfusion.

Cardiomyopathy
Streptococcal exotoxins,[49] and some clostridial toxins,[102] have direct myocardial depressant activity. In streptococcal toxic shock syndrome, such activity likely contributes to global hypokinesia as measured by echocardiography and cardiac outputs.[50] Among survivors, cardiomyopathy is reversible, fully resolving in 3 to 24 months after infection. Some patients have survived with the use of cardiac assist devices. Management is difficult because the use of vasopressors increases afterload, resulting in decreased peripheral perfusion and decreased cardiac output. Symmetric gangrene resulting in the loss of 1 to 4 limbs has been described. Careful monitoring and maintenance of mean arterial pressure to not more than 65 mm Hg in this infection seems prudent, though no clinical studies have been performed to support this recommendation.

Adjunctive Measures

Hyperbaric oxygen
A 2003 review of 57 studies from 1997 to 2003 concluded that hyperbaric oxygen (HBO) was not useful for NF,[103] a finding similar to other studies.[55,104,105] In contrast, a significant survival benefit of HBO in NF was demonstrated in recent studies from the United States and Australia (4.2%–12.0% mortality among patients receiving HBO vs 23%–24.3% in non–HBO-treated controls).[7,106] Other studies have also suggested a beneficial role for HBO in gas gangrene,[103,105] although experimental studies showed no benefit.[107] A new clinical study was initiated in 2015 to evaluate HBO's impact on

inflammatory and vasoactive biomarkers in necrotizing infections[108]; results have not yet been published. Thus, the use and benefits of HBO remain controversial. The absolute necessity of surgical debridement should not be delayed while pursuing HBO treatment.

Intravenous immune globulin

Although its use remains somewhat controversial, we favor administration of intravenous immune globulin (IVIG) for patients with necrotizing soft tissue infection caused by GAS The rationale for its use is based on its ability to neutralize key extracellular toxins that mediate shock and organ failure (reviewed in[109]). Although prior retrospective studies and statistically underpowered prospective trials on the efficacy of IVIG for NSTIs proved inconclusive,[110–112] newer studies support its use in the setting of streptococcal toxic shock syndrome and NF. For example, a 2018 meta-analysis that included 5 studies of patients with streptococcal toxic shock syndrome treated with clindamycin (1 randomized and 4 nonrandomized) demonstrated that use of IVIG was associated with a significant reduction in 30-day mortality (33.7%–15.7%).[113] This outcome was likely attributable to the ability of clindamycin and IVIG to decrease the production and/or activity of circulating GAS toxins. Similarly, in a subsequent prospective observational study of patients with necrotizing soft tissue infection caused by GAS, the use of IVIG was associated with reduced 90-day mortality.[114] However, the 2018 meta-analysis discussed elsewhere in this article excluded a recent, multicenter retrospective study involving a large, propensity-matched cohort of patients with NF and vasopressor-dependent shock owing largely to GAS and/or S aureus.[111] The authors found that adjunctive IVIG was not associated with survival or hospital length-of-stay benefits in patients with NF shock who received aggressive surgical management and antibiotics. Furthermore, there was no benefit, even when IVIG was initiated within the first 2 days of hospital admission. Thus, the value of IVIG in NF and TSS remains to be fully demonstrated.

In summary, necrotizing soft tissue infections share many clinical and pathologic features, but in each case, early diagnosis and treatment are essential to reduce morbidity and ensure survival. Diagnostic pitfalls should be recognized and early surgical consultation sought for suspected cases.

CLINICS CARE POINTS

- Skin sloughing, ecchymoses, and purple violaceous bullae are classic signs of necrotizing infection but may be absent early in the course of infection. This presents a diagnostic dilemma particularly for patients with group A streptococcal infections lacking a defined portal of entry, those with spontaneous gas gangrene caused by Clostridium septicum or those with Clostridium sordellii infections.
- Severe pain and fever are associated with necrotizing infections but both may be masked by early self- administration of NSAIDS or other anti-pyretics such as acetaminophen and also in those patients who develop necrotizing infections following surgical procedures such as bowel resection etc.
- Severe pain following muscle strain or blunt trauma that progressively intensifies over 24-72 hrs may be an early sign of spontaneous group A streptococcal infection and requires diagnostic testing and not just administration of narcotics in the Emergency Department.
- Severe capillary leak, intravascular hemolysis and acute cardiomyopathy may complicate ICU management. Thus, transfusion and colloid replacement may be useful in conjunction with crystalloid. Bedside echocardiography may define those with reduced cardiac outputs due to myocardial dysfunction and in whom

potent vasoconstrictors may further reduce cardiac output by increasing afterload.

- Source control by surgical debridement is critically important and resected tissue should be sent for immediate Gram stain and culture to define appropriate antibiotic treatment.

DISCLOSURE

The authors have nothing to disclose.

REFERENCES

1. Glass GE, Sheil F, Ruston JC, et al. Necrotising soft tissue infection in a UK metropolitan population. Ann R Coll Surg Engl 2015;97(1):46–51.
2. Khamnuan P, Chongruksut W, Jearwattanakanok K, et al. Necrotizing fasciitis: epidemiology and clinical predictors for amputation. Int J Gen Med 2015;8: 195–202.
3. Suzuki K, Hayashi Y, Otsuka H, et al. [Case report; a case of Lemierre's syndrome associated with necrotizing fasciitis and septic embolization]. Nihon Naika Gakkai Zasshi 2016;105(1):99–104.
4. Tawa A, Larmet R, Malledant Y, et al. Severe sepsis associated with Lemierre's syndrome: a rare but life-threatening disease. Case Rep Crit Care 2016;2016: 1264283.
5. Luckett WH. VII. Large phagedenic ulcer of the abdomen. Ann Surg 1909;50(3): 605–8.
6. Meleney FL. Bacterial synergism in disease processes: with a confirmation of the synergistic bacterial etiology of a certain type of progressive gangrene of the abdominal wall. Ann Surg 1931;94(6):961–81.
7. Devaney B, Frawley G, Frawley L, et al. Necrotising soft tissue infections: the effect of hyperbaric oxygen on mortality. Anaesth Intensive Care 2015;43(6): 685–92.
8. Miller LG, Perdreau-Remington F, Rieg G, et al. Necrotizing fasciitis caused by community-associated methicillin-resistant *Staphylococcus aureus* in Los Angeles. N Engl J Med 2005;352(14):1445–53.
9. Stevens DL. Streptococcal Infections. In: Goldman L, Bennett JC, editors. Cecil textbook of medicine. 21st edition. Philadelphia: WB Saunders; 2000. p. 1619–24.
10. Nelson GE, Pondo T, Toews KA, et al. Epidemiology of Invasive Group A Streptococcal Infections in the United States, 2005-2012. Clin Infect Dis 2016;63(4): 478–86.
11. Hamilton SM, Stevens DL, Bryant AE. Pregnancy-related group a streptococcal infections: temporal relationships between bacterial acquisition, infection onset, clinical findings, and outcome. Clin Infect Dis 2013;57(6):870–6.
12. Stevens DL. Invasive group A streptococcus infections. Clin Infect Dis 1992; 14:2–13.
13. Adams EM, Gudmundsson S, Yocum DE, et al. Streptococcal myositis. Arch Intern Med 1985;145:1020–3.
14. Stevens DL, Tanner MH, Winship J, et al. Reappearance of scarlet fever toxin A among streptococci in the Rocky Mountain West: severe group A streptococcal infections associated with a toxic shock-like syndrome. N Engl J Med 1989; 321(1):1–7.

15. Nuwayhid ZB, Aronoff DM, Mulla ZD. Blunt trauma as a risk factor for group A streptococcal necrotizing fasciitis. Ann Epidemiol 2007;17(11):878–81.

16. Stevens DL, Bryant AE. Severe group A streptococcal infections. In: Ferretti JJ, Stevens DL, Fischetti VA, editors. Streptococcus pyogenes: basic biology to clinical manifestations. NCBI e-book; Bookshelf ID: NBK333425; 2016:PMID: 26866227.

17. Bisno AL, Stevens DL. Streptococcal infections in skin and soft tissues. N Engl J Med 1996;334:240–5.

18. Schurr M, Engelhardt S, Helgerson R. Limb salvage for streptococcal gangrene of the extremity. Am J Surg 1998;175(3):213–7.

19. Efstratiou A, Lamagni T. Epidemiology of Streptococcus pyogenes. In: Ferretti J, Stevens DL, Fischetti VA, editors. Streptococcus pyogenes : basic biology to clinical manifestations [Internet]. Oklahoma City (OK): University of Oklahoma Health Sciences Center; 2016.

20. Bryant AE, Bayer CR, Aldape MJ, et al. The roles of injury and nonsteroidal anti-inflammatory drugs in the development and outcomes of severe group A streptococcal soft tissue infections. Curr Opin Infect Dis 2015;28(3):231–9.

21. Aronoff DM, Bloch KC. Assessing the relationship between the use of nonsteroidal antiinflammatory drugs and necrotizing fasciitis caused by group A streptococcus. Medicine (Baltimore) 2003;82(4):225–35.

22. Demeslay J, De BG, Vairel B, et al. Possible role of anti-inflammatory drugs in complications of pharyngitis. A retrospective analysis of 163 cases. Eur Ann Otorhinolaryngol Head Neck Dis 2014;131(5):299–303.

23. Feasson T, Debeaupte M, Bidet C, et al. Impact of anti-inflammatory drug consumption in peritonsillar abscesses: a retrospective cohort study. BMC Infect Dis 2016;16(1):432.

24. Lepelletier D, Pinaud V, Le CP, et al. Is there an association between prior anti-inflammatory drug exposure and occurrence of peritonsillar abscess (PTA)? A national multicenter prospective observational case-control study. Eur J Clin Microbiol Infect Dis 2017;36(1):57–63.

25. Hamilton SM, Bayer CR, Stevens DL, et al. Effects of selective and nonselective nonsteroidal anti-inflammatory drugs on antibiotic efficacy of experimental group A streptococcal myonecrosis. J Infect Dis 2014;209(9):1429–35.

26. Weng TC, Chen CC, Toh HS, et al. Ibuprofen worsens Streptococcus pyogenes soft tissue infections in mice. J Microbiol Immunol Infect 2011;44(6):418–23.

27. Ture Z, Demiraslan H, Kontas O, et al. The role of nonsteroidal anti-inflammatory drugs intramuscular injection in the development and severity of deep soft tissue infection in mice. Fundam Clin Pharmacol 2017;32(2):147–54.

28. Hamilton SM, Bayer CR, Stevens DL, et al. Muscle injury, vimentin expression, and nonsteroidal anti-inflammatory drugs predispose to cryptic group A streptococcal necrotizing infection. J Infect Dis 2008;198(11):1692–8.

29. Stevens DL, Laposky LL, Montgomery P, et al. Recurrent gas gangrene at a site of remote injury: localization due to circulating antitoxin. West J Med 1988;148: 204–5.

30. Stevens DL. Clostridial myonecrosis and other clostridial diseases. In: Bennett JC, Plum F, editors. Cecil textbook of medicine. 20th edition. Philadelphia: W.B. Saunders Co.; 1996. p. 2090–3.

31. Fleming A. On the bacteriology of septic wounds. Lancet 1915;186(4803): 638–43.

32. MacLennan JD. The histotoxic clostridial infections of man. Bacteriol Rev 1962; 26:177–276.

33. Stewart JC. Anaerobic cellulitis. JAMA 1905;45:528–35.
34. Qvist G. Anaerobic cellulitis and gas gangrene. Br Med J 1941;2(4206):217–21.
35. Bodey GP, Rodriguez S, Fainstein V, et al. Clostridial bacteremia in cancer patients. A 12-year experience. Cancer 1991;67(7):1928–42.
36. Stevens DL, Musher DM, Watson DA, et al. Spontaneous, nontraumatic gangrene due to *Clostridium septicum*. Rev Infect Dis 1990;12(2):286–96.
37. Aldape MJ, Bryant AE, Stevens DL. *Clostridium sordellii* infection: epidemiology, clinical findings, and current perspectives on diagnosis and treatment. Clin Infect Dis 2006;43(11):1436–46.
38. Bryant AE. Biology and pathogenesis of thrombosis and procoagulant activity in invasive infections caused by group A streptococci and Clostridium perfringens. Clin Microbiol Rev 2003;16(3):451–62.
39. Bryant AE, Bayer CR, Aldape MJ, et al. *Clostridium perfringens* phospholipase C-induced platelet/leukocyte interactions impede neutrophil diapedesis. J Med Microbiol 2006;55(Pt 5):495–504.
40. Norrby-Teglund A, Basma H, Andersson J, et al. Varying titres of neutralizing antibodies to streptococcal superantigens in different preparations of normal polyspecific immunoglobulin G (IVIG): implications for therapeutic efficacy. Clin Infect Dis 1998;26(3):631–8.
41. Hackett SP, Stevens DL. Superantigens associated with staphylococcal and streptococcal toxic shock syndromes are potent inducers of tumor necrosis factor beta synthesis. J Infect Dis 1993;168(1):232–5.
42. Fast DJ, Schlievert PM, Nelson RD. Toxic shock syndrome-associated staphylococcal and streptococcal pyrogenic toxins are potent inducers of tumor necrosis factor production. Infect Immun 1989;57:291–4.
43. Norrby-Teglund A, Newton D, Kotb M, et al. Superantigenic properties of the group A streptococcal exotoxin SpeF (MF). Infect Immun 1994;62(12):5227–33.
44. Norrby-Teglund A, Norgren M, Holm SE, et al. Similar cytokine induction profiles of a novel streptococcal exotoxin, MF, and pyrogenic exotoxins A and B. Infect Immun 1994;62(9):3731–8.
45. Kotb M, Majumdar G, Hackett SP, et al. Temporal relationship of cytokine release by peripheral blood mononuclear cells stimulated by the streptococcal superantigen, pepM5. American Society for Microbiology 1992;New Orleans, LA.
46. Kotb M, Norrby-Teglund A, McGeer A, et al. An immunogenetic and molecular basis for differences in outcomes of invasive group A streptococcal infections. Nat Med 2002;8(12):1398–404.
47. Stevens DL, Bryant AE, Hackett SP, et al. Group A streptococcal bacteremia: the role of tumor necrosis factor in shock and organ failure. J Infect Dis 1996;173(3):619–26.
48. Herwald H, Cramer H, Morgelin M, et al. M protein, a classical bacterial virulence determinant, forms complexes with fibrinogen that induce vascular leakage. Cell 2004;116(3):367–79.
49. Bolz DD, Li Z, McIndoo ER, et al. Cardiac myocyte dysfunction induced by streptolysin O is membrane pore and calcium dependent. Shock 2015;43(2):178–84.
50. Stevens DL, Shelly MP, Stiller R, Villasenor-S.A., Bryant AE. Acute reversible cardiomyopathy in patients with streptococcal toxic shock syndrome. Proceedings of the XVIIth Lancefield International Symposium on Streptococci and Streptococcal Diseases, 179. Porto Heli, Greece, 2008. Ref Type: Abstract.
51. Li Z, Bryant AE, Hamilton SM, et al. Do cardiomyocytes mount an immune response to Group A Streptococcus? Cytokine 2011;54(3):258–65.

52. Li Z, Bryant AE, Parimon T, et al. Cardiac dysfunction in StrepTSS: group A streptococcus disrupts the directional cardiomyocyte-to-macrophage crosstalk that maintains macrophage quiescence. Cytokine 2012;59(1):191–4.

53. Bryant AE, Bayer CR, Huntington JD, et al. Group A streptococcal myonecrosis: increased vimentin expression after skeletal-muscle injury mediates the binding of *Streptococcus pyogenes*. J Infect Dis 2006;193(12):1685–92.

54. Vaittinen S, Lukka R, Sahlgren C, et al. The expression of intermediate filament protein nestin as related to vimentin and desmin in regenerating skeletal muscle. J Neuropathol Exp Neurol 2001;60(6):588–97.

55. McHenry CR, Piotrowski JJ, Petrinic D, et al. Determinants of mortality for necrotizing soft-tissue infections. Ann Surg 1995;221(5):558–63.

56. Alayed KA, Tan C, Daneman N. Red flags for necrotizing fasciitis: a case control study. Int J Infect Dis 2015;36:15–20.

57. Carbonetti F, Cremona A, Carusi V, et al. The role of contrast enhanced computed tomography in the diagnosis of necrotizing fasciitis and comparison with the Laboratory Risk Indicator for Necrotizing Fasciitis (LRINEC). Radiol Med 2016;121(2):106–21.

58. Stamenkovic I, Lew PD. Early recognition of potentially fatal necrotizing fasciitis. The use of frozen-section biopsy. N Engl J Med 1984;310:1689–93.

59. Majeski J, Majeski E. Necrotizing fasciitis: improved survival with early recognition by tissue biopsy and aggressive surgical treatment. South Med J 1997; 90(11):1065–8.

60. Chelsom J, Halstensen A, Haga T, et al. Necrotising fasciitis due to group A streptococci in western Norway: incidence and clinical features. Lancet 1994; 344:1111–5.

61. Wall DB, Klein SR, Black S, et al. A simple model to help distinguish necrotizing fasciitis from nonnecrotizing soft tissue infection. J Am Coll Surg 2000;191(3): 227–31.

62. Wong CH, Khin LW, Heng KS, et al. The LRINEC (Laboratory Risk Indicator for Necrotizing Fasciitis) score: a tool for distinguishing necrotizing fasciitis from other soft tissue infections. Crit Care Med 2004;32(7):1535–41.

63. Burner E, Henderson SO, Burke G, et al. Inadequate sensitivity of laboratory risk indicator to rule out necrotizing fasciitis in the emergency department. West J Emerg Med 2016;17(3):333–6.

64. Holland MJ. Application of the Laboratory Risk Indicator in Necrotising Fasciitis (LRINEC) score to patients in a tropical tertiary referral centre. Anaesth Intensive Care 2009;37(4):588–92.

65. Putnam LR, Richards MK, Sandvall BK, et al. Laboratory evaluation for pediatric patients with suspected necrotizing soft tissue infections: a case-control study. J Pediatr Surg 2016;51(6):1022–5.

66. van Stigt SF, de VJ, Bijker JB, et al. Review of 58 patients with necrotizing fasciitis in the Netherlands. World J Emerg Surg 2016;11:21.

67. Wilson MP, Schneir AB. A case of necrotizing fasciitis with a LRINEC score of zero: clinical suspicion should trump scoring systems. J Emerg Med 2013; 44(5):928–31.

68. Fernando SM, Tran A, Cheng W, et al. Necrotizing soft tissue infection: diagnostic accuracy of physical examination, imaging, and LRINEC score: a systematic review and meta-analysis. Ann Surg 2019;269(1):58–65.

69. Freischlag JA, Ajalat G, Busuttil RW. Treatment of necrotizing soft tissue infections. The need for a new approach. Am J Surg 1985;149(6):751–5.

70. Bucca K, Spencer R, Orford N, et al. Early diagnosis and treatment of necro-tizing fasciitis can improve survival: an observational intensive care unit cohort study. ANZ J Surg 2013;83(5):365–70.
71. Hadeed GJ, Smith J, O'Keeffe T, et al. Early surgical intervention and its impact on patients presenting with necrotizing soft tissue infections: a single academic center experience. J Emerg Trauma Shock 2016;9(1):22–7.
72. Clinical and Laboratory Standards Institute. Performance Standards for antimi-crobial susceptibility testing; 30th edition. CLSI Supplement M100 2020.
73. Goldstein EJ, Citron DM, Goldman RJ, et al. United States National Hospital Sur-vey of anaerobic culture and susceptibility methods, II. Anaerobe 1995;1(6): 309–14.
74. Goldstein EJC, Merriam CV, Citron DM. The in vitro activity of tedizolid compared to linezolid and five other antimicrobial agents against 332 anaerobic isolates including Bacteroides fragilis group spp., Prevotella, Porphyromonas and Veillonella spp. Antimicrob Agents Chemother 2020;64(9):e01088-20.
75. Goldstein EJC, Citron DM, Tyrrell KL. In vitro activity of eravacycline and comparator antimicrobials against 143 recent strains of Bacteroides and Para-bacteroides species. Anaerobe 2018;52:122–4.
76. Goldstein EJC, Citron DM, Tyrrell KL, et al. Comparative in vitro activities of rel-ebactam, imipenem, the combination of the two, and six comparator antimicro-bial agents against 432 strains of anaerobic organisms, including imipenem-resistant strains. Antimicrob Agents Chemother 2018;62(2). e01992-17.
77. Snydman DR, Jacobus NV, McDermott LA, et al. Trends in antimicrobial resis-tance among Bacteroides species and Parabacteroides species in the United States from 2010-2012 with comparison to 2008-2009. Anaerobe 2017;43:21–6.
78. Brook I, Wexler HM, Goldstein EJ. Antianaerobic antimicrobials: spectrum and susceptibility testing. Clin Microbiol Rev 2013;26(3):526–46.
79. Stevens DL, Bisno AL, Chambers HF, et al. Practice guidelines for the diagnosis and management of skin and soft-tissue infections. Clin Infect Dis 2005;41(10): 1373–406.
80. Stevens DL, Bisno AL, Chambers HF, et al. Practice guidelines for the diagnosis and management of skin and soft tissue infections: 2014 update by the Infec-tious Diseases Society of America. Clin Infect Dis 2014;59(2):e10–52.
81. Lipsky BA, Berendt AR, Cornia PB, et al. 2012 Infectious Diseases Society of America clinical practice guideline for the diagnosis and treatment of diabetic foot infections. J Am Podiatr Med Assoc 2013;103(1):2–7.
82. Zimbelman J, Palmer A, Todd J. Improved outcome of clindamycin compared with beta-lactam antibiotic treatment for invasive Streptococcus pyogenes infection. Pediatr Infect Dis J 1999;18(12):1096–100.
83. Carapetis JR, Jacoby P, Carville K, et al. Effectiveness of clindamycin and intra-venous immunoglobulin, and risk of disease in contacts, in invasive group a streptococcal infections. Clin Infect Dis 2014;59(3):358–65.
84. Linner A, Darenberg J, Sjolin J, et al. Clinical efficacy of polyspecific intravenous immunoglobulin therapy in patients with streptococcal toxic shock syndrome: a comparative observational study. Clin Infect Dis 2014;59(6):851–7.
85. Stevens DL, Bryant-Gibbons AE, Bergstrom R, et al. The Eagle effect revisited: efficacy of clindamycin, erythromycin, and penicillin in the treatment of strepto-coccal myositis. J Infect Dis 1988;158:23–8.
86. Maruyama S, Yoshioka H, Fujita K, et al. Sensitivity of group A streptococci to antibiotics. Prevalence of resistance to erythromycin in Japan. Am J Dis Child 1979;133(11):1143–5.

87. Richter SS, Heilmann KP, Dohrn CL, et al. Increasing telithromycin resistance among Streptococcus pyogenes in Europe. J Antimicrob Chemother 2008; 61(3):603–11.

88. Bingen E, Bidet P, Mihaila-Amrouche L, et al. Emergence of macrolide-resistant Streptococcus pyogenes strains in French children. Antimicrob Agents Chemother 2004;48(9):3559–62.

89. Zhou W, Jiang YM, Wang HJ, et al. Erythromycin-resistant genes in group A beta-haemolytic Streptococci in Chengdu, Southwestern China. Indian J Med Microbiol 2014;32(3):290–3.

90. DeMuri GP, Sterkel AK, Kubica PA, et al. Macrolide and clindamycin resistance in group a streptococci isolated from children with pharyngitis. Pediatr Infect Dis J 2017;36(3):342–4.

91. York MK, Gibbs L, Perdreau-Remington F, et al. Characterization of antimicrobial resistance in Streptococcus pyogenes isolates from the San Francisco Bay area of northern California. J Clin Microbiol 1999;37(6):1727–31.

92. Chen I, Kaufisi P, Erdem G. Emergence of erythromycin- and clindamycin-resistant Streptococcus pyogenes emm 90 strains in Hawaii. J Clin Microbiol 2011;49(1):439–41.

93. Bryant AE, Bayer CR, Aldape MJ, et al. Emerging erythromycin and clindamycin resistance in group A streptococcus: efficacy of linezolid and tedizolid in experimental necrotizing infection. J Glob Antimicrob Resist 2020;22:601–7.

94. Stevens DL, Laine BM, Mitten JE. Comparison of single and combination antimicrobial agents for prevention of experimental gas gangrene caused by *Clostridium perfringens*. Antimicrob Agents Chemother 1987;31:312–6.

95. Stevens DL, Maier KA, Laine BM, et al. Comparison of clindamycin, rifampin, tetracycline, metronidazole, and penicillin for efficacy in prevention of experimental gas gangrene due to *Clostridium perfringens*. J Infect Dis 1987;155: 220–8.

96. Khanna N. Clindamycin-resistant Clostridium perfringens cellulitis. J Tissue Viability 2008;17(3):95–7.

97. Salido AJ, Tarrago AC, Casas CO, et al. Spontaneous abscess of the anterior abdominal wall caused by Clostridium perfringens resistant to clindamycin. Surg Infect (Larchmt) 2012;13(4):276–7.

98. Leal J, Gregson DB, Ross T, et al. Epidemiology of Clostridium species bacteremia in Calgary, Canada, 2000-2006. J Infect 2008;57(3):198–203.

99. Liu CY, Huang YT, Liao CH, et al. Increasing trends in antimicrobial resistance among clinically important anaerobes and Bacteroides fragilis isolates causing nosocomial infections: emerging resistance to carbapenems. Antimicrob Agents Chemother 2008;52(9):3161–8.

100. Marchand-Austin A, Rawte P, Toye B, et al. Antimicrobial susceptibility of clinical isolates of anaerobic bacteria in Ontario, 2010-2011. Anaerobe 2014;28:120–5.

101. Rhodes A, Evans LE, Alhazzani W, et al. Surviving sepsis campaign: international guidelines for management of sepsis and septic shock: 2016. Intensive Care Med 2017;43(3):304–77.

102. Stevens DL, Troyer BE, Merrick DT, et al. Lethal effects and cardiovascular effects of purified alpha- and theta-toxins from *Clostridium perfringens*. J Infect Dis 1988;157:272–9.

103. Wang C, Schwaitzberg S, Berliner E, et al. Hyperbaric oxygen for treating wounds: a systematic review of the literature. Arch Surg 2003;138(3):272–9.

104. Jallali N, Withey S, Butler PE. Hyperbaric oxygen as adjuvant therapy in the management of necrotizing fasciitis. Am J Surg 2005;189(4):462–6.

105. Willy C, Rieger H, Vogt D. [Hyperbaric oxygen therapy for necrotizing soft tissue infections: contra]. Chirurg 2012;83(11):960–72.
106. Shaw JJ, Psoinos C, Emhoff TA, et al. Not just full of hot air: hyperbaric oxygen therapy increases survival in cases of necrotizing soft tissue infections. Surg Infect (Larchmt) 2014;15(3):328–35.
107. Stevens DL, Bryant AE, Adams K, et al. Evaluation of hyperbaric oxygen therapy for treatment of experimental *Clostridium perfringens* infection. Clin Infect Dis 1993;17:231–7.
108. Hansen MB, Simonsen U, Garred P, et al. Biomarkers of necrotising soft tissue infections: aspects of the innate immune response and effects of hyperbaric oxygenation-the protocol of the prospective cohort BIONEC study. BMJ Open 2015;5(5):e006995.
109. Stevens DL. The toxic shock syndromes. Infect Dis Clin North Am 1996;10(4): 727–46.
110. Madsen MB, Hjortrup PB, Hansen MB, et al. Immunoglobulin G for patients with necrotising soft tissue infection (INSTINCT): a randomised, blinded, placebo-controlled trial. Intensive Care Med 2017;43(11):1585–93.
111. Kadri SS, Swihart BJ, Bonne SL, et al. Impact of intravenous immunoglobulin on survival in necrotizing fasciitis with vasopressor-dependent shock: a propensity score-matched analysis from 130 US Hospitals. Clin Infect Dis 2017;64(7): 877–85.
112. Darenberg J, Ihendyane N, Sjolin J, et al. Intravenous immunoglobulin G therapy in streptococcal toxic shock syndrome: a European randomized, double-blind, placebo-controlled trial. Clin Infect Dis 2003;37(3):333–40.
113. Parks T, Wilson C, Curtis N, et al. Polyspecific intravenous immunoglobulin in clindamycin-treated patients with streptococcal toxic shock syndrome: a systematic review and meta-analysis. Clin Infect Dis 2018;67(9):1434–6.
114. Bruun T, Rath E, Bruun MM, et al. Risk factors and predictors of mortality in streptococcal necrotizing soft-tissue infections: a multicenter prospective study. Clin Infect Dis 2020. https://doi.org/10.1093/cid/ciaa027.

Gram-Negative Skin and Soft Tissue Infections

Jean-Francois Jabbour, MD, MSc, Souha S. Kanj, MD, FIDSA, FRCP, FESCMID, FECMM*

KEYWORDS

- Gram-negative • Skin and soft tissue infections • Epidemiology • Diagnosis
- Treatment

KEY POINTS

- The incidence of skin and soft tissue infections (SSTIs) caused by gram-negative bacilli (GNB) is increasing globally and is correlated with the rise in antibacterial drug resistance.
- It is important to determine the patient and epidemiologic risk factors for the prompt and proper initiation of therapy.
- Novel antibiotics against multidrug-resistant/extensively drug-resistant GNB have been introduced recently and should be considered in the management of SSTIs.

INTRODUCTION

Skin and soft tissue infections (SSTIs) commonly are encountered in the hospital and the community settings and are on the rise. According to the Global Burden of Disease Study in 2013, SSTIs were the fourth leading cause of disability worldwide.[1] US national trends for patient visits for SSTIs reflected a 50% increase in the overall rate of visits from 1997 to 2005, reaching 14.2 million visits.[2] A more recent population-based study from the United States estimates that the rate of clinically diagnosed SSTIs is approximately 500 per 10,000 person-years.[3] One study from 86 medical centers in the United States, however, noted a decrease in the rate of SSTIs among patients living with human immunodeficiency virus,[4] but most studies on the epidemiology of SSTIs point toward an increasing trend.[5]

The Infectious Diseases Society of America (IDSA) classifies SSTIs according to skin extension as either complicated, where deep tissues are involved and surgical intervention often is required, or uncomplicated, where the infection is limited to the superficial layers and can be managed with antibiotic therapy or incision.[6] Additional parameters, including rate of progression and tissue necrosis also are used to classify SSTIs.[6] For the purpose of this review, SSTIs are stratified further according to the causative class of pathogens: either gram-positive bacteria (GPB) or gram-negative

Division of Infectious Diseases, Department of Internal Medicine, American University of Beirut Medical Center, PO Box 11-0236, Riad El Solh, Beirut 1107 2020, Lebanon
* Corresponding author.
E-mail address: sk11@aub.edu.lb

Infect Dis Clin N Am 35 (2021) 157–167
https://doi.org/10.1016/j.idc.2020.10.008
0891-5520/21/© 2020 Elsevier Inc. All rights reserved.

bacilli (GNB). Although GPB, notably *Staphylococcus aureus* and group A ß-hemolytic streptococci, comprise the majority of SSTI-causative pathogens, GNB play an under-rated role.

The aim of this review is to discuss the importance of GNB SSTIs while looking into their epidemiology, risk factors, diagnosis, prognosis, and clinical management.

EPIDEMIOLOGY AND RISK FACTORS OF GRAM-NEGATIVE SKIN AND SOFT TISSUE INFECTIONS

GNB generally are the less common culprits for SSTIs compared with GPB. It is diffi-cult to accurately define the incidence of GNB SSTIs because they usually are not the focus of most studies. Over the past decade, GNB have been garnering more attention because their incidence seems to be on the rise.[7] Microbiologic testing of SSTIs from a subgroup of patients with culture-positive specimens in the US revealed that *S aureus* was the predominant organism among 108,243 isolates (81%) and GNB were the second most commonly isolated organisms (14%).[3] It has been observed that GNB SSTIs are encountered more frequently in the hospital setting.[8] Among hospital-acquired infections, GNB SSTIs mostly are associated with surgical site in-fections (SSIs) and constitute a big portion of polymicrobial infections, such as in dia-betic foot infections.[8] A study on SSIs from patients with secondary and tertiary peritonitis in the intensive care unit (ICU) in Spain showed that *Escherichia coli* (20.4%) and *Pseudomonas* spp (19.3%) were the most commonly isolated organisms, whereas GPB collectively added up to 29.7% of all organisms.[9] In a retrospective study from Greece in patients admitted for SSTIs, GNB were the organisms isolated most frequently, including *E coli* (28.4%), *P aeruginosa* (24.3%), *Proteus* spp (20.3%), *Klebsiella pneumoniae* (17.6%), and others.[10] The predominance of GNB was linked to patients' characteristics and history, because the cohort was of an older age group and most patients had a high comorbidity rate as well as previous hospital-izations and prior antibiotic exposure.[10]

A more recent study from the United States found that GNB constituted approxi-mately 12% of SSTIs from adult patients admitted for primary SSTIs, whereas approx-imately 24% were mixed infections of GPB and GNB.[11] In a review article looking at global studies on diabetic foot infections, GNB, especially *P aeruginosa*, were more prevalent in subtropical and less-developed countries.[12] In diabetic foot infections, chronicity of the disease is helpful in determining the infection's microbiological pro-file. Unlike the acute phase of the infection that usually is caused by GPB, chronic dia-betic foot infections often are polymicrobial and mostly caused by aerobic GNB and obligate anaerobic bacteria.[12] Although diabetic foot infections mainly are recognized as polymicrobial infections (66%), studies allude to a shift in the microbiology as more GNB seem to be the causative pathogens (14% in monomicrobial infections vs 9% for monomicrobial GPB infections).[13] In necrotizing fasciitis, 70% to 90% of infections are polymicrobial and consist of mixed GPB and GNB obligate and facultative anaer-obes.[14] Another common subtype of necrotizing fasciitis consists of mixed *Clos-tridium* spp and GNB, such as *Aeromonas* spp.[14]

The increase in GNB SSTIs coincides with the rise of multidrug-resistant (MDR) pathogens. Although not specific to SSTIs, MDR pathogens, as defined by Magior-akos and colleagues,[15] are resistant to at least 1 antibiotic agent in 3 or more anti-microbial categories, and extensively drug-resistant (XDR) are resistant to at least 1 agent in all but 2 or fewer antimicrobial categories. Carbapenem-resistant Entero-bacteriaceae (CRE) and Carbapenem-resistant *P aeruginosa* (CRPA) are trouble-some in SSTIs and are difficult to treat. In the International Network for Optimal

Resistance Monitoring (INFORM) surveillance program, the frequency of MDR Enterobacteriaceae reached 7% from 3289 isolates of SSTIs, whereas XDR Entero-bacteriaceae and CRE represented 1% of SSTIs each.[16] As for *P aeruginosa*, MDR isolates were found in approximately 12% of 845 isolates of SSTIs, XDR species in 3%, and piperacillin-tazobactam–resistant species in approximately 4%.[16] *Acineto-bacter baumannii* can be a causative pathogen in SSTIs in patients with burns, com-bat wounds, obesity, immunosuppression, and cirrhosis, as well as diabetes mellitus.[17,18]

In an effort to characterize the epidemiology of GNB SSTIs, recent data from the Consortium on Resistance Against Carbapenem in *Klebsiella* and Other Enterobacteri-aceae (CRACKLE-1) showed that GNB SSTIs were most common in pressure ulcers (34%) and SSIs (30%).[19] The anatomic site in wound infections is an important deter-minant of the etiology. Wounds located in the abdominal and anal/perianal regions, as well as after urinary tract surgeries, most likely harbor GNB.[20] In CRACKLE-1, the most common locations for GNB wound infections were the extremities (27.5%) and the sacrum (24.6%).[19] It also was found that admission from long-term care facil-ities is a significant predictor of CRE SSTIs (*P* value = .04).[19] Other risk factors for GNB SSTIs include inappropriate antibiotic treatment,[21] breast implant SSIs,[21] prolonged hospital stay,[22] uncontrolled diabetes mellitus,[22] and traumatic injury from fresh or saltwater.[22] **Table 1** lists the specific SSTI types related to Enterobacteriaceae, *P aer-uginosa*, and *A baumannii* with their shared risk factors for the acquisition of resistant strains (see **Table 1**).

DIAGNOSIS

A diagnosis of SSTIs often is challenging, because the microbiologic yield usually is low and does not always reflect the true etiology of the infection.[5] Swab cultures from a superficial wound or exudates from a fistula can be misleading because they

Table 1
The most common Gram-negative bacilli that cause specific types of skin and soft tissue infections and the risk factors for the acquisition of resistant strains

Gram-Negative Pathogen	Specific Skin and Soft Tissue Type	Risk Factors for the Acquisition of Multidrug-Resistant or Extensively Drug-Resistant Strains[19]
P aeruginosa	• Ecthyma gangrenosum • Burn wound infections • Hot tub folliculitis • Foot infection due to nail puncture • Toe web infection • Green nail syndrome • Perichondritis of the ear	• Diabetes • Neutropenia • Burn wounds • Pressure ulcers • Immunocompromised state • Long-term care facility resident • Prior hospitalization • ICU length of stay
A baumannii	• Postsurgical wound infection, especially in the presence of prosthetics • War-related injuries	• Recent broad-spectrum antibiotic therapy • Prior colonization with MDR and XDR GNB
Enterobacteriaceae	• Breast implant SSIs • SSIs after surgery on urinary tract • Abdominal/perianal SSIs	• The presence of indwelling devices

might represent colonizers rather than true pathogens.[23] Cultures from needle aspiration of the affected skin in cellulitis are positive in up to only 40% of cases and in up to only 30% of samples from a punch biopsy.[5] In cellulitis and erysipelas, blood cultures have a yield of less than or equal to 5%.[5] Because cultures in these relatively uncomplicated cases do not aid in the diagnosis, clinical reasoning is key in guiding therapy, and microbiologic testing is not required in the absence of a complicated course. Clinical judgment should be based on a patient's risk factors, severity of illness, source of admission, local and institutional epidemiology, history of prior antibiotic therapy, and characteristics of the SSTI when considering whether or not to obtain cultures. Cultures can be very useful in purulent infections where specimens are obtained after drainage or from deep tissues during surgical débridement.[6] Blood cultures and biopsy or aspiration also can be helpful in uncomplicated SSTIs, particularly in cancer patients or in cases of suspected fungal infections and an immunocompromised state.[24] A Gram stain from any specimen can guide therapy and cultures on aerobic and anaerobic media are needed to make the definitive microbiologic diagnosis whenever possible. Matrix-assisted laser desorption ionization–time-of-flight imaging mass spectrometry shortens the time to definitive microbiologic identification in SSTIs.[25] In addition, rapid diagnostics are being used for the identification of SSTI pathogens, including molecular patterns of resistance. These can be of tremendous help in implementing antimicrobial stewardship efforts with rapid initiation of proper therapy and de-escalation of broad-spectrum antibiotics when not needed. Currently, there is no evidence that 16S RNA has any added benefit in the diagnosis of cellulitis as it was not found to be more sensitive than cultures.[26]

Imaging might have an added role in the diagnosis of SSTIs, especially the complicated ones. Plain radiographs can be useful to identify necrosis or the presence of gas, especially in necrotizing fasciitis.[27] Ultrasound can assess the presence of abscesses and computed tomography can assess deeper infections and guide the drainage procedure.[27] The IDSA recommends magnetic resonance imaging as the radiographic modality of choice for pyomyositis.[6] It also is the most sensitive noninvasive method to investigate necrotizing infections and the extent of involvement.[27] Recently, whole-body positron emission tomography using fluorodeoxyglucose F 18 also has been found to be of help in diagnosing deep soft tissue infections when done as part of a work-up for fever.[28]

PROGNOSIS

The overall mortality of SSTIs is relatively low in the United States, reaching approximately only 0.46% in 2011.[29] There are no direct studies that address mortality among GNB causing SSTIs per se, however, SSTIs caused by MDR GNB have a worse prognosis. In CRACKLE-1, 16% of patients admitted with CRE SSTIs died, and of the patients who survived, 34% required high-level supportive care after discharge.[19] In some conditions, the mortality rate of CRE SSTIs reaches up to 33%, such as in postsurgical mediastinitis.[30] Predictors of mortality were an immunosuppressed state, Pitt bacteremia score greater than 3, and prolonged hospitalization prior to the first positive culture.[19] Despite residence in a long-term care facility being a risk factor for CRE SSTI acquisition, long-term care facility residents were less likely to die.[19]

SSTIs of mixed GPB and GNB etiology are associated with a worse outcome. In 1 study from 42 US hospitals on 5156 SSTIs, patients with mixed infections (18.8%) had a significantly higher mortality rate, longer length of hospital stay, and higher charges.[31] Worse outcomes also were associated with SSTIs due to P aeruginosa. Inappropriate initial treatment is recognized as one of the most important prognostic factors for SSTIs. A study on hospital-acquired complicated SSTIs found that SSTIs of a mixed etiology were more likely to be treated inappropriately than nonmixed SSTIs.[32] This was supported by another study where 23% of complicated SSTIs were treated with an inappropriate initial antibiotic regimen.[33]

CLINICAL MANAGEMENT OF GRAM-NEGATIVE SKIN AND SOFT TISSUE INFECTIONS

Current treatment of GNB SSTIs is becoming more challenging as the rate of antimicrobial resistance is increasing. Appropriate and prompt initiation of antibiotic therapy is crucial, because delay is associated with increase in mortality and inappropriate therapy gives rise to more resistant pathogens.[21,34] The IDSA guidelines generally have addressed some aspects of uncomplicated GNB SSTIs treatment, in particular SSIs, where a cephalosporin or fluoroquinolone in combination with anaerobic coverage, such as metronidazole, is recommended.[6] **Table 2** represents the available antibiotics that are used in the treatment of SSTIs and their activity against *P aeruginosa, A baumannii,* and Enterobacteriaceae, along with their doses (see **Table 2**). Amoxicillin-clavulanate or ampicillin-sulbactam is recommended for animal and human bites to target *Pasteurella multocida*, as well as other microbes of the oral flora, but alternatives, such as doxycycline and carbapenems, are warranted in cases of clinical deterioration as MDR GNB are becoming more prevalent.[6] For Enterobacteriaceaeproducing extended-spectrum β-lactamases (ESBLs), treatment with carbapenems, tigecycline, fluoroquinolones, or trimethoprim/sulfamethoxazole can be chosen according to susceptibility results, extent of infection, and need for intravenous versus oral therapy.[35,36] Note that the ESBL-producing Enterobacteriaceae also often are resistant to trimethoprim/sulfamethoxazole and fluoroquinolones. Ceftolozane-tazobactam can be used as a carbapenem-sparing agent.[36] In suspected or confirmed *P aeruginosa* infection, treatment with a fluoroquinolone, ceftazidime, cefepime, piperacillin-tazobactam, or a carbapenem other than ertapenem can be used. Adjunctive to antibiotic therapy, drainage and surgical débridement are necessary in purulent, necrotizing, and complicated SSTIs.

Whenever the suspicion for SSTIs with MDR or XDR GNB is high, conventional antibiotics play a minor role in the management. Several novel antibiotics are being investigated for the management of MDR infections and can be used in SSTI treatment. For the management of CRE SSTIs, ceftazidime-avibactam is a suitable choice, especially for *K pneumoniae* carbapenemase (KPC) or OXA-48 producers, as proved in the REPRISE trial.[37] Another option includes ceftaroline-avibactam.[22] Meropenem-vaborbactam and imipenem/cilastatin-relebactam are active against KPC producers, yet have an unreliable activity against OXA-48 producers.[22,38] For CREs producing metallo-β-lactamases (MBLs), aztreonam-avibactam was shown to be safe and effective.[39,40] Although not preferable to be used as a first-line agent, some novel antibiotics are active against both KPC-producing and MBL-producing CREs. These include cefiderocol and plazomicin, and omadacycline for *K pneumoniae*.[22] If need be, novel agents can be combined with older antibiotics, such as polymyxins, tigecycline, gentamicin, or fosfomycin, although this is controversial because some experts believe that combination therapy adds cost and toxicity and might induce more resistance.[41,42] Combination therapy was found to be one of the highest factors that expose patients with SSTIs to avoidable antibiotics.[41] When novel antibiotics are not available, high-dose tigecycline and the extended infusion of carbapenems can be used to treat certain CRE SSTIs.[22] Monotherapy with aminoglycosides or polymyxins should only be considered when no other options are available.

Table 2
Antibiotic agents used for the treatment of the most common Gram negative pathogens causing skin and soft tissue infections based on susceptibility results

Class	Antibiotic Agent	Dose Recommended[a]	Pseudomonas aeruginosa	Acinetobacter baumannii	Enterob- acteriaceae
Penicillin-β-lactamase combinations	Amoxicillin-clavulanate	Oral: 875 mg, every 12 h	−	−	±[b]
	Ampicillin-sulbactam	3 g, every 6 h	−	±[c]	±[b]
	Piperacillin-tazobactam	4.5 g, every 6 h	+	−	±[b]
Cephalosporins	Cefuroxime	Oral: 500 mg, every 12 h Intravenous: 750 mg, every 12 h	−	−	±[b]
	Cefotaxime	1–2 g, every 6 h	−	−	±[b]
	Ceftazidime	1–2 g, every 8 h	+	±[c]	±[b]
	Ceftriaxone	1–2 g, once daily	−	−	±[b]
	Cefepime	1–2 g, every 8 h	+	±[c]	±[b]
	Cefiderocol	2 g, every 8 h	+	±[c]	+
Monobactams	Aztreonam	1–2 g, every 8 h	±	−	±[b]
Fluoroquinolones	Ciprofloxacin	• Intravenous: 400 mg, every 8–12 h • Oral: 500–750 mg, every 12 h	±	±[c]	±[b]
	Levofloxacin	500–750 mg, once daily (intravenous or oral)	±	±[c]	±[b]
Phosphonic acid derivative	Fosfomycin	Intravenous: 4–6 g, every 6 h	±	−	±[b]
Carbapenems	Doripenem	500 mg, every 8 h	+	±[c]	+
	Ertapenem	1 g, once daily	−	−	+
	Imipenem/cilastatin	500 mg, every 6 h – 1 g every 8 h	+	±[c]	+
	Meropenem	1 g, every 8 h	+	±[c]	+
Novel β-lactams with β-lactamase inhibitors	Ceftazidime–avibactam	2.5 g, every 8 h	+	−	+
	Ceftolozane/tazobactam	1.5 g, every 8 h	+	−	+
	Imipenem/cilastatin–relebactam	1.25 g, every 6 h	+	±[c]	+
	Meropenem–vaborbactam	4 g, every 8 h	+	±[c]	+
Aminoglycosides	Tobramycin	5 mg/kg/d, every 8 h	+	±[c]	±[b]
	Gentamicin	5–7 mg/kg, every 24 h	+	±[c]	±[b]
	Amikacin	5 mg/kg, every 8 h	+	±[c]	+
	Plazomicin	15 mg/kg, every 24 h	−	−	+

		Dose			
Tetracyclines	Doxycycline	Oral: 100 mg, every 12 h	−	±c	±b
	Eravacycline[d]	1 mg/kg, every 12 h	−	±c	+
	Minocycline	100 mg, every 12 h	−	±c	±b
	Omadacycline	• Intravenous: 100 mg, every 24 h[e] • Oral: 300 mg, every 24 h[f]	−	−	+
Glycylcycline	Tigecycline	50–100 mg, every 12 h[g]	−	±c	±c
Polymyxins	Colistin	9 million units, as loading doses, followed by 4.5 million units, every 12 h	+	±c	±h
	Polymyxin B	15,000–25,000 units/kg, every 24 h	+	±c	+h

+ indicates activity against the respective organism; − indicates that the drug is not active against the organism; and ± indicates variable activity or acquired resistance that can be problematic.

^a Dosing is for intravenous formulation unless otherwise specified. Doses are for normal kidney function and should be adjusted according to creatinine clearance.

^b Acquired resistance occurs for ESBL-producing organisms.

^c Resistance in *Acinetobacter* spp is highly problematic with no antibiotic having reliable activity.

^d Eravacycline is not FDA approved for the treatment of acute bacterial SSTIs.

^e Loading dose: 200 mg as a single dose.

^f Loading dose: 450 mg as a single dose for the first 2 days

^g Loading dose: 100 mg as a single dose.

^h Polymyxins are not active against *Proteus* spp, *Morganella* spp, *Providencia* spp, and *Serratia* spp due to intrinsic resistance.

When suspecting CRPA SSTI, ceftolozane-tazobactam, ceftazidime-avibactam, imipenem-relebactam, and cefiderocol are agents with potent antipseudomonal activity.[22] In addition, the novel fluoroquinolones, finafloxacin and delafloxacin, have a promising role in the future management of CRPA SSTI, especially that fluoroquinolones are the only oral antipseudomonal agents. The US Food and Drug Administration (FDA) approved the use of delafloxacin in 2017 for the treatment of acute SSTIs.[43] Murepavadin is an outer-membrane protein targeting drug that showed success in the treatment of CRPA infections yet remains under investigation because it has severe nephrotoxic effects (ClinicalTrials.gov identifiers NCT02096315 and NCT02096328). A topical formulation of the drug could be useful in the treatment of SSTIs and is under development.[44]

Carbapenem-resistant *A baumannii* (CRAB) typically are XDR, with few options to treat. Polymyxins are considered the backbone of treatment in combination with older antibiotics according to in vitro susceptibility.[22] Cefiderocol has shown potent inhibition in 1 in vitro study and may play a role in the treatment of CRAB SSTIs.[45]

Duration of therapy should be guided by underlying host factors and clinical response. Long durations of therapy are highly discouraged in the era of increased resistance. In a study assessing the avoidable exposure of antibiotics in patients with SSTIs, 42% of subjects received antibiotics for greater than or equal to 10 days.[41] In line with antimicrobial stewardship principles, shorter monotherapy would have reduced the antibiotic exposure in these patients by 19% to 55%.[41]

SUMMARY

GNB are becoming an increasing cause of SSTIs worldwide and the role of MDR and XDR GNB pathogens in these infections is more recognized. Because initial antimicrobial therapy is crucial for the prognosis of patients with resistant or mixed SSTIs, empiric treatment must be guided by a patient's risk factors and epidemiologic cues. Rapid diagnostics improve care and outcome.

Although new antibiotics are introduced and can be used in the treatment, management decisions should be guided by antimicrobial stewardship principles using the narrow-spectrum agents whenever possible while promptly initiating the novel antimicrobial agents whenever MDR and XDR pathogens are suspected. To date, data on GNB SSTIs are limited. More clinical studies that focus on the burden, risk factors, outcomes, duration of therapy, and treatment with the novel agents are needed.

CLINICS CARE POINTS

- The rate of SSTIs caused by GNB is increasing globally.
- Risk factors for the acquisition of multidrug and XDR GNB SSTIs include diabetes, neutropenia, burn wounds, pressure ulcers, immunosuppression, prior antibiotic exposure and hospitalization, and long-term facility care residency.
- Microbiological cultures of blood and skin or soft tissue are indicated, including in uncomplicated cases of SSTIs in the setting of immunosuppression and when fungal infections are suspected.
- SSTIs with MDR GNB or mixed infections have a worse outcome.
- The use of novel antibiotics is encouraged when suspecting SSTIs with MDR GNB.
- The combination of novel antibiotics with conventional antibiotics should be used sparsely to avoid the added toxicity and increase in resistance.

DISCLOSURE

The authors have nothing to disclose.

REFERENCES

1. Karimkhani C, Dellavalle RP, Coffeng LE, et al. Global skin disease morbidity and mortality: an update from the global burden of disease study 2013. JAMA Dermatol 2017;153(5):406–12.
2. Hersh AL, Chambers HF, Maselli JH, et al. National trends in ambulatory visits and antibiotic prescribing for skin and soft-tissue infections. Arch Intern Med 2008;168(14):1585–91.
3. Ray GT, Suaya JA, Baxter R. Incidence, microbiology, and patient characteristics of skin and soft-tissue infections in a U.S. population: a retrospective population-based study. BMC Infect Dis 2013;13:252.
4. Morgan E, Hohmann S, Ridgway JP, et al. Decreasing Incidence of Skin and Soft-tissue Infections in 86 US Emergency Departments, 2009-2014. Clin Infect Dis 2019;68(3):453–9.
5. Kaye KS, Petty LA, Shorr AF, et al. Current Epidemiology, Etiology, and Burden of Acute Skin Infections in the United States. Clin Infect Dis 2019;68(Suppl 3): S193–9.
6. Stevens DL, Bisno AL, Chambers HF, et al. Executive summary: practice guidelines for the diagnosis and management of skin and soft tissue infections: 2014 Update by the Infectious Diseases Society of America. Clin Infect Dis 2014;59(2):147–59.
7. Del Giacomo P, Losito AR, Tumbarello M. The role of carbapenem-resistant pathogens in cSSTI and how to manage them. Curr Opin Infect Dis 2019;32(2): 113–22.
8. Dryden MS. Complicated skin and soft tissue infection. J Antimicrob Chemother 2010;65(Suppl 3):iii35–44.
9. Ballus J, Lopez-Delgado JC, Sabater-Riera J, et al. Surgical site infection in critically ill patients with secondary and tertiary peritonitis: epidemiology, microbiology and influence in outcomes. BMC Infect Dis 2015;15(1):304.
10. Ioannou P, Tsagkaraki E, Athanasaki A, et al. Gram-negative bacteria as emerging pathogens affecting mortality in skin and soft tissue infections. Hippokratia 2018;22(1):23–8.
11. Mcginnis E, Cammarata S, Tan R-D, et al. Characteristics of Patients Hospitalized for Acute Bacterial Skin and Skin Structure Infections (ABSSSI) From 2009 to 2013. Open Forum Infect Dis 2016;3(suppl_1). https://doi.org/10.1093/ofid/ofw172.145.
12. Uçkay I, Gariani K, Pataky Z, et al. Diabetic foot infections: state-of-the-art. Diabetes Obes Metab 2014;16(4):305–16.
13. Ramakant P, Verma AK, Misra R, et al. Changing microbiological profile of pathogenic bacteria in diabetic foot infections: time for a rethink on which empirical therapy to choose? Diabetologia 2011;54(1):58–64.
14. Misiakos EP, Bagias G, Patapis P, et al. Current concepts in the management of necrotizing fasciitis. Front Surg 2014;1. https://doi.org/10.3389/fsurg.2014.00036.
15. Magiorakos A-P, Srinivasan A, Carey RB, et al. Multidrug-resistant, extensively drug-resistant and pandrug-resistant bacteria: an international expert proposal for interim standard definitions for acquired resistance. Clin Microbiol Infect 2012;18(3):268–81.

16. Sader HS, Castanheira M, Duncan LR, et al. Antimicrobial Susceptibility of Enterobacteriaceae and Pseudomonas aeruginosa Isolates from United States Medical Centers Stratified by Infection Type: Results from the International Network for Optimal Resistance Monitoring (INFORM) Surveillance Program, 2015–2016. Diagn Microbiol Infect Dis 2018;92(1):69–74.

17. Guerrero DM, Perez F, Conger NG, et al. Acinetobacter baumannii-associated skin and soft tissue infections: recognizing a broadening spectrum of disease. Surg Infect 2010;11(1):49–57.

18. Ali A, Botha J, Tiruvoipati R. Fatal skin and soft tissue infection of multidrug resistant Acinetobacter baumannii: A case report. Int J Surg Case Rep 2014;5(8): 532–6.

19. Henig O, Cober E, Richter SS, et al. A prospective observational study of the epidemiology, management, and outcomes of skin and soft tissue infections due to carbapenem-resistant enterobacteriaceae. Open Forum Infect Dis 2017; 4(3). https://doi.org/10.1093/ofid/ofx157.

20. Pulido-Cejudo A, Guzmán-Gutierrez M, Jalife-Montaño A, et al. Management of acute bacterial skin and skin structure infections with a focus on patients at high risk of treatment failure. Ther Adv Infect Dis 2017;4(5):143–61.

21. Brink AJ, Richards GA. The role of multidrug and extensive-drug resistant Gam-negative bacteria in skin and soft tissue infections. Curr Opin Infect Dis 2020; 33(2):93–100.

22. Jabbour J-F, Sharara SL, Kanj SS. Treatment of multidrug-resistant Gram-negative skin and soft tissue infections. Curr Opin Infect Dis 2020;33(2):146–54.

23. Poulakou G, Lagou S, Tsiodras S. What's new in the epidemiology of skin and soft tissue infections in 2018? Curr Opin Infect Dis 2019;32(2):77–86.

24. Navarro-San Francisco C, Ruiz-Garbajosa P, Cantón R. The what, when and how in performing and interpreting microbiological diagnostic tests in skin and soft tissue infections. Curr Opin Infect Dis 2018;31(2):104–12.

25. Perez KK, Olsen RJ, Musick WL, et al. Integrating rapid pathogen identification and antimicrobial stewardship significantly decreases hospital costs. Arch Pathol Lab Med 2013;137(9):1247–54.

26. Johnson KE, Kiyatkin DE, An AT, et al. PCR offers no advantage over culture for microbiologic diagnosis in cellulitis. Infection 2012;40(5):537–41.

27. Esposito S, Bassetti M, Borre' S, et al. Diagnosis and management of skin and soft-tissue infections (SSTI): a literature review and consensus statement on behalf of the Italian Society of Infectious Diseases and International Society of Chemotherapy. J Chemother Florence Italy 2011;23(5):251–62.

28. Arnon-Sheleg E, Israel O, Keidar Z. PET/CT Imaging in Soft Tissue Infection and Inflammation—An Update. Semin Nucl Med 2020;50(1):35–49.

29. Kaye KS, Patel DA, Stephens JM, et al. Rising United States hospital admissions for acute bacterial skin and skin structure infections: recent trends and economic impact. PLoS One 2015;10(11):e0143276.

30. Abboud CS, Monteiro J, Stryjewski ME, et al. Post-surgical mediastinitis due to carbapenem-resistant Enterobacteriaceae: Clinical, epidemiological and survival characteristics. Int J Antimicrob Agents 2016;47(5):386–90.

31. Itani KMF, Merchant S, Lin S-J, et al. Outcomes and management costs in patients hospitalized for skin and skin-structure infections. Am J Infect Control 2011;39(1):42–9.

32. Zilberberg MD, Shorr AF, Micek ST, et al. Epidemiology and outcomes of hospitalizations with complicated skin and skin-structure infections: implications of

healthcare-associated infection risk factors. Infect Control Hosp Epidemiol 2009; 30(12):1203–10.

33. Lipsky BA, Napolitano LM, Moran GJ, et al. Inappropriate initial antibiotic treatment for complicated skin and soft tissue infections in hospitalized patients: incidence and associated factors. Diagn Microbiol Infect Dis 2014;79(2):273–9.

34. Bassetti M, Carnelutti A, Peghin M. Patient specific risk stratification for antimicrobial resistance and possible treatment strategies in gram-negative bacterial infections. Expert Rev Anti Infect Ther 2017;15(1):55–65.

35. Eckmann C, Dryden M. Treatment of complicated skin and soft-tissue infections caused by resistant bacteria: value of linezolid, tigecycline, daptomycin and vancomycin. Eur J Med Res 2010;15(12):554–63.

36. Karaiskos I, Giamarellou H. Carbapenem-Sparing Strategies for ESBL producers: when and how. Antibiotics (Basel) 2020;9(2). https://doi.org/10.3390/antibiotics9020061.

37. Carmeli Y, Armstrong J, Laud PJ, et al. Ceftazidime-avibactam or best available therapy in patients with ceftazidime-resistant Enterobacteriaceae and Pseudomonas aeruginosa complicated urinary tract infections or complicated intraabdominal infections (REPRISE): a randomised, pathogen-directed, phase 3 study. Lancet Infect Dis 2016;16(6):661–73.

38. Stewart A, Harris P, Henderson A, et al. Treatment of Infections by OXA-48-Producing *Enterobacteriaceae*. Antimicrob Agents Chemother 2018;62(11). e01195-18.

39. Jayol A, Nordmann P, Poirel L, et al. Ceftazidime/avibactam alone or in combination with aztreonam against colistin-resistant and carbapenemase-producing Klebsiella pneumoniae. J Antimicrob Chemother 2018;73(2):542–4.

40. Shaw E, Rombauts A, Tubau F, et al. Clinical outcomes after combination treatment with ceftazidime/avibactam and aztreonam for NDM-1/OXA-48/CTX-M-15-producing Klebsiella pneumoniae infection. J Antimicrob Chemother 2018; 73(4):1104–6.

41. Hurley HJ, Knepper BC, Price CS, et al. Avoidable antibiotic exposure for uncomplicated skin and soft tissue infections in the ambulatory care setting. Am J Med 2013;126(12):1099–106.

42. Leong HN, Kurup A, Tan MY, et al. Management of complicated skin and soft tissue infections with a special focus on the role of newer antibiotics. Infect Drug Resist 2018;11:1959–74.

43. Baxdela (delafloxacin) Tablets and Injection. Available at: https://www.accessdata.fda.gov/drugsatfda_docs/nda/2017/208610Orig1s000,208611Orig1s000TOC.cfm. Accessed June 27, 2020.

44. Tümmler B. Emerging therapies against infections with Pseudomonas aeruginosa. F1000Research 2019;8. https://doi.org/10.12688/f1000research.19509.1.

45. Hsueh SC, Lee YJ, Huang YT, et al. In vitro activities of cefiderocol, ceftolozane/tazobactam, ceftazidime/avibactam and other comparative drugs against imipenem-resistant Pseudomonas aeruginosa and Acinetobacter baumannii, and Stenotrophomonas maltophilia, all associated with bloodstream infections in Taiwan. J Antimicrob Chemother 2019;74(2):380–6.

Skin and Soft Tissue Infections in Persons Who Inject Drugs

Henry F. Chambers, MD

KEYWORDS

- Injection drug use • Staphylococcus aureus • Streptococcus pyogenes
- Clostridium perfringens • Clostridium sordellii • Cutaneous abscess • Cellulitis
- Necrotizing fasciitis

KEY POINTS

- Skin and soft tissue infections are the most common reason for persons who inject drugs to seek medical care.
- Cellulitis and abscess account for the majority of skin and soft tissue infections.
- Necrotizing fasciitis and other necrotizing soft tissue infections, although relatively uncommon, have high rates of morbidity and mortality and are medical and surgical emergencies.
- Rarely encountered causes of skin and soft tissue infections include nonperfringens clostridial species, *Bacillus* species, and nontoxigenic strains of *Corynebacterium diphtheria*.
- Harm reductions strategies such as needle exchange programs and opioid substitution may decrease the frequency of skin and soft tissue infections in persons who inject drugs.

SCOPE OF THE PROBLEM AND ITS EPIDEMIOLOGY

Injection drug use constitutes a heavy social, economic, and health burden in the United States with an estimated lifetime proportion of persons who inject drugs (PWID) at 2.6% of the US population[1] and with 1 million active users in 2011.[2] These estimates are almost certainly on the low side, given the opioid and substance abuse crisis of the past several years. The National Survey on Drug Use and Health estimated that in 2018 5.5 million people aged 12 and older had used cocaine, 808,000 had used heroin, 1.9 million had used methamphetamine, and 10.3 million had misused opioids.[3] Skin and soft tissue infection (SSTI) is the most common acute infectious complication of injection drug use with 64% of PWID reporting at least one episode in the prior year in one study.[4] SSTI accounts for 37.5% to 58% of hospitalizations[5]

Division of HIV, Infectious Diseases and Global Medicine, Department of Medicine, Zuckerberg San Francisco General Hospital, University of California, San Francisco, 1001 Potrero Avenue, Building 30, Room 3400, San Francisco, CA 94110, USA
E-mail address: henry.chambers@ucsf.edu

Infect Dis Clin N Am 35 (2021) 169–181
https://doi.org/10.1016/j.idc.2020.10.006
0891-5520/21/© 2020 Elsevier Inc. All rights reserved.
id.theclinics.com

of PWID at a cost of more than $190 million in 2001 dollars.[6] Cellulitis and abscess account for one-half or more of these infections.[7]

RISK FACTORS FOR SKIN AND SOFT TISSUE INFECTION

The precise mechanisms responsible for development of SSTIs in PWID are not well-defined, but include venous thrombosis, microvascular damage, local tissue injury, ischemia, necrosis, a disrupted cutaneous barrier, chronic inflammation, and impaired lymphatic and venous drainage as a result of repeated, frequent, and nonsterile injection. These factors create an ideal milieu for bacterial colonization and tissue invasion. Other contributing factors and practices are the drug itself, the diluents and processes used to prepare and administer the drug, direct inoculation of bacteria at the site of injection, bacterial contamination of the drug product or injection equipment, reuse and sharing of needles and syringes, frequency of injection, route of injection, and medical comorbidities such as human immunodeficiency virus (HIV) infection, diabetes, and hepatitis C. PWID who are homelessness also are at high risk of SSTIs.[8] Injection drug use is associated with increased rates of *Staphylococcus aureus* colonization,[9] which in turn increases the risk of *S aureus* infection.[10,11]

Cocaine or cocaine mixed with heroin (referred to as a "speedball") is a potent vasoconstrictor that can cause local ischemia[12] and tissue injury and necrosis that, when contaminated by bacteria and in the presence of an impaired local host response, can progress to infection. Methamphetamine use has been associated with methicillin-resistant *S aureus* (MRSA) colonization, a potential risk factor for MRSA SSTI.[13] Methamphetamine promotes biofilm formation and can impair wound healing processes and innate immune function, further exacerbating susceptibility to infection.[14] Heroin use seems to be associated with a higher risk of SSTI compared with amphetamines or other drugs.[8] Use of black tar heroin, originating from Mexico and the predominant form available on the US west coast, has been associated with more extensive vein loss and soft tissue abscesses than powder heroin and with clostridial infections including wound botulism, tetanus, and necrotizing soft tissue infections.[15–17] These infections may be due to lower purity and bacterial contamination of black tar heroin or as a consequence of deliberate or unintentional subcutaneous injection because of scarred veins.[15]

Behavioral practices such as needle licking before injection, use of another person's injection equipment, use of nonpowder drugs, assisted injection, and frequent injection increase the risk of SSTI.[12,18–20] Subcutaneous or intradermal injection ("skin popping") and intramuscular injection ("muscling") and use of dirty needles have also been associated with an increased risk of SSTIs.[12,21,22] Application of alcohol to skin before injection may be protective.[12]

TYPES OF INFECTIONS
Cutaneous Abscess and Cellulitis

Cutaneous abscess is the most common SSTI in PWID accounting for almost three-quarters of those presenting for medical care at 1 center.[23] Two cross-sectional studies of PWID in the community found that 18% to 29% had an active abscess.[21,22] In a cohort study of PWID in Vancouver 21.5% of participants reported having an abscess within the prior 6 months.[24] Skin popping in particular is associated with increased risk of cutaneous abscess.[21,22,25] These infections present with typical signs and symptoms of swelling with surrounding induration, overlying erythema, pain, and tenderness. Abscesses may be single or multiple, although a single abscess is the norm.[23] Abscess distribution reflects the pattern of injection into multiple body sites, arms, legs, and buttocks being the most common followed by neck, groin, and torso. Fever is often absent with only about one-third reporting subjective fevers and less than 10% have a documented fever at presentation in 1 case series.[23] Fluctuance is not always apparent. Differentiating between abscess and cellulitis can be difficult, particularly for deeper abscesses located in the fascia or muscle, or if significant induration is present. Bedside ultrasound imaging may be helpful in establishing the diagnosis.[26,27] Computed tomography (CT) scans or MRI can be useful if the results are equivocal and also enable evaluation for involvement of deeper tissues. A high index of suspicion for extension of infection into adjacent tissues or for necrotizing SSTI is warranted, particularly for patients with an apparent abscess accompanied by high fevers, severe pain out of proportion to findings on physical examination, and signs and symptoms of systemic toxicity.

Incision and drainage of the abscess should be performed. This procedure may be performed on an out-patient basis for a single, simple abscess on an extremity. Criteria for hospitalization are not well-defined, but indications include infections involving the face, hand, groin, or neck, any of which can involve deeper tissues; severe infection with signs and symptoms of systemic toxicity; hemodynamic instability; an immunocompromising condition; and failure of out-patient therapy.

The Infectious Diseases Society of America guidelines[28] recommend culturing the abscess, although the value of doing so has been questioned because culture results infrequently affect management.[29] Indeed, the microbiology of cutaneous abscesses in PWID is rather predictable and stereotypical, similar to that of persons who do not inject drugs, but with some differences.[30] S aureus is the predominant organism in both groups, with MRSA accounting for a large proportion of isolates. Streptococcal species, both viridans group and beta-hemolytic, infrequently isolated from abscesses of persons who do not inject drugs, are commonly isolated from abscesses of PWID. Polymicrobial infection and anaerobic organisms are also more common in PWID, although their clinical relevance is questionable because these entities rarely require specific therapy. Although it may be reasonable not to obtain cultures in out-patients, provided that an appropriate empirical regimen covering gram-positive organisms including MRSA is prescribed, culture of the abscess should obtained from patients admitted to the hospital to allow for specific pathogen-directed antimicrobial therapy, particularly if an oral, step-down agent is prescribed.[28] Culture of the abscess is also advisable in the case of treatment failure. Blood cultures should be obtained from patients who have fever and other systemic signs and symptoms of infection to assess for the presence of bacteremia, which could signify a more serious infection, such as a concomitant endocarditis.

Two double-blind, randomized, placebo-controlled trials[31,32] have shown that adjunctive antimicrobial therapy in addition to incision and drainage improves outcomes, even for patients with small abscesses. Empirical therapy should cover both S aureus, including MRSA, and streptococci. Oral options are trimethoprim–sulfamethoxazole and clindamycin. More limited data indicate that doxycycline or minocycline is also effective.[33,34] Vancomycin is preferred for empirical intravenous therapy. Five to 7 days of antimicrobial therapy is sufficient in most patients.

Cellulitis with or without an abscess is the second most common SSTI in PWID. These infections typically occur on the extremities at sites of prior injection. The microbiology of cellulitis is poorly characterized because of the absence of purulent material for culture. As with cutaneous abscess, the usefulness of blood cultures in cases of cellulitis has been questioned because these results rarely change therapy.[35–37] In general blood cultures when obtained in cases of cellulitis are usually negative and, if positive, far and away the most common organisms are S aureus and beta-hemolytic streptococci.[29,36,38] The limited data that are available indicate that the microbiology of cellulitis in PWID is similar. Whether positive cultures of blood accurately reflects the microbiology of blood culture-negative cases is an open question based on 1 small study owing to the inability of culture and molecular diagnostics performed on skin to establish the cause of cellulitis.[39] Results of clinical trials indicate that oral agents effective for the treatment of uncomplicated abscesses, for example, trimethoprim–sulfamethoxazole and clindamycin, are also effective for uncomplicated cellulitis.[40,41] The need to cover MRSA in cases of uncomplicated cellulitis in PWID is an unresolved issue. A randomized, double-blind trial of cefalexin as a single agent compared with cefalexin in combination with trimethoprim–sulfamethoxazole to cover MRSA for treatment of uncomplicated cellulitis in out-patients found that cures rates were similar in both treatment arms.[41] Of note, patients with a history of injection drug use within the prior month and fever were excluded from this study. Given that the prevalence of MRSA among PWID is high, that S aureus is in general an important cause of SSTI in these individuals, and that S aureus is not uncommonly isolated in blood cultures of patients with more complicated infections, blood culture and coverage both for S aureus, including MRSA, and streptococci are recommended for initial management of cellulitis in PWID who have fever, hemodynamic instability, or systemic signs of systemic infection. Vancomycin is the preferred intravenous empirical agent. Linezolid, daptomycin, and dalbavancin are acceptable alternatives.

Necrotizing Skin and Soft Tissue Infections

Injection drug use is a major risk factor for necrotizing fasciitis and other necrotizing soft tissue infections. Necrotizing fasciitis accounts for approximately 1% of SSTIs in PWID.[42,43] Classic findings such as soft tissue edema, erythema, severe pain and tenderness of the affected area, fever, skin necrosis, crepitus, anesthesia of overlying skin, and bullae, which may be hemorrhagic, are not always present.[44] Necrotizing fasciitis can present in association with an abscess or cellulitis, belying the severity and seriousness of infection of deeper tissues and at times with surprisingly little involvement of overlying skin. Clues to the diagnosis are marked systemic toxicity and pain out of proportion to the physical findings. In cases where the diagnosis is uncertain on clinical grounds, plain radiography may be useful for ruling in the diagnosis if there is gas present along fascial planes, although this finding in present in only one-half or fewer cases.[45] CT scans and MRI provide much better visualization and resolution of deep tissues and have sensitivities of approximately 80% and 90%, respectively. Findings include presence of deep abscess; soft tissue gas; fascial thickening, nonenhancement on CT scans or enhancement on MRI, subfascial fluid, and subcutaneous edema and fat stranding. Although CT scans and MRI have excellent sensitivities, definitively excluding the diagnosis of necrotizing fasciitis requires surgical exploration and biopsy to demonstrate normal adherence of the fascia to muscle and a lack of involvement of deeper tissues.

Necrotizing fasciitis is a surgical disease. Antimicrobial therapy is important but adjunctive to surgery. Early surgical debridement, the earlier the better,[44] is indicated to determine the extent of the infection and to remove devitalized tissue, which may include amputation. Repeated surgical exploration and debridement every day or two may be needed to ensure that all devitalized tissue has been removed and that progression of the infection has been arrested.

Necrotizing fasciitis in PWID may be polymicrobial (type 1) or monomicrobial (type 2).[44] Indistinguishable on clinical grounds, the 2 types are microbiologically distinct. Type 1 infections are mixed infections caused by aerobic and anaerobic organisms, both gram positive and gram negative, whereas type 2 infections are predominantly caused by *S pyogenes* or *S aureus*, including MRSA.[46] The use of black tar heroin is a risk factor for necrotizing fasciitis, both monomicrobial and polymicrobial, caused by clostridial species.[47] Empirical antimicrobial therapy pending results of Gram stain and culture should be broad to cover both gram-positive organisms including MRSA, gram-negative organisms, and anaerobes. Vancomycin plus a carbapenem, vancomycin plus a third-generation or fourth-generation cephalosporin plus metronidazole, or vancomycin plus piperacillin-tazobactam provide the required coverage. Definitive therapy should be based on results of Gram stain, culture, and susceptibility testing. Adjunctive clindamycin is recommended for necrotizing fasciitis caused by *S pyogenes* for its antitoxin effect as a protein synthesis inhibitor. The role of intravenous gamma globulin (IVIG) is not entirely clear. A retrospective cohort study of necrotizing fasciitis of 161 IVIG-treated patients propensity matched to 161 patients who were not treated with IVIG found no mortality benefit or effect on length of hospital stay with IVIG beyond that observed with debridement and antimicrobial therapy.[48] A meta-analysis of 5 studies including 165 patients suggested that IVIG may decrease mortality by about one-half in patients with streptococcal toxic shock syndrome or necrotizing fasciitis.[49]

Clostridial myonecrosis (gas gangrene) owing to *Clostridium perfringens* or *C sordellii* is a rare but aggressive and life-threatening infection.[17,47,50] It is associated with the use of black tar heroin and direct injection into muscle. The presentation is acute with onset of severe pain, thought to be due to toxin-mediated ischemia, over the site of injection. The overlying skin is initially pale then progresses to purple or red discoloration and bullae, and becomes tense and exquisitely tender. Severe sepsis and septic shock are common complications. Primary therapy of these infections is surgical debridement and amputation if necessary. A 10- to 14-day course of penicillin (vancomycin in penicillin-allergic patients) plus clindamycin is the recommended antimicrobial therapy.

Pyomyositis

Pyomyositis is a purulent infection of skeletal muscle, usually with abscess formation. It may arise hematogenously, by direct extension from a contiguous focus, or as a consequence of direct injection.[51] These infections present as focal pain, tenderness, induration, and swelling of the affected muscle. Fluctuance and other signs of frank abscess may be present in later stages of infection, but these indicators are absent early on. The overlying skin may seem to be normal or erythematous. Any muscle may be involved but gluteal, thigh, or calf muscles are most commonly involved. More than 1 focus of infection is present in 13% to 24% of cases.[52] Fever is usually, but not always, present. A variety of noninfectious process, such as contusion, muscle strain, hematoma, and neoplasm, and other infectious processes, including necrotizing skin and soft tissue and bone and joint infections, may resemble pyomyositis in their presentation.

Unless a deep tissue abscess is evident clinically, a CT scan or MRI of the affected muscle is the best way to make the diagnosis of pyomyositis and advisable in any case to define the extend of infection. Blood cultures are positive in up to one-third of cases. *S aureus*, including strains of MRSA, is the most common pathogen, isolated in about two-thirds of cases, followed by streptococcal species. Gram-negative bacteria, anaerobes, and other gram-positive organisms may also cause pyomyositis and 5% or less are polymicrobial. Vancomycin or a suitable alternative, such as linezolid or daptomycin, is appropriate for initial empirical therapy with additional gram-negative and anaerobic coverage for patients with severe sepsis or hemodynamic instability. If an abscess is present, it should be drained percutaneously or by incision and surgical drainage along with pathogen-directed antimicrobial therapy based on results of culture and Gram stain. Early infection without abscess formation can be managed with antimicrobial therapy alone. The duration of therapy is not well-defined, guided by clinical and radiographic response, and is typically 2 to 4 weeks.

Skin and Soft Tissue Infections Caused by Unusual Organisms

Sporadic cases and outbreaks of rarely encountered organisms, often associated with use of black tar heroin, skin-popping, and direct injection into muscle, have been reported to cause SSTIs in PWID. These are toxin-mediated infections in which clostridial species predominate.[53,54] Necrotizing fasciitis and myonecrosis caused by C sordellii,[17,47,50] is a rapidly progressive, often fatal infection resembling that caused by C perfringens. These infections arise at sites of injection of black tar heroin. The close temporal proximity of cases and molecular analysis demonstrating clonal relatedness of isolates from patients and drug paraphernalia suggest contaminated drug as the source of the organism.

Clostridium novyi caused a large outbreak of necrotizing soft tissue infections in Scotland, England, and Ireland over a 5-month period in 2000.[55] As with other clostridial infections, the clinical course was characterized by marked soft tissue edema, minimal pus, and irreversible septic shock with a median time to death of 4 days in fatal cases.

Injection drug use is a risk factor for tetanus. Injection drug use accounted for 8% of the 264 cases of tetanus reported in the United States from 2009 to 2017.[56] Clostridium tetani can also cause necrotizing soft tissue infection[56] in addition[57] to focal or generalized tetanus in the absence of a clear source of infection. Patients with generalized tetanus present with trismus, difficulty in swallowing, muscles spasms, hypertonia, and signs of autonomic overactivity, including sweating and tachycardia. In addition to airway management, controlling muscle spasms, and supportive care, the initial therapy is directed toward halting and neutralizing tetanus toxin production. Primary therapy is administration of human tetanus immune globulin to neutralize unbound toxin that has already been produced and wound debridement to remove devitalized tissue and the source of toxin production. Antimicrobial therapy with either penicillin or metronidazole is adjunctive to wound debridement. Tetanus does not confer natural immunity. Patients with tetanus should receive the full 3-dose series of tetanus toxoid. The immunization status of PWIDs should be reviewed whenever these individuals present for care.

Wound botulism[53] is caused by elaboration of toxin produced by C botulinum present within the anaerobic environment of an infected wound. Of the 8 types of botulinum toxin, A through H, types A and B have been associated with wound botulism.[58] Presenting signs and symptoms include bulbar nerve palsy, diplopia, extraocular muscle weakness, burry vision, dysphonia, dysarthria, shortness of breath and respiratory failure, and symmetric descending weakness. In contrast with foodborne botulism, gastrointestinal symptoms are typically absent. Fever and leukocytosis may be absent and the accompanying wound, if present, may not be particularly impressive in appearance. Heptavalent botulin antitoxin, which contains antibodies to toxins A through G, should be administered immediately to neutralize unbound toxin and wounds should undergo incision and drainage to eliminate the source of toxin production. Antimicrobial therapy with penicillin or metronidazole (any one of a variety of agents with activity against clostridial species should also be effective) is recommended, although its role in treatment is not established.

Other gram-positive species have been rarely reported to cause SSTIs in PWID. Case reports have described *Bacillus cereus* as a cause of SSTI, bacteremia, and endocarditis in PWID.[59,60] *Bacillus anthracis* caused outbreaks of SSTI, bacteremia, and severe sepsis in the UK and Germany in 2009 and 2010.[61,62] Cutaneous infections, generally polymicrobial, owing to nontoxigenic strains of *C diphtheria* have been associated with injection drug use.[63]

Chronic Cutaneous Ulcers

Chronic cutaneous or venous ulcers, usually affecting the lower extremities, are a common complication of injection drug use and can persist even after cessation of active drug use.[51,64,65] These ulcers are the consequence of repeated and accumulated damage to skin, subcutaneous tissues, and lymphatics from recurrent infections, venous thrombosis and thrombophlebitis, and the inflammatory and sclerotic effects of drugs and adulterants. These chronic wounds typically have irregular borders and are accompanied by pain and serous, bloody, or purulent drainage, which is at times malodorous. Ulcers can be multiple and extend into deeper tissues. Primary therapy consists of debridement of necrotic tissue and eschar, drainage of purulent fluid collections, elevation of the extremity to relieve edema, and local wound care with wet-to-dry and compression dressings to promote wound healing and closure of the ulcer. Skin grafting may be required to close large defects.

Topical or systemic antimicrobial therapy probably has no role in promoting wound healing,[66,67] unless the wound becomes secondarily infected. These wounds are colonized and the presence of bacteria alone is not a reliable indication of infection. Clinical signs and symptoms of secondary infection are fever, increased pain, purulent drainage, and evidence of cellulitis of skin surrounding the wound. If there is evidence of infection, swab or tissue cultures should be obtained to direct antimicrobial therapy, which may be either oral or parenteral. The duration of antimicrobial therapy is not well defined and will depend on the severity of the infection, but a 5- to 10-day course is usually sufficient.

PREVENTION AND HARM REDUCTION

Obviously, the most effective means of preventing SSTIs in PWID is to abstain from injecting drugs. Short of this, several of the factors known to increase the risk of infection—sharing and reuse of needles, syringes, and paraphernalia; use of nonsterile needles and syringes; lack of aseptic technique; and frequency of drug injection—are modifiable through harm reduction strategies, which seek to reduce the behavior and thus lower the risk of infection. These strategies include provision of sterile needles and syringes, exchange of used needles and syringes for sterile equipment, and opioid substitution (eg, methadone).

Data on the effectiveness of harm reduction strategies in PWID comes mainly from studies of HIV and hepatitis C virus (HCV) transmission. A systematic review and meta-analysis of twelve studies by Aspinall and colleagues[68] found that needle and syringe exchange was associated with a decrease in HIV transmission. A review of 13 systematic reviews and meta-analyses by Fernandes and colleagues[69] found that overall needle exchange reduced the risk behavior and HIV transmission and to a lesser extent HCV transmission, but in conjunction with opioid replacement. A Cochrane review[70] of effectiveness of needle exchange programs and opioid substitution therapy found that opioid substitution was associate with a reduction in HCV transmission, particularly combined with needle exchange.

Evidence for effectiveness of needle exchange was weaker. A cost-effectiveness analysis of the impact of needle exchange programs in the UK found that these programs decrease HCV transmission, were cost effective, and in some cases cost saving.[71] A systematic review of pharmacy-based needle exchange found that, although there was a reduction in risk behavior, an effect on HIV or HCV transmission was unclear.[72]

Evidence that harm reduction strategies reduce risk of SSTIs in PWID is limited. Failure to aseptically clean the injection site has been associated with increased risk of skin and soft tissues[12] in PWID. A small time-series study found an inverse correlation between the number of abscesses treated in community facilities and the number of visits to a needle exchange program and the number of needles exchanged.[73] A cross-sectional study of 1876 participants recruited in 2013 to 2014 from the Needle Exchange Surveillance Initiative in Scotland[74] found that participation of PWID in needle exchange programs and current participation in opioid substitution therapy each reduced the risk of SSTI. Combined participation in needle exchange and opioid substitution therapy had the greatest impact, decreasing the risk of infection by almost 40%.

SUMMARY

Injection drug use causes tissue injury and carries a significant risk of SSTI. The types of infections range from uncomplicated abscess and cellulitis to serious and potentially lethal necrotizing soft tissue infections. The vast majority of these infections are caused by gram-positive organisms, *S aureus*, and streptococcal species in particular. Chronic skin ulcers, usually of the lower extremities, are long-term complications of injection drug use. Strategies to encourage abstinence, decrease the frequency of drug use, and modify risk behaviors may be effective in preventing SSTIs in PWID.

CLINICS CARE POINTS

- Cellulitis and abscess, which account for the majority of SSTIs, can often be managed in the out-patient setting.
- Abscesses should undergo surgical incision and drainage.
- Cultures of blood, abscess, purulent drainage, and, if available, debrided tissue should be obtained in patients who are hospitalized for treatment of SSTIs.
- Abscesses can masquerade as a cellulitis, particularly if there is significant overlying induration and inflammation and if these involve deeper tissues, or if the infection has not improved on antibiotics. Ultrasound examination, CT scans, or MRI are useful in differentiating cellulitis from abscess.
- Necrotizing fasciitis and other necrotizing soft tissue infections may not be readily apparent at presentation and these infections should be considered and ruled out in patients with pain out of proportion to physical findings, severe systemic toxicity, or hemodynamic instability.

DISCLOSURE

The author has nothing to disclose.

REFERENCES

1. Lansky A, Finlayson T, Johnson C, et al. Estimating the number of persons who inject drugs in the United States by meta-analysis to calculate national rates of HIV and hepatitis C virus infections. PLoS One 2014;9(5):e97596.
2. Ropelewski LR, Mancha BE, Hulbert A, et al. Correlates of risky injection practices among past-year injection drug users among the US general population. Drug Alcohol Depend 2011;116(1–3):64–71 [Erratum appears in: Drug Alcohol Depend. 2011;119(3):239].
3. Key substance use and mental health indicators in the United States: results from the 2018 National Survey on Drug Use and Health. Available at: https://www.samhsa.gov/data/sites/default/files/cbhsq-reports/NSDUHNationalFindingsReport2018/NSDUHNationalFindingsReport2018.pdf. Accessed August 11, 2020.
4. Monteiro J, Phillips KT, Herman DS, et al. Self-treatment of skin infections by people who inject drugs. Drug Alcohol Depend 2020;206:107695.
5. Marks M, Pollock E, Armstrong M, et al. Needles and the damage done: reasons for admission and financial costs associated with injecting drug use in a Central London Teaching Hospital. J Infect 2013;66(1):95–102.
6. Takahashi TA, Maciejewski ML, Bradley K. US hospitalizations and costs for illicit drug users with soft tissue infections. J Behav Health Serv Res 2010;37(4):508–18.
7. Jenkins TC, Sabel AL, Sarcone EE, et al. Skin and soft-tissue infections requiring hospitalization at an academic medical center: opportunities for antimicrobial stewardship. Clin Infect Dis 2010;51(8):895–903.
8. Dahlman D, Berge J, Björkman P, et al. Both localized and systemic bacterial infections are predicted by injection drug use: a prospective follow-up study in Swedish criminal justice clients. PLoS One 2018;13(5):e0196944.
9. Bassetti S, Battegay M. Staphylococcus aureus infections in injection drug users: risk factors and prevention strategies. Infection 2004;32(3):163–9.
10. Kluytmans J, van Belkum A, Verbrugh H. Nasal carriage of Staphylococcus aureus: epidemiology, underlying mechanisms, and associated risks. Clin Microbiol Rev 1997;10(3):505–20.
11. Sakr A, Brégeon F, Mège JL, et al. Staphylococcus aureus nasal colonization: an update on mechanisms, epidemiology, risk factors, and subsequent infections. Front Microbiol 2018;9:2419.
12. Murphy EL, DeVita D, Liu H, et al. Risk factors for skin and soft-tissue abscesses among injection drug users: a case-control study. Clin Infect Dis 2001;33(1):35–40.
13. Popovich KJ, Snitkin ES, Zawitz C, et al. Frequent methicillin-resistant Staphylococcus aureus introductions into an inner-city jail: indications of Community Transmission Networks. Clin Infect Dis 2020;71(2):323–31.
14. Mihu MR, Roman-Sosa J, Varshney AK, et al. Methamphetamine alters the antimicrobial efficacy of phagocytic cells during methicillin-resistant Staphylococcus aureus skin infection. mBio 2015;6(6). e01622–15.
15. Ciccarone D. Heroin in brown, black and white: structural factors and medical consequences in the US heroin market. Int J Drug Policy 2009;20(3):277–82.
16. Summers PJ, Struve IA, Wilkes MS, et al. Injection-site vein loss and soft tissue abscesses associated with black tar heroin injection: a cross-sectional study of two distinct populations in USA. Int J Drug Policy 2017;39:21–7.
17. Kimura AC, Higa JI, Levin RM, et al. Outbreak of necrotizing fasciitis due to Clostridium sordellii among black-tar heroin users. Clin Infect Dis 2004;38(9):e87–91.

18. Dahlman D, Håkansson A, Kral AH, et al. Behavioral characteristics and injection practices associated with skin and soft tissue infections among people who inject drugs: a community-based observational study. Subst Abus 2017;38(1):105–12.

19. Phillips KT, Anderson BJ, Herman DS, et al. Risk factors associated with skin and soft tissue infections among hospitalized people who inject drugs. J Addict Med 2017;11(6):461–7.

20. Lee WK, Ti L, Hayashi K, et al. Assisted injection among people who inject drugs in Thailand. Subst Abuse Treat Prev Policy 2013;8:32.

21. Binswanger IA, Kral AH, Bluthenthal RN, et al. High prevalence of abscesses and cellulitis among community-recruited injection drug users in San Francisco. Clin Infect Dis 2000;30(3):579–81.

22. Smith ME, Robinowitz N, Chaulk P, et al. High rates of abscesses and chronic wounds in community-recruited injection drug users and associated risk factors. J Addict Med 2015;9(2):87–93.

23. Takahashi TA, Merrill JO, Boyko EJ, et al. Type and location of injection drug use-related soft tissue infections predict hospitalization. J Urban Health 2003;80(1):127–36.

24. Lloyd-Smith E, Kerr T, Hogg RS, et al. Prevalence and correlates of abscesses among a cohort of injection drug users. Harm Reduct J 2005;2:24.

25. Fink DS, Lindsay SP, Slymen DJ, et al. Abscess and self-treatment among injection drug users at four California syringe exchanges and their surrounding communities. Subst Use Misuse 2013;48(7):523–31.

26. Mower WR, Crisp JG, Krishnadasan A, et al. Effect of initial bedside ultrasonography on emergency department skin and soft tissue infection management. Ann Emerg Med 2019;74(3):372–80.

27. Abrahamian FM, Talan DA, Moran GJ. Management of skin and soft-tissue infections in the emergency department. Infect Dis Clin North Am 2008;22(1):89–116, vi.

28. Stevens DL, Bisno AL, Chambers HF, et al. Infectious Diseases Society of America. Practice guidelines for the diagnosis and management of skin and soft tissue infections: 2014 update by the Infectious Diseases Society of America. Clin Infect Dis 2014;59(2):e10–52 [Erratum appears in: Clin Infect Dis. 2015;60(9):1448. Dosage error in article text].

29. Torres J, Avalos N, Echols L, et al. Low yield of blood and wound cultures in patients with skin and soft-tissue infections. Am J Emerg Med 2017;35(8):1159–61.

30. Jenkins TC, Knepper BC, Jason Moore S, et al. Microbiology and initial antibiotic therapy for injection drug users and non-injection drug users with cutaneous abscesses in the era of community-associated methicillin-resistant Staphylococcus aureus. Acad Emerg Med 2015;22(8):993–7.

31. Talan DA, Mower WR, Krishnadasan A, et al. Trimethoprim-sulfamethoxazole versus placebo for uncomplicated skin abscess. N Engl J Med 2016;374(9):823–32.

32. Daum RS, Miller LG, Immergluck L, et al. DMID 07-0051 team. a placebo-controlled trial of antibiotics for smaller skin abscesses. N Engl J Med 2017;376(26):2545–55.

33. Cenizal MJ, Skiest D, Luber S, et al. Prospective randomized trial of empiric therapy with trimethoprim- sulfamethoxazole or doxycycline for outpatient skin and soft tissue infections in an area of high prevalence of methicillin-resistant Staphylococcus aureus. Antimicrob Agents Chemother 2007;51(7):2628–30.

34. Carris NW, Pardo J, Montero J, et al. Minocycline as A substitute for doxycycline in targeted scenarios: a systematic review. Open Forum Infect Dis 2015;2(4): ofv178.
35. Coburn B, Morris AM, Tomlinson G, et al. Does this adult patient with suspected bacteremia require blood cultures? JAMA 2012;308(5):502–11.
36. Bauer S, Aubert CE, Richli M, et al. Blood cultures in the evaluation of uncomplicated cellulitis. Eur J Intern Med 2016;36:50–6.
37. Klotz C, Courjon J, Michelangeli C, et al. Adherence to antibiotic guidelines for erysipelas or cellulitis is associated with a favorable outcome. Eur J Clin Microbiol Infect Dis 2019;38(4):703–9.
38. Gunderson CG, Martinello RA. A systematic review of bacteremias in cellulitis and erysipelas. J Infect 2012;64(2):148–55.
39. Crisp JG, Takhar SS, Moran GJ, et al. EMERGEncy ID Net Study Group. Inability of polymerase chain reaction, pyrosequencing, and culture of infected and uninfected site skin biopsy specimens to identify the cause of cellulitis. Clin Infect Dis 2015;61(11):1679–87.
40. Miller LG, Daum RS, Creech CB, et al. DMID 07-0051 Team. Clindamycin versus trimethoprim-sulfamethoxazole for uncomplicated skin infections. N Engl J Med 2015;372(12):1093–103.
41. Moran GJ, Krishnadasan A, Mower WR, et al. Effect of cephalexin plus trimethoprim-sulfamethoxazole vs cephalexin alone on clinical cure of uncomplicated cellulitis: a randomized clinical trial. JAMA 2017;317(20):2088–96.
42. Lewer D, Hope VD, Harris M, et al. Incidence and treatment costs of severe bacterial infections among people who inject heroin: a cohort study in South London. Engl Drug Alcohol Depend 2020;212:108057.
43. Callahan TE, Schecter WP, Horn JK. Necrotizing soft tissue infection masquerading as cutaneous abscess following illicit drug injection. Arch Surg 1998;133(8):812–7 [discussion: 817–9].
44. Stevens DL, Bryant AE. Necrotizing soft-tissue infections. N Engl J Med 2017; 377(23):2253–65.
45. Tso DK, Singh AK. Necrotizing fasciitis of the lower extremity: imaging pearls and pitfalls. Br J Radiol 2018;91(1088):20180093.
46. Miller LG, Perdreau-Remington F, Rieg G, et al. Necrotizing fasciitis caused by community-associated methicillin-resistant Staphylococcus aureus in Los Angeles. N Engl J Med 2005;352(14):1445–53.
47. Dunbar NM, Harruff RC. Necrotizing fasciitis: manifestations, microbiology and connection with black tar heroin. J Forensic Sci 2007;52(4):920–3.
48. Kadri SS, Swihart BJ, Bonne SL, et al. Impact of intravenous immunoglobulin on survival in necrotizing fasciitis with vasopressor-dependent shock: a propensity score-matched analysis from 130 US hospitals. Clin Infect Dis 2017;64(7): 877–85.
49. Parks T, Wilson C, Curtis N, et al. Polyspecific intravenous immunoglobulin in clindamycin-treated patients with streptococcal toxic shock syndrome: a systematic review and meta-analysis. Clin Infect Dis 2018;67(9):1434–6.
50. Bangsberg DR, Rosen JI, Aragón T, et al. Clostridial myonecrosis cluster among injection drug users: a molecular epidemiology investigation. Arch Intern Med 2002;162(5):517–22.
51. Ebright JR, Pieper B. Skin and soft tissue infections in injection drug users. Infect Dis Clin North Am 2002;16(3):697–712.
52. Crum NF. Bacterial pyomyositis in the United States. Am J Med 2004;117(6): 420–8.

53. Gonzales y Tucker RD, Frazee B. View from the front lines: an emergency medicine perspective on clostridial infections in injection drug users. Anaerobe 2014; 30:108–15.
54. Finn SP, Leen E, English L, et al. Autopsy findings in an outbreak of severe systemic illness in heroin users following injection site inflammation: an effect of Clostridium novyi exotoxin? Arch Pathol Lab Med 2003;127(11):1465–70.
55. Brett MM, Hood J, Brazier JS, et al. Soft tissue infections caused by spore-forming bacteria in injecting drug users in the United Kingdom. Epidemiol Infect 2005;133(4):575–82.
56. Faulkner AE, Tiwari TSP. Manual for surveillance of vaccine-preventable diseases. tetanus. Available at: https://www.cdc.gov/vaccines/pubs/surv-manual/chpt16-tetanus.pdf. Accessed August 13, 2020.
57. Cardinal PR, Henry SM, Joshi MG, et al. Fatal necrotizing soft-tissue infection caused by Clostridium tetani in an injecting drug user: a case report. Surg Infect (Larchmt) 2020;21(5):457–60.
58. Centers for Disease Control and Prevention. National Center for Infectious Diseases, Division of Bacterial and Mycotic Diseases. Botulism in the United States, 1899-1996. Handbook for Epidemiologists, Clinicians, and Laboratory Workers. 1998. Available at: https://www.cdc.gov/botulism/pdf/bot-manual.pdf. Accessed August 13, 2020.
59. Benusic MA, Press NM, Hoang LM, et al. A cluster of Bacillus cereus bacteremia cases among injection drug users. Can J Infect Dis Med Microbiol 2015;26(2): 103–4.
60. Schaefer G, Campbell W, Jenks J, et al. Persistent Bacillus cereus Bacteremia in 3 Persons Who Inject Drugs, San Diego, California, USA. Emerg Infect Dis 2016; 22(9):1621–3.
61. Hicks CW, Sweeney DA, Cui X, et al. An overview of anthrax infection including the recently identified form of disease in injection drug users. Intensive Care Med 2012;38(7):1092–104.
62. Veitch J, Kansara A, Bailey D, et al. Severe systemic Bacillus anthracis infection in an intravenous drug user. BMJ Case Rep 2014;2014. bcr2013201921.
63. Lowe CF, Bernard KA, Romney MG. Cutaneous diphtheria in the urban poor population of Vancouver, British Columbia, Canada: a 10-year review. J Clin Microbiol 2011;49(7):2664–6.
64. Pieper B, Kirsner RS, Templin TN, et al. Injection drug use: an understudied cause of venous disease. Arch Dermatol 2007;143(10):1305–9.
65. Coull AF, Atherton I, Taylor A, et al. Prevalence of skin problems and leg ulceration in a sample of young injecting drug users. Harm Reduct J 2014;11:22.
66. Nelson EA, Jones J. Venous leg ulcers. BMJ Clin Evid 2008;2008:1902.
67. Nelson EA, Adderley U. Venous leg ulcers. BMJ Clin Evid 2016;2016:1902.
68. Aspinall EJ, Nambiar D, Goldberg DJ, et al. Are needle and syringe programmes associated with a reduction in HIV transmission among people who inject drugs: a systematic review and meta-analysis. Int J Epidemiol 2014;43(1):235–48.
69. Fernandes RM, Cary M, Duarte G, et al. Effectiveness of needle and syringe Programmes in people who inject drugs - an overview of systematic reviews. BMC Public Health 2017;17(1):309.
70. Platt L, Minozzi S, Reed J, et al. Needle syringe programmes and opioid substitution therapy for preventing hepatitis C transmission in people who inject drugs. Cochrane Database Syst Rev 2017;9(9):CD012021.

71. Sweeney S, Ward Z, Platt L, et al. Evaluating the cost- effectiveness of existing needle and syringe programmes in preventing hepatitis C transmission in people who inject drugs. Addiction 2019;114(3):560–70.
72. Sawangjit R, Khan TM, Chaiyakunapruk N. Effectiveness of pharmacy-based needle/syringe exchange programme for people who inject drugs: a systematic review and meta-analysis. Addiction 2017;112(2):236–47.
73. Tomolillo CM, Crothers LJ, Aberson CL. The damage done: a study of injection drug use, injection related abscesses and needle exchange regulation. Subst Use Misuse 2007;42(10):1603–11.
74. Dunleavy K, Munro A, Roy K, et al. Association between harm reduction intervention uptake and skin and soft tissue infections among people who inject drugs. Drug Alcohol Depend 2017;174:91–7.

Skin and Soft Tissue Infections in Patients with Diabetes Mellitus

Christopher Polk, MD[a,1], Mindy M. Sampson, DO[a,1],
Danya Roshdy, PharmD[b], Lisa E. Davidson, MD[c,*]

KEYWORDS

- Diabetic • Foot • Infection • Wound • Charcot

KEY POINTS

- Patients with diabetes are at high risk for skin and soft tissue infections because of end-organ damage from hyperglycemia.
- Diabetic foot wounds should be assessed for cause and treated accordingly with either offload from pressure or vascular assessment if due to ischemia.
- When antibiotics are used for treatment of wounds that are secondarily infected or have associated cellulitis, they should be selected with consideration for methicillin-resistant *Staphylococcus aureus*, *Pseudomonas*, and other antibiotic-resistant pathogens.
- Concern for osteomyelitis, Charcot foot, or underlying skin and soft tissue infections of the diabetic foot is driven by clinical presentation. MRI is helpful for assessment of these conditions only in the correct context.

INTRODUCTION AND EPIDEMIOLOGY

Diabetes is one of the most common diseases worldwide, with an estimated 422 million adults living with diabetes.[1] The global prevalence of diabetes has nearly doubled over the last 25 years, representing 8.5% of the world's adult population.[1] Patients with diabetes are significantly more likely to develop skin and soft tissue infections (SSTI), including cellulitis, osteomyelitis, and postoperative wound infections.[2] In a large retrospective, multiyear study of more than 2 million patients with SSTI, 10% occurred in diabetics.[3] The SSTI complication rate in ambulatory patients was more than 5 times higher in diabetics than nondiabetics.[3] Similarly, in patients hospitalized with SSTI, the rate of complications was almost 5% in diabetics versus 1% in

a Division of Infectious Diseases, Department of Medicine, Atrium Health, Charlotte, NC, USA;
b Antimicrobial Support Network, Division of Pharmacy, Atrium Health, 1000 Blythe Boulevard, Charlotte, NC 28203, USA; c Division of Infectious Diseases, Department of Medicine, Atrium Health, 1540 Garden Terrace, Suite 211, Charlotte, NC 28203, USA
1 Present address: 4539 Hedgemore Drive, Charlotte, NC 28209.
* Corresponding author.
E-mail address: Lisa.Davidson@atriumhealth.org

Infect Dis Clin N Am 35 (2021) 183–197
https://doi.org/10.1016/j.idc.2020.10.007
0891-5520/21/© 2020 Elsevier Inc. All rights reserved.
id.theclinics.com

nondiabetics.[3] Patients with diabetes admitted to the hospital with SSSI were more likely to have complications, such as bacteremia, endocarditis, and sepsis.[3]

The costs of SSTIs in diabetics are a huge burden to patients and the health care system. In 2011, it was estimated that inpatient care for diabetics with infections would cost approximately $48 billion.[4] Patients with diabetes and SSTIs have a longer hospital length of stay, higher rates of clinical failure, increased rates of readmission, and higher mortality when compared with nondiabetics.[5,6] Patients with diabetic foot infection are 55% more likely to require hospitalization and 154% more likely to require amputation, compared with diabetics without foot infection.[7] Once a patient is admitted with a diabetic foot infection, more than 50% will require surgery.[8]

PATHOPHYSIOLOGY AND HOST FACTORS

Multiple host factors in diabetics combine to cause increased risk of SSTI (**Box 1**). The primary driver of infection in diabetics is uncontrolled hyperglycemia. Infections and related complications (including mortality) are higher in type 1 versus type 2 diabetics, correlating with rates of glycemic control.[2] Hyperglycemia promotes mitochondrial dysfunction and the formation of reactive oxygen species, resulting in oxidative stress.[9] Prolonged oxidative stress on a cellular level ultimately results in blocking insulin signaling pathways and increased inflammation. Increased oxidative stress also affects the cells of the immune system, activating proinflammatory cytokines. Long-term exposure of cells to high levels of glucose, oxidative stress, free radicals, and an inflammatory state then results in end-organ damage.[9]

Disruption of the normal skin barrier and poor vascularization in diabetics (especially in the lower extremities) lead to increased risk of bacterial invasion.[10] With loss of this critical barrier to invasion, the most common bacteria causing diabetic SSTIs are gram-positive skin organisms that may normally colonize the skin.[11] In superficial ulcerations and cellulitis, *Streptococcus* species and *Staphylococcus aureus* (both methicillin-susceptible and methicillin-resistant) predominate. Diabetes is a known risk factor associated with increased risk of colonization with methicillin-resistant *Staphylococcus aureus* (MRSA).[12] More recent molecular analysis suggests that other gram-positive organisms, such as *Corynebacterium* species and *Finegoldia* species, may play an important role in biofilm formation.[13] Gram-negative organisms are less common but predominate in deep tissue infections, such as diabetic foot infection. Gram-negative organisms, including *Pseudomonas aeruginosa* and Enterobacteriaceae, are common in deep tissue infections, including diabetic foot infections.[14]

Box 1
Host risk factors associated with skin and soft tissue infection in patients with diabetes mellitus

- Uncontrolled hyperglycemia
- Disruption of skin barrier
- Sensory neuropathy
- Autonomic neuropathy
- Trauma/pressure
- Venous or arterial insufficiency
- Immune system dysfunction

Although superficial cellulitis or abscesses are usually monomicrobial, infected lower-extremity ulcers and wounds are more likely to be polymicrobial.[14] Significant antibiotic exposure and prolonged hospitalization are both associated with increased risk of multidrug-resistant infections.[15] Anerobic organisms are often present in biofilm and more recently are recognized to be present in diabetic ulcers by 16s RNA analysis.[16] Although there has been some debate of the clinical significance of anaerobic organisms in superficial infections, such as diabetic ulcers, anaerobes are important pathogens in deep tissue and necrotic infections.[17]

CLINICAL EVALUATION OF DIABETIC PATIENTS WITH SKIN AND SOFT TISSUE INFECTION

Many patients with diabetes are often unaware that an infection or wound is present. Clinical history should include review of any recent falls or trauma. A complete skin evaluation should occur in both routine visits and hospitalizations because patients with severe neuropathic and vascular complications may not manifest traditional symptoms of SSTIs. Skin infections usually manifest with 2 or more clinical signs and symptoms, including erythema, tenderness, pain, warmth, or induration.[17] Patients may also present with purulent drainage or presence of rash, boils, furuncles, or carbuncles. All diabetic patients should have a thorough foot examination, focusing on sensation and distal circulation.[18] Patients with active cellulitis should be evaluated for criteria such as edema, erythema, and purulent discharge. If ulcerations are present, it is important to evaluate depth, ulcer margins, and undermining lesions. In patients with large necrotic pressure ulcers or diabetic foot ulcers, evaluation of depth of infection is critical to determine if there is underlying bone involvement.[19]

Peripheral vascular disease is extremely common in diabetic patients.[20] Clinical examination should include evaluation of peripheral circulation for evidence of arterial disease (poor pulses in distal extremities) and venous insufficiency (chronic edema with associated skin hyper pigmentation). It is important to differentiate on clinical examination between chronic edema with erythema and active cellulitis.[20] An examination of the cardiovascular system is also warranted in patients admitted to the hospital with SSTIs. Chen and colleagues[21] found that in patients admitted with diabetic foot infections complicated by remote-site invasive, nonfoot infections, 64% had had a concomitant bacteremia and 7% had endocarditis. Therefore, evaluation of the heart and lungs is critical to the early detection of systemic disease.

Diabetic patients with SSTIs, both superficial and deep, can present with systemic inflammatory response syndrome (SIRS) and septic shock. Although fever and leukocytosis may be less common in superficial infection, the presence of these clinical findings should alert the provider for presence of deep tissue or disseminated infection.[19] Complicating factors include acute kidney injury, peripheral arterial disease, puncture wounds, trauma, immunosuppressive medications, and progressive infection despite antibiotic therapy.[20] Clinical laboratory tests that are recommended on admission for moderate to severe infections include white blood cell count, C-reactive protein (CRP), erythrocyte sedimentation rate (ESR), and procalcitonin (PCT). However, these are not necessarily diagnostic, and some studies have shown they may be normal in patients presenting with severe diabetic infections.[19]

DIABETIC FOOT INFECTION

Most wounds of the diabetic foot initially develop as pressure ulcerations (**Fig. 1**) because of a combination of loss of sensation from neuropathy, impaired immunity from glucose dysregulation, and angiopathy from vascular disease.[22] Approximately

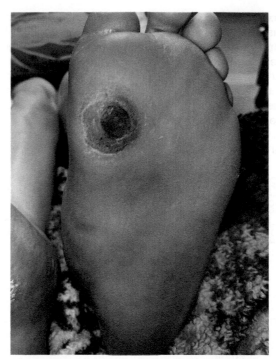

Fig. 1. Pressure ulcer that demonstrates no signs or symptoms of secondary infection.

half of diabetic foot ulcers become secondarily infected.[22] Infection is defined as the presence of purulence and inflammatory changes in or around the ulcer.[17] Having patients with diabetes monitor their feet daily to identify any sign of infection early, especially in light of diminished sensation, helps to improve outcomes.[23]

In the absence of infection, the mainstays of treatment are debridement of surrounding callus and offloading pressure from the foot.[17] A full contact cast to ensure that offloading is achieved is the gold-standard therapy, but has the drawback of loss of ability for daily foot monitoring for development of infection.[24] Close medical follow-up is also indicated for any diabetic foot wound given that any infectious complication can quickly progress in this area and result in limb loss.

A variety of wound dressings are available for treatment of diabetic foot wounds: alginates, growth factors, honey-impregnated dressing, hydrocolloids, hydrogels, polyurethane foams, silver or antibiotic impregnated dressings, and topical enzymes dressings.[22] Choice of dressing varies based on wound type and depth, including presence of wound tissue necrosis or slough requiring debridement.[22] Wounds with necrosis or slough may benefit from a dressing with topical enzymatic debridement, hydrocolloids, or hydrogels promoting autolytic debridement. Honey, silver, or antibiotic-impregnated dressings can be used for infected wounds. Alginate may be a good choice for deep wounds, and growth factor dressings may speed healing of an epithelizing wound.[22]

Distinguishing between an uninfected and infected diabetic foot wound that requires antibiotic therapy in addition to offloading and wound dressing is a clinical diagnosis. Prophylactic antibiotics or antibiotics to "reduce bioburden of bacteria" in patients with diabetic wounds are not helpful in wound healing and increase risk of colonization and infection with multidrug-resistant pathogens.[17] The underlying cause of wound development should be the focus of interventions to heal noninfected wounds: revascularization if possible for ischemia, off-loading of pressure, and improvement in glycemic control. If infection is present, it should also be treated to allow healing. Infection can be assessed clinically by the presence of erythema, warmth, and edema surrounding the wound and excessively purulent drainage and macerated tissue breakdown of the wound. If the ulcer has eroded down to bone palpable at the base of the wound, then underlying osteomyelitis is likely present by this probe-to-bone test. If presence of infection cannot be distinguished definitively on physical examination, then inflammatory markers such as CRP and PCT may be helpful. Antibiotics would be indicated for treatment of infection if these markers are elevated.

Multiple classifications systems can be used to stage diabetic wounds. All assess for presence and severity of infection and presence of ischemia (**Table 1**). Best choice and route of antibiotic therapy for infected wounds can be guided by these classifications, with deeper and more severe infections, particularly osteomyelitis, often requiring parenteral antibiotic therapy. Osteomyelitis also requires a longer duration of therapy than isolated superficial SSTIs. Deeper infections involving bone or vascular compromise are more difficult to treat. Wound classifications can be predictive of clinical outcomes.[25]

Selection of appropriate antibiotic therapy for treatment of diabetic foot wounds requires consideration of microbial flora typical for this location. Diabetics are at higher risk of both MRSA and pseudomonal infections, which is a consideration in antibiotic selection.[17] Past cultures from a particular patient may be predictive of pathogen colonization and helpful in empiric antibiotic selection.[26] If a patient has recently been documented to not have MRSA nasal carriage through a surveillance swab, then risk of an MRSA pathogen in any foot infection is less than 10%.[27,28] Local prevalence of MRSA should also be considered in the empiric setting or for definitive therapy in the absence of culture data; national guidelines previously recommended anti-MRSA therapy if the local prevalence is greater than 50% for mild and 30% for moderate soft tissue infections.[17]

Before initiation of empiric antibiotic therapy, cultures can be obtained from the diabetic wound to guide therapy. Superficial swabs from wounds are unlikely to be useful. Recommended culture technique for diabetic wounds is to first clean the wound with iodine or chlorhexidine and then scrape deep tissue to obtain cultures. If bone is palpable at the wound base, then debrided bone fragments can be sent for culture.[17] Traditional culture techniques allowing assessment of growth of one or 2 predominant organisms may be preferred over direct molecular pathogen identification. Molecular methods of pathogen identification are more sensitive than traditional culture techniques but cannot distinguish between live and dead organisms or low colony count colonization and true pathogens in this context of a nonsterile site.[29,30]

DIABETIC FOOT INFECTIONS OWING TO ISCHEMIA

Peripheral arterial disease is found in 40% of diabetic foot infections as another important consideration in diabetic wounds.[31] Diabetic pressure wounds discussed thus far are usually on plantar foot surfaces, especially under the great toe. These pressure wounds differ from ischemic foot wounds, which usually start on the distal toe tips or calcaneus and can be distinguished clinically on examination (**Figs. 2 and 3**).[31] The authors are often perplexed by the difficulty that some providers may have in recognizing ischemic foot changes, as failure to do so in order to manage the underlying vascular disease inevitably results in treatment failure. Ischemic changes of the

Table 1
Classification systems used to stage diabetic wounds

Clinical Classification of Infection	PEDIS/IWGDF* Grade	IDSA Infection Severity	Texas Classification	
			Texas Stage	Texas Grade
No signs or symptoms of infection. Infection determined by the presence of 2 or more of the following items: • Local swelling or induration • Erythema • Local tenderness or pain • Local increased warmth • Purulent discharge	1	Uninfected	A C: Ischemia without infection	0: epithelized preulcer or postulcer 1: Superficial ulcer 2: Ulcer penetration to tendon or capsule 3: Ulcer penetration to bone or joint
Local infection with no systemic manifestations (as described in later discussion) involving: • Only the skin or subcutaneous tissue (with no involvement of deeper tissue) • If present, erythema does not extend beyond 2 cm from the rim of the wound in any direction • Exclude other causes of inflammatory skin response (eg, trauma, gout, acute Charcot neuroosteoarthropathy, fracture, thrombosis, or venous stasis)	2	Mild	B: Infection D: Infection with ischemia	0 or 1 possible 0 or 1 possible
Local infection with no systemic manifestations (as described in later discussion) involving: • Erythema extending 2 or more centimeters from the wound, or • Structures deeper than skin and subcutaneous tissues (eg, tendon, muscle, joint, and bone)	3	Moderate	B D: Infection with ischemia	2 or 3 possible 2 or 3 possible

Local infection with signs of SIRS, as manifested by 2 or more of the following: • Temperature >38°C or <36°C • Heart rate exceeds 90 beats/min • Respiratory rate >20 breaths/min or $Paco_2$ <4.3 kPa (32 mm Hg) • White blood cell count >12,000 or <4000 cells/uL or ≥10% immature (band) forms Note severe ischemia often involves severe infection	4	Severe	B D: Infection with ischemia	0–3 possible 0–3 possible
Infection involving bone (osteomyelitis): • If <2 SIRS criteria are present, classify as 3(O) under IWGDF classification If 2 or more SIRS criteria are present, classify as 4(O) under IWGDF classification	Add "O" after 3 or 4		D: Infection with ischemia	3 most likely 3 most likely

* Perfusion, Extent, Depth, Infection, and Sensation Classification / International Working Group on the Diabetic Foot.

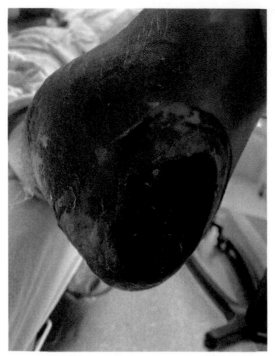

Fig. 2. Black necrotic eschar of the heel.

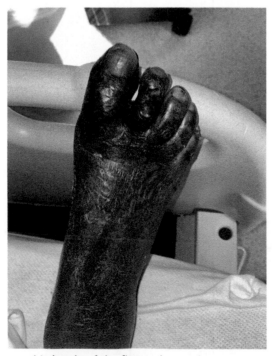

Fig. 3. Dry gangrene and ischemia of the first and second toes.

foot often will cause an area of mild erythema and edema but with much more pronounced tissue pain and tenderness unless neuropathy is present. The tell-tale presence of a black necrotic eschar plus the location is a definitive examination finding of ischemic foot ulcers.

Dry gangrene or uninfected foot ischemia must be distinguished from wet or infected gangrene. Wet gangrene or the grossly infected ischemic foot can often be identified by smell even before visualization. On inspection, devitalized necrotic tissue with purulent discharge and a fluctuant area or crepitus is often found (**Figs. 4** and **5**). Soft tissue gas may be present on imaging by plain films or computed tomography scan. Without surgical debridement and removal of necrotic tissue when wet gangrene is present, cytokines released into the bloodstream can result in sepsis, including renal and other organ dysfunction. Infected gangrene can be life threatening even with systemic antibiotic therapy and requires urgent surgical intervention.

For dry gangrene, it may be reasonable to withhold antibiotic therapy while interventions for the underlying vascular disease are underway. The role of antibiotic treatment for the ischemic diabetic foot is to prevent proximal spread of infection and systemic illness or sepsis. If there is an area of soft tissue infection at the margin of vascular perfusion though a short course of oral antibiotics while awaiting demarcation of devitalized tissue for eventual debridement is usually a reasonable approach. Antibiotics alone are ineffective for treatment of ischemic foot wounds because poor tissue perfusion prevents their penetration into the lesion. Interventions to address the underlying vascular disease and surgical debridement of the devitalized tissue are required.[17]

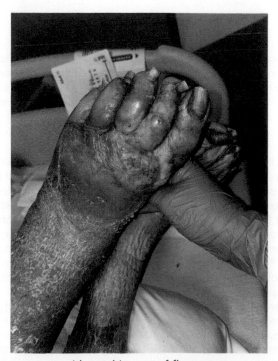

Fig. 4. Wet gangrene present with notable area of fluctuance.

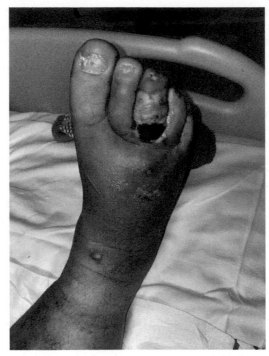

Fig. 5. Erythema and pustules are present on the dorsum of the foot, indicating the presence of a SSTI necessitating antibiotics.

OSTEOMYELITIS

A common concern for both pressure and ischemic wounds in the diabetic foot is that underlying osteomyelitis may develop. Osteomyelitis should be suspected if a deep ulcer is present or if probing the wound contacts bone.[17] Guidelines suggest obtaining a plain radiograph in all patients presenting with a new diabetic foot infection to screen for osteomyelitis. Elevated CRP, PCT, and ESR may also suggest the presence of osteomyelitis but are not specific and can be elevated in superficial infections as well.[19]

If osteomyelitis is suspected, MRI of the foot is the preferred diagnostic imaging modality. Bone scan combined with a leukocyte scan may also be used if MRI cannot be obtained.[17] MRI is the most sensitive modality for diagnosis of osteomyelitis in diabetic foot infection with a good negative predictive value but a specificity of less than 80%.[26,32] At times reactive bone changes under the area of soft tissue infection may be present on MRI, which may limit its utility in assessing for osteomyelitis in these acute presentations. Charcot foot may also be difficult to distinguish from infection on imaging.[33] Unless needed by the surgeon to determine margins of debridement, the utility of MRI is also limited in an ischemic foot in which healing will be determined by reperfusion.

In the case of an acute onset of foot cellulitis, if there is uncertainty whether an underlying osteomyelitis is present, a reasonable approach is to treat with antibiotics and observe for improvement. A short course of antibiotics may be prescribed and the foot reassessed for osteomyelitis with further imaging or cultures off antibiotics once the soft tissue infection is treated.

OTHER INFECTIONS OF THE DIABETIC FOOT

Cellulitis with or without an associated diabetic wound may develop in the diabetic foot. If a diabetic wound is present, then the microbial pathogen may be cultured from the wound, and antibiotics can be tailored accordingly.[10] If no wound is present, then cellulitis can be divided into purulent and nonpurulent presentations as at other sites. Purulent cellulitis should have any area of abscess drained, cultured, and treated empirically for S aureus with consideration for MRSA. Nonpurulent cellulitis is usually streptococcal.[10] In addition to appropriate antibiotic therapy, tremendous benefit is gained through leg elevation and control of edema.[34] The foot should always be assessed for conditions predisposing to cellulitis: wounds, tinea infection resulting in skin breaks, and edema. Management of these is key to prevention of recurrences. Tinea pedis is usually a chronic management challenge with successful treatment focusing on keeping the foot dry and using topical or, in cases of severe infection, systemic antifungals.[35]

Finally, it is important to note that the changes owing to Charcot foot are not from infection. It may be particularly difficult to distinguish infection from acute Charcot foot when edema, remodeling changes, and warmth of the foot may develop over a relatively short time course.[36,37] Use of MRI to distinguish between Charcot foot and osteomyelitis may also be problematic; clinicians may need to obtain fluid or bone cultures to determine if infection is present.[37] Treatment with antibiotics with lack of improvement should lead to increased suspicion of this diagnosis. Treatment should focus on offloading of the foot with involvement of an orthopedic specialist.[36]

THERAPEUTIC OPTIONS FOR DIABETIC SKIN AND SOFT TISSUE INFECTIONS

Although comparative studies have been performed, no single antiblotic or combination of agents appears to be superior to others. Antibiotic selection should be based on the severity of infection; patient-specific risk factors for MRSA or Pseudomonas, or other multidrug-resistant organism; available culture and susceptibility information; and likely duration of therapy with consideration of potential adverse effects. In addition, pharmacokinetic and pharmacodynamic properties should be considered, as antibiotics vary in ability to achieve therapeutic concentrations in infected tissue.[38]

For mild infections, oral therapies are recommended.[17] For patients without risk factors or cultures indicating MRSA, therapy can be targeted toward gram-positive cocci, such as staphylococci (methicillin-sensitive Staphylococcus aureus) and streptococci. Oral options include dicloxacillin, cephalexin, amoxicillin/clavulanate, and clindamycin. If MRSA is present or suspected, options include doxycycline, trimethoprim/sulfamethoxazole, or clindamycin. Frequency of dosing should be taken into account in patients with known compliance issues, as medication adherence decreases with increasing dosing frequency.[39] Medication compliance can be especially problematic with oral beta-lactams, such as dicloxacillin and cephalexin, which must be given 4 times daily. Fluoroquinolones are appealing given the ability for daily dosing, but ciprofloxacin lacks activity against streptococci and S aureus, and levofloxacin is suboptimal against S aureus.

Several new antimicrobials have been developed since the last iteration of the Infectious Diseases Society of America (IDSA) guidelines were published. Delafloxacin is an attractive new antibiotic with more robust activity against gram-positive organisms, specifically MRSA, because of more balanced inhibitory activities against both DNA gyrase (the target in gram-negative organisms) and topoisomerase (the target in gram-positive organisms), limiting selection and emergence of resistance. In addition, this agent may be particularly useful for diabetic foot infections, as it has increased intracellular update and enhanced efficacy in acidic environments because of its unique anionic state at neutral pH.[40] Omadacycline was Food and Drug Administration (FDA) approved in 2018 for acute bacterial skin and skin structure infections and is available orally.[41] This agent has a broad spectrum of in vitro activity, including vancomycin-resistant enterococci, multidrug-resistant gram-negative organisms such as ESBL (Extended spectrum beta-lactamase) producers, and *Acinetobacter baumanii*. These agents are unnecessarily broad in their activity for mild infections, and they are significantly higher in cost compared with other agents and may be subject to formulary restrictions. Also, use of these agents for diabetic foot infections is off-label given that such patients were largely excluded from phase 3 registrational trials based on FDA guidance for studies of acute bacterial skin and skin structure infections.[42]

SUMMARY

SSTIs in diabetics span a wide range of presentations from pressure and ischemic wounds to cellulitis with concern for underlying osteomyelitis or Charcot foot. These infections can progress rapidly with significant morbidity if not treated promptly and often require a multidisciplinary care team, including surgeons and infectious disease physicians. Glycemic control is also key for achieving good outcomes. MRSA, pseudomonas, and other antibiotic-resistant pathogens may be more prevalent in skin and soft tissue infections in the diabetic foot compared with in other sites and populations. All of these factors drive choice for appropriate antibiotic selection in this situation.

CLINICS CARE POINTS

- End-organ damage from prolonged hyperglycemia makes diabetic patients more at risk for skin and soft tissue infection, especially in the lower extremities.
- Diabetic ulcers and foot wounds should be assessed for disease severity, with several grading scales available, including assessment for infection and vascular perfusion status. Treatment should be tailored to wound origin and should include an evaluation of the need for pressure off-loading or reperfusion therapy, in addition to antimicrobial therapy.
- All diabetic foot infections need to be assessed for development of osteomyelitis with a plain film with consideration of MRI or further imaging if clinically indicated.
- Choice of antibiotic therapy in diabetic foot infections depends on past cultures and patient risks factors for methicillin-resistant *Staphylococcus aureus*, pseudomonas, and multidrug-resistant organisms as well as severity and depth of infection.
- Patients should be counseled on the importance of control of hyperglycemia, pedal edema, and tinea pedis in prevention of diabetic foot infections.

DISCLOSURE

C. Polk has received research funding from Merck, United States.

REFERENCES

1. World Health Organization. Global report on diabetes. 2016. Available at: https://www.who.int/publications/i/item/9789241565257. Accessed August 3, 2020.
2. Carey IM, Critchley JA, DeWilde S, et al. Risk of infection in type 1 and type 2 diabetes compared with the general population: a matched cohort study. Diabetes Care 2018;41(3):513–21.

3. Suaya JA, Eisenberg DF, Fang C, et al. Skin and soft tissue infections and associated complications among commercially insured patients aged 0-64 years with and without diabetes in the U.S. PLoS One 2013;8(4):e60057.

4. Korbel L, Spencer JD. Diabetes mellitus and infection: an evaluation of hospital utilization and management costs in the United States. J Diabetes Complications 2015;29(2):192–5.

5. Lipsky BA, Itani KM, Weigelt JA, et al. The role of diabetes mellitus in the treatment of skin and skin structure infections caused by methicillin-resistant Staphylococcus aureus: results from three randomized controlled trials. Int J Infect Dis 2011;15(2):e140–6.

6. Raya-Cruz M, Payeras-Cifre A, Ventayol-Aguilo L, et al. Factors associated with readmission and mortality in adult patients with skin and soft tissue infections. Int J Dermatol 2019;58(8):916–24.

7. Lavery LA, Armstrong DG, Wunderlich RP, et al. Risk factors for foot infections in individuals with diabetes. Diabetes Care 2006;29(6):1288–93.

8. Tan TW, Shih CD, Concha-Moore KC, et al. Disparities in outcomes of patients admitted with diabetic foot infections. PLoS One 2019;14(2):e0211481.

9. Daryabor G, Atashzar MR, Kabelitz D, et al. The effects of type 2 diabetes mellitus on organ metabolism and the immune system. Front Immunol 2020;11:1582.

10. Lipsky BA, Silverman MH, Joseph WS. A proposed new classification of skin and soft tissue infections modeled on the subset of diabetic foot infection. Open Forum Infect Dis 2017;4(1):ofw255.

11. Benavent E, Murillo O, Grau I, et al. The impact of gram-negative bacilli in bacteremic skin and soft tissue infections among patients with diabetes. Diabetes Care 2019;42(7):e110–2.

12. Torres K, Sampathkumar P. Predictors of methicillin-resistant Staphylococcus aureus colonization at hospital admission. Am J Infect Control 2013;41(11): 1043–7.

13. Johani K, Fritz BG, Bjarnsholt T, et al. Understanding the microbiome of diabetic foot osteomyelitis: insights from molecular and microscopic approaches. Clin Microbiol Infect 2019;25(3):332–9.

14. Citron DM, Goldstein EJ, Merriam CV, et al. Bacteriology of moderate-to-severe diabetic foot infections and in vitro activity of antimicrobial agents. J Clin Microbiol 2007;45(9):2819–28.

15. Henig O, Pogue JM, Cha R, et al. Epidemiology of diabetic foot infection in the Metro-Detroit area with a focus on independent predictors for pathogens resistant to recommended empiric antimicrobial therapy. Open Forum Infect Dis 2018; 5(11):ofy245.

16. Sloan TJ, Turton JC, Tyson J, et al. Examining diabetic heel ulcers through an ecological lens: microbial community dynamics associated with healing and infection. J Med Microbiol 2019;68(2):230–40.

17. Lipsky BA, Berendt AR, Cornia PB, et al. 2012 Infectious Diseases Society of America clinical practice guideline for the diagnosis and treatment of diabetic foot infections. Clin Infect Dis 2012;54(12):e132–73.

18. Wukich DK, Armstrong DG, Attinger CE, et al. Inpatient management of diabetic foot disorders: a clinical guide. Diabetes Care 2013;36(9):2862–71.

19. Lipsky BA, Senneville E, Abbas ZG, et al. Guidelines on the diagnosis and treatment of foot infection in persons with diabetes (IWGDF 2019 update). Diabetes Metab Res Rev 2020;36(Suppl 1):e3280.

20. Stevens DL, Bisno AL, Chambers HF, et al. Practice guidelines for the diagnosis and management of skin and soft tissue infections: 2014 update by the Infectious Diseases Society of America. Clin Infect Dis 2014;59(2):e10–52.

21. Chen SY, Giurini JM, Karchmer AW. Invasive systemic infection after hospital treatment for diabetic foot ulcer: risk of occurrence and effect on survival. Clin Infect Dis 2017;64(3):326–34.

22. Ramirez-Acuna JM, Cardenas-Cadena SA, Marquez-Salas PA, et al. Diabetic foot ulcers: current advances in antimicrobial therapies and emerging treatments. Antibiotics (Basel) 2019;8(4):193.

23. Bonner T, Foster M, Spears-Lanoix E. Type 2 diabetes-related foot care knowledge and foot self-care practice interventions in the United States: a systematic review of the literature. Diabet Foot Ankle 2016;7:29758.

24. Messenger G, Masoetsa R, Hussain I. A narrative review of the benefits and risks of total contact casts in the management of diabetic foot ulcers. J Am Coll Clin Wound Spec 2017;9(1–3):19–23.

25. Oyibo SO, Jude EB, Tarawneh I, et al. A comparison of two diabetic foot ulcer classification systems: the Wagner and the University of Texas wound classification systems. Diabetes Care 2001;24(1):84–8.

26. Barwell ND, Devers MC, Kennon B, et al. Diabetic foot infection: antibiotic therapy and good practice recommendations. Int J Clin Pract 2017;71(10). https://doi.org/10.1111/ijcp.13006.

27. Mergenhagen KA, Croix M, Starr KE, et al. Utility of methicillin-resistant Staphylococcus aureus nares screening for patients with a diabetic foot infection. Antimicrob Agents Chemother 2020;64(4). e02213-19.

28. Lavery LA, Fontaine JL, Bhavan K, et al. Risk factors for methicillin-resistant Staphylococcus aureus in diabetic foot infections. Diabet Foot Ankle 2014;5. https://doi.org/10.3402/dfa.v5.23575.

29. Lavigne JP, Sotto A, Dunyach-Remy C, et al. New molecular techniques to study the skin microbiota of diabetic foot ulcers. Adv Wound Care (New Rochelle) 2015; 4(1):38–49.

30. Noor S, Raghav A, Parwez I, et al. Molecular and culture based assessment of bacterial pathogens in subjects with diabetic foot ulcer. Diabetes Metab Syndr 2018;12(3):417–21.

31. Prompers L, Schaper N, Apelqvist J, et al. Prediction of outcome in individuals with diabetic foot ulcers: focus on the differences between individuals with and without peripheral arterial disease. The EURODIALE Study. Diabetologia 2008; 51(5):747–55.

32. Kapoor A, Page S, Lavalley M, et al. Magnetic resonance imaging for diagnosing foot osteomyelitis: a meta-analysis. Arch Intern Med 2007;167(2):125–32.

33. Al-Khawari HA, Al-Saeed OM, Jumaa TH, et al. Evaluating diabetic foot infection with magnetic resonance imaging: Kuwait experience. Med Princ Pract 2005; 14(3):165–72.

34. Sullivan T, de Barra E. Diagnosis and management of cellulitis. Clin Med (Lond) 2018;18(2):160–3.

35. Gupta AK, Cooper EA. Update in antifungal therapy of dermatophytosis. Mycopathologia 2008;166(5–6):353–67.

36. Pitocco D, Scavone G, Di Leo M, et al. Charcot neuroarthropathy: from the laboratory to the bedside. Curr Diabetes Rev 2019;16(1):62–72.

37. Vopat ML, Nentwig MJ, Chong ACM, et al. Initial diagnosis and management for acute Charcot neuroarthropathy. Kans J Med 2018;11(4):114–9.

38. Ray GT, Suaya JA, Baxter R. Incidence, microbiology, and patient characteristics of skin and soft-tissue infections in a U.S. population: a retrospective population-based study. BMC Infect Dis 2013;13:252.
39. Srivastava K, Arora A, Kataria A, et al. Impact of reducing dosing frequency on adherence to oral therapies: a literature review and meta-analysis. Patient Prefer Adherence 2013;7:419–34.
40. Jorgensen SCJ, Mercuro NJ, Davis SL, et al. Delafloxacin: place in therapy and review of microbiologic, clinical and pharmacologic properties. Infect Dis Ther 2018;7(2):197–217.
41. Paratek Pharmaceuticals I. NUZYRA. Package insert. 2020.
42. Food and Drug Administration Center for Drug Evaluation Research. Guidance for Industry Acute Bacterial Skin and Skin Structure Infections: Developing Drugs for Treatment. 2013.

68. Ray GT, Suaya JA, Baxter R. Incidence, microbiology, and patient characteristics of skin and soft-tissue infections in a U.S. population: a retrospective population-based study. *BMC Infect Dis.* 2013;13:252.

Skin and Soft Tissue Infections in Non–Human Immunodeficiency Virus Immunocompromised Hosts

Shivan Shah, MD, Samuel Shelburne, MD, PhD*

KEYWORDS

- Skin infection • Immunocompromised host • Necrotizing fasciitis • Fungal infection
- Antimicrobial resistance

KEY POINTS

- The type and severity of host immunosuppression are a key factor in the development and treatment outcomes of immunosuppressed patients with skin and soft tissue infections.
- Environmental factors are important considerations in the etiology of skin and soft tissue infections in the immunocompromised population, with particular pathogens being acquired after exposure to water, debris, or flora.
- Immunosuppressed patients have a higher risk of infection with antimicrobial-resistant pathogens owing to an increased use of prophylactic anti-infectives, recurrent infections, and nosocomial pathogen acquisition.
- Empiric treatment must acknowledge the broad variety of organisms and the risk of antimicrobial resistance to optimize appropriate anti-infective therapy.
- Skin and soft tissue infections in this population can result from disseminated disease such that additional workup may be needed.

INTRODUCTION

In the non–human immunodeficiency virus (HIV)-infected immunocompromised host, skin and soft tissue infections (SSTIs) are among the most common infectious causes of morbidity and mortality.[1] Decreased function of both the innate and acquired immune systems places patients at increased risk for infections from the commensal microflora or from pathogens encountered in the environment.[2] The outcomes of immunocompromised patients with SSTIs are generally worse compared with immunocompetent patients, even with the same causative organism.[3,4] Moreover, these patients often have significant breakdown of the skin integument, including changes

Department of Infectious Diseases, MD Anderson Cancer Center, 1515 Holcombe Boulevard, Box 1460, Houston, TX 77030, USA
* Corresponding author.
E-mail address: sshelburne@mdanderson.org

Infect Dis Clin N Am 35 (2021) 199–217
https://doi.org/10.1016/j.idc.2020.10.009
0891-5520/21/© 2020 Elsevier Inc. All rights reserved.

relating to surgical procedures, in-dwelling venous catheters, and chronic wounds, further predisposing them to cutaneous infections. Finally, with the increased use of a diverse array of immunosuppressive medications, there has been augmented recognition of atypical and antimicrobial resistant infections that makes managing these infections increasingly challenging.[5–7] There have been several excellent overviews of this complex subject either in its entirety or addressing particular facets.[2,8–10] Herein, we focus on the diagnostic and treatment approaches to immunocompromised patients with SSTIs in patients with underlying hematologic malignancy and/or those undergoing hematopoietic stem cell transplantation.Although immunocompromised patients do develop SSTIs due to typical pathogens such as staphylococci and streptococci, this review will highlight organisms that do not routinely cause SSTI's in the immunocompetent population.

IMMUNE DEFICITS PREDISPOSING PATIENTS TO SKIN AND SOFT TISSUE INFECTIONS

Although human immune function is composed of complex, interlocking aspects, for the purposes of considering risk to particular pathogens causing SSTIs it can be useful to separately consider the innate and acquired immune systems. Defects in the innate immune system, such as neutropenia seen after cytotoxic chemotherapy, typically initially increase the risk of invasive bacterial infections, such as those caused by staphylococci, streptococci, and gram-negative bacteria.[11,12] With pronounced and profound defects in the innate immune system, patients become susceptible to disseminated fungal infections that can involve the skin such as fusariosis or *Candida* species.[6,9] Defects in the acquired immune system can arise from a variety of causes such as an underlying malignancy (eg, multiple myeloma) or treatment with a broad array of medications such cytokine blockers, tyrosine kinase inhibitors, corticosteroids, or monoclonal antibodies.[13] Patients with deficiencies in the acquired immune system are susceptible to SSTIs caused by a wide variety of pathogens ranging from herpes viruses to mycobacteria to endemic fungi.[14–16] By combining a knowledge of exposure history, underlying immune defects, and clinical presentation, practitioners can generate differential diagnoses of causative agents of SSTIs permitting both optimization of empiric therapy and diagnostic approaches.[2]

BACTERIAL INFECTIONS
Pseudomonas aeruginosa

Classically *P aeruginosa* has been the most feared bacteria causing disease among neutropenic patients with 50% to 70% mortality rates in the absence of active therapy.[17] Localized *P aeruginosa* SSTIs can result from cutaneous inoculation typically involving moist areas such as the groin or axilla or can result from oropharyngeal

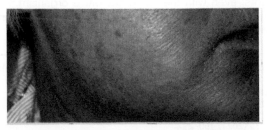

Fig. 1. Facial SSTI owing to *P aeruginosa* in a patient with acute myelogenous leukemia and profound neutropenia.

spread to adjacent tissues of the face[18] (**Fig. 1**). More severe forms of infections such as necrotizing fasciitis or pyomyositis can also be caused by *P aeruginosa* in immunocompromised patients.[19,20] Ecthyma gangrenosum, a necrotizing vasculitis of the skin primarily caused by *P aeruginosa*, is reflective of disseminated infection and generally limited to patients with hematologic malignancy.[21] The diagnosis of *P aeruginosa* SSTI is based on culture either of blood or the infection site.

β-Lactams are the cornerstones of anti–*P aeruginosa* therapy with ceftazidime, cefepime, imipenem, and meropenem generally having activity. Unfortunately, the last several years have seen the rise of multidrug-resistant *Pseudomonas*, which is becoming more prevalent in the oncological population, at least in part owing to widespread fluoroquinolone prophylaxis.[22,23] The rise of multidrug-resistant *P aeruginosa* has been somewhat mitigated by newer β-lactams, specifically ceftolozane–tazobactam.[24] In light of its pathogenic nature and ability to develop antimicrobial resistance, *P aeruginosa* infections are always a concern, which in turn can lead to prolonged therapy, particularly given the increased recurrence rates in immunocompromised patients.[25] A recent observational study of *P aeruginosa* bacteremia showed no difference in recurrence rates for short (8–10 days) versus long (14–16 days) durations of therapy, but recurrence rates were 13% to 14% in both groups, highlighting the need for vigilance whenever treating serious *P aeruginosa* infections.[26]

Stenotrophomonas maltophilia

S maltophilia is a glucose nonfermentative, gram-negative bacillus that can colonize the respiratory tract and surfaces of medical devices.[27] *S maltophilia* possesses inherent resistance to several antibiotics, including carbapenems, and the increasing use of antibiotics has allowed this bacterium to become a predominant nosocomial pathogen.[28] Although *S maltophilia* is rarely a cause of SSTIs in immunocompetent patients, it can cause a range of devastating SSTIs in the immunocompromised host, particularly those with profound neutropenia[29] (**Fig. 2**).

SSTIs owing to *S maltophilia* usually occur from hematogenous spread of the bacteria and typically are reported in patients with central venous catheters, although catheters may or may not be the actual infection source.[30] Lesions can either be localized or involve various body sites, including the extremities.[29] Initially, lesions typically are tender and are annular in shape, with a violaceous center. The

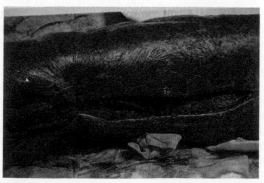

Fig. 2. Necrotizing soft tissue of the leg owing to *S maltophilia* in patient with acute myelogenous leukemia and profound neutropenia.

violaceous center subsequently undergoes necrosis, and the lesions can resemble ecthyma gangrenosum.[31] Diagnosis of *S maltophilia* SSTI is culture based, often of blood.

Given that most antimicrobials used empirically in immunocompromised patients are not active against *S maltophilia*, identifying the risk for *S maltophilia* could help with optimal empiric therapy.[32] However, risk factors with sufficient predictive values to be actionable have not been identified. Given its inherent resistance to carbapenems, exposure to these agents may perpetuate overgrowth and facilitate subsequent superinfection more so than other agents.[30,33] There are no comparative clinical outcomes data to guide treatment of *S maltophilia* SSTIs. Based on in vitro studies, trimethoprim–sulfamethoxazole is the recommended treatment.[27] Levofloxacin, minocycline, and tigecyline typically also have good in vitro activity, although resistance can develop to any or all of these agents.[27,34] The new β-lactam cefidericol seems to have good in vitro activity against *S maltophilia*, but clinical data are lacking.[35] The role of combination therapy such as trimethoprim–sulfamethoxazole and a fluoroquinolone is not clear and is not routinely recommended, although it is advocated by some.[36] Venous catheter removal seems to be an important part of optimizing outcomes, given that catheter retention has been associated with further metastatic skin lesions forming.[30]

Enterobacterales

The *Enterobacterales* are an order of gram-negative bacteria that includes *Escherichia coli*, *Klebsiella*, *Enterobacter*, *Salmonella*, and *Shigella*. These bacteria are generally the leading cause of bacteremia in immunocompromised patients.[37–39] Although rarely causative agents of SSTIs in immunocompetent persons, *Enterobacterales* SSTIs can be particularly severe in the immunosuppressed population.[20,40,41] Moreover, increasing rates of antimicrobial resistance in *Enterobacterales* complicates management.[42] The majority of serious *Enterobacterales* SSTIs in immunocompromised patients to date have been caused by *E coli*,[5,20,43] although *Klebsiella pneumoniae* necrotizing fasciitis is being increasingly appreciated.[44]

Systematic descriptions of clinical presentations of *Enterobacterales* SSTIs in immunocompromised patients are rather scant and have primarily focused on severe, deep infections such as necrotizing fasciitis and pyomyositis.[5,45] The origin of *Enterobacterales* SSTIs can either be at the infection site (particularly after surgical procedures) or from hematogenous spread, presumably after gastrointestinal translocation.[45] With more severe *Enterobacterales* SSTIs, patients are typically neutropenic and bacteremic.[45] Thus, *Enterobacterales* should be suspected as potential causative agents of severe, deep-seated SSTIs in patients with profound innate immune system deficits. The diagnosis of *Enterobacterales* SSTIs is based on site specific culture, whereas blood cultures may or may not be positive.

The treatment of *Enterobacterales* SSTIs depends on the causative organism with empiric therapy guided by rates of antimicrobial resistant organisms in specific facilities. Third- and fourth-generation cephalosporins have long been the primary treatments for *Enterobacterales* infection, but increasing resistance rates to these agents have been well-documented.[46] A recent randomized, controlled trial showed improved outcomes with a carbapenem compared with piperacillin–tazobactam for bacteremia with ceftriaxone resistant *Enterobacterales* (*E coli* and *Klebsiella* specifically).[47] AmpC-producing *Enterobacterales* (eg, *Enterobacter* spp.) are generally treated with either cefepime or a carbapenem.[48] Newer combination β-lactam/β-lactamase inhibitor combinations, such as ceftazidime–avibactam and meropenem–

vaborbactam, have been used for carbapenem-resistant *Enterobacterales*, although susceptibility to individual agents should be confirmed.[49,50] Given the high rates of fluoroquinolone and trimethoprim–sulfamethoxazole resistance among *Enterobacterales* causing infections in immunosuppressed patients, the use of these agents is not routinely recommended until susceptibility is confirmed.[51,52]

NONTUBERCULOUS MYCOBACTERIA

Nontuberculous mycobacteria (NTM) most commonly cause chronic lung infections.[53] However, the incidence of NTM causing SSTIs is increasing, particularly in patients with decreased adaptive immune function, such as those who have undergone hematopoietic stem cell transplantation.[54–56] There are more than 190 NTM species and species-specific infection rates vary greatly depending on geographic location.[57] Population-based surveillance for NTMs is currently limited to pulmonary disease, so the species composition of NTMs causing SSTI are not clear. Based on limited studies,[15,54,58] members of the *Mycobacterium abscessus* complex seem to be the most common cause of NTM SSTI, with several other species featuring prominently, such as *Mycobacterium chelonae*, *Mycobacterium avium-intracellulare*, and *M fortuitum*. Cutaneous disease owing to *Mycobacterium haemophilum* is primarily limited to immunocompromised patients.[59,60]

NTM SSTIs in immunocompromised patients can result from direct inoculation or owing to disseminated disease.[55] The characteristics of NTM skin lesions are different depending on the type of mycobacterium.[55] *Mycobacterium avium-intracellulare* and rapidly growing NTM can cause red nodules that form large ulcerated lesions or sinus tracts (**Fig. 3**). Depending on the species and host immunosuppression level, the bacteria can disseminate and cause multiple painful plaques, papules, and pustules.[55] *Mycobacterium marinum* SSTIs are typically sportrichoid-like disease following the lymphatic tracts in both immunocompromised and immunocompetent individuals, particularly in association with water exposure.[56] For all NTM SSTIs, diagnosis is based on culture of the infected site, although low organism burden and fastidious growth requirements can be problematic.[55] The presence of granulomas on skin biopsy should alert practitioners to the possibility of an NTM infection, although immunocompromised patients may not mount a granulomatous response.[61]

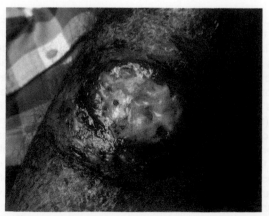

Fig. 3. Necrotic lesion of the forearm owing to *Mycobacterium avium* complex in patient with chronic lymphocytic leukemia.

Treatments for NTM SSTI differ depending on the particular species and presence of dissemination with recent guidelines published for pulmonary NTM disease.[62] Ideally, patients are treated with 2 or more agents to which the particular organism is susceptible, because the development of resistance on monotherapy is high.[55] The duration of treatment is typically from 3 to 4 months for localized infections and 6 to 12 months or more for disseminated disease.[55] In cases where there are foreign bodies, prompt removal is important when feasible.[63]

Nocardia spp.

Nocardia are aerobic, gram-positive, partially acid-fast filamentous bacteria found predominantly in the soil. Primary cutaneous Nocardia infections typically occur by inoculation owing to trauma. In immunocompromised patients, cutaneous Nocardia infection is primarily a manifestation of disseminated disease with pulmonary and central nervous systems involvement being common.[64] Transplant recipients, either hematopoietic or solid organ, are at particular risk for Nocardia infections, with disease usually occurring months to years after transplantation.[65] SSTIs owing to Nocardia in immunocompromised patients typically manifest as slow grow erythematous or subcutaneous nodules that can eventually have a lymphocutaneous or sporotrichosis form.[64] The diagnosis is made by culture of involved sites, which can take longer to turn positive than typical bacterial cultures, and thus consultation with the microbiology laboratory is recommended when Nocardia is considered as a causative agent. Filamentous, branching gram-positive rods are observed on direct examination in some 70% of cases.[66]

There are more than 100 Nocardia species, although the relationship between species identification and specific treatment protocols is not well-established.[65] For severe or disseminated infection, typically 3 active antimicrobials are recommended, such as trimethoprim–sulfamethoxazole, imipenem, and amikacin for the first several weeks.[65] Isolated cutaneous disease can often be treated with single agent trimethoprim–sulfamethoxazole.[64] Susceptibility to other antimicrobials is variable and should be confirmed by susceptibility testing. Linezolid has excellent in vitro activity, and there are emerging data regarding clinical effectiveness although linezolid often cannot be tolerated for long periods of time, particularly in transplant recipients.[67,68] Disseminated nocardiosis is typically treated for 1 to 2 years compared with 3 to 6 months if localized.

Candida spp.

Candida spp. are the most common cause of fungal infection in immunosuppressed patients.[69,70] SSTIs involving candida are uncommon but can occur in immunocompromised patients as part of disseminated disease, particularly in patients with hematologic malignancy and neutropenia.[6] A recent systematic review identified 100 published cases of disseminated candidiasis with skin lesions.[6] The most commonly identified Candida species were Candida tropicalis (68%), Candida krusei (15%), and Candida albicans (10%). C tropicalis tended to cause disseminated maculopapular lesions in patients not receiving fluconazole prophylaxis (**Fig. 4**), whereas Candida kruzei infections occurred more commonly in patients receiving fluconazole and were often nodular in nature. In accordance with its virulent nature, C tropicalis can cause severe SSTIs such as necrotizing cellulitis and pyomyositis.[71] Diagnosis of Candida SSTI is made by biopsy and culture of the involved site; blood cultures may or may not also be positive for Candida.[72]

Management guidelines for candidiasis have been published,[73] herein, we focus on aspects particular to immunocompromised patients. Over the past several years,

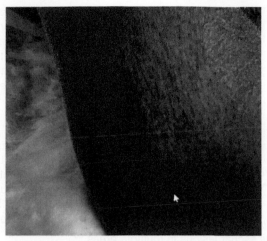

Fig. 4. Subcutaneous nodule on the leg of a patient with acute myelogenous leukemia and profound neutropenia. Biopsy showed *Candida tropicalis* resistant to fluconazole.

triazole-resistant *Candida* has become increasingly common in profoundly immuno-compromised patients, particularly *Candida glabrata*.[74] Infections owing to triazole-resistant *Candida* generally should be treated with an echinocandin. Profoundly immunocompromised patients can develop meningitis as a part of disseminated candidiasis,[75] and for these patients it is recommended to use liposomal amphotericin B or a triazole antifungal (if susceptible), given that echinocandins have poor penetration into the central nervous system.[73] *Candida auris* is a recently emerging, multidrug-resistant *Candida* species. Immunosuppression is a risk for *C auris* infection, and treatment is based on infection site and susceptibility testing results.[76]

CUTANEOUS MOLD INFECTIONS

In patients with marked neutrophil deficiencies, molds can cause SSTIs, with the majority of cases caused by *Aspergillus*, *Zygomycetes* (*Rhizopus* and *Mucor*), and *Fusarium* spp.[77] Patients are generally exposed to these environmental molds via the respiratory tract with progression to deep tissue invasion and dissemination as a result of their angioinvasive nature. Cutaneous mold infections tend to present as tender nodules that progress to necrotic lesions, in contrast with cutaneous candidiasis, in which necrosis is much less common.[77]

Aspergillus spp. are ubiquitous in the environment, but invasive aspergillosis is almost invariably encountered in immunocompromised patients. Primary cutaneous aspergillosis typically occurs after trauma, such as venipuncture or at catheter sites.[78] Lesions develop into red papules or plaque that evolve into a central black eschar. Cutaneous involvement secondary to dissemination is rarely observed in aspergillosis but has been described to involve multiple subcutaneous nodules that can progress to ulceration.[7]

Nontraumatic *Fusarium* SSTIs are almost exclusively found in neutropenic patients and transplant recipients through hematogenous spread.[79] Unlike aspergillosis and mucormycosis, skin involvement is common in fusariosis, occurring in some 75% of cases.[77] Fusarium-induced mycotoxicosis leads to thrombus formation, angioinvasive disease, and disseminated infection (**Fig. 5**). Fusarium skin lesions can resemble those

Fig. 5. Early hemorrhagic lesion owing to *Fusarium* spp. on the leg of a patient with acute myelogenous leukemia.

caused by *Aspergillus*, but typically are more numerous and invade through blood vessels to create small eschar lesions in multiple areas.[80]

The zygomycetes family are composed of many different molds, but the two most common causing infections are *Rhizopus* spp. and *Mucor* spp.[78] Skin soft tissue infections are relatively rarely seen in zygomycosis but can result from hematogenous spread or via direct inoculation from contaminated elastic, gauze, or areas of venipuncture. The heterogeneous nature of skin lesions in zygomycosis, ranging from small papules to rapidly progressive full-thickness necrosis, likely results from the diverse species involved and host immunosuppression status (**Fig. 6**).[78]

The diagnosis of mold SSTIs is generally is made by biopsy of the affected site with blood cultures rarely being positive except for fusariosis.[81] Treatment for mold SSTIs ideally consists of both antifungal agents and surgical debridement of devitalized tissue.[81] Medical therapy of mold SSTI varies depending on the infecting agent and whether the infection developed while taking antifungal prophylaxis.[82] In general, *Aspergillus* and *Fusarium* infections are treated with mold-active triazoles such as voriconazole or posaconazole, whereas Mucorales infections are initially treated with amphotericin B products.[81,83] After improvement with amphotericin B, consolidation therapy for Mucorales consists of either posaconazole or isavuconazole with detailed species-specific treatments provided in.[81] Given the suboptimal outcomes observed in mold SSTIs with associated neutropenia,[80] leukocyte transfusions have been used

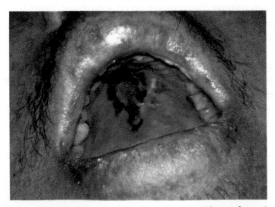

Fig. 6. Necrotic palate lesion to zygomycetes in patient with profound neutropenia.

with anecdotal success.[84] Once patients have a mold SSTI, they are at risk until they are no longer immunosuppressed and should be considered for secondary prophylaxis.

DIMORPHIC FUNGI (ENDEMIC MYCOSIS)

The major endemic mycoses in the United States are histoplasmosis, blastomycosis, and coccidioidomycosis. Most data on SSTIs caused by these organisms come from persons with AIDS, with data on non-HIV immunocompromised patients mainly limited to case reports.[85] Infections due to these organisms are acquired from the environment primarily through inhalation of the mold phase. All 3 of these mycoses have historically had distinct geographic areas, but recent studies and epidemiologic data indicate that these are more widespread than previously thought.[86] Thus, testing for the different endemic mycoses should be considered if a patient has compatible clinical features regardless of geographic location.

Known as a "great imitator," the cutaneous lesions of histoplasmosis are highly variable ranging from polymorphic plaques, to papules, pustules, nodules, ulcers, molluscum-like lesions, acneiform eruptions, exfoliative erythroderma, abscesses, and cellulitis.[86] Cutaneous lesions of histoplasmosis in Latin America seem to more prevalent compared with North America and present as crusted papuloulcerative lesions, perhaps because of geographic differences in *Histoplasma capsalatum* species.[87] Biopsy of lesions can show necrotizing granulomas and yeast forms of the fungi. Additionally, antibody and antigen tests can be useful in diagnosis of histoplasmosis, although antibody testing may be of limited value in immunosuppressed patients such as transplant recipients.[88] Additionally, antigen tests for histoplasmosis can cross-react with other endemic mycoses such as blastomycosis.[89]

Blastomycosis generally produces a pulmonary form of the disease and, to a lesser extent, extrapulmonary forms, such as cutaneous, osteoarticular, and genitourinary. Both immunocompetent and immunocompromised individuals can be infected, but more severe disease occurs in the immunocompromised.[90] Some 60% of patients with blastomycosis have cutaneous involvement, typically from disseminated disease.[85] Lesions usually are a painless ulcer or verrucous plaques, and occur on the head, neck, and extremities, although a purely pustular form has been described.[91] Diagnosis is made by skin biopsy with antigen and antibody testing of limited value in immunocompromised patients.[88] Similar to histoplasmosis, the *Blastomyces* antigen test will commonly be positive in patients with other endemic mycoses.[92]

Reactive skin manifestations of coccidioidomycosis do not contain visible microorganisms and occur during acute primary pulmonary infection in up to 50% of patients.[93] Lesions can present as erythema nodosum, erythema multiforme, acute generalized exanthema, reactive interstitial granulomatous dermatitis, and Sweet's syndrome.[93] Patients with deficits in acquired immunity are at risk for disseminated coccidioidomycosis, with the skin being one of the major sites of involvement.[93] The most common skin manifestation of disseminated coccidioidomycosis is nodules, but a wide variety of skin involvement can be seen ranging from plaques to abscesses.[93] Diagnosis is primarily made based on skin biopsy, although serologic assays can be helpful.[88]

Treatment guidelines for all 3 of these mycoses have been published.[94–96] Given that SSTIs owing to these organisms in immunocompromised patients reflect disseminated disease, treatment primarily involves induction with amphotericin-based products before switching to triazole therapy after a few weeks. Itraconazole is considered the first-line maintenance therapy for histoplasmosis and blastomycosis, whereas fluconazole is optimal for coccidioidomycosis.[88]

Cryptococcocus spp.

Cutaneous manifestations occur in up to 15% of cryptococcosis and can be the first sign of systemic disease, which mainly affects persons with deficits in acquired immune function.[97] Alternatively, primary cutaneous cryptococcal infection can occur in both immunocompetent and immunocompromised hosts.[16] Cutaneous manifestations of cryptococcosis are heterogeneous and include papules, pustules, vesicles, nonhealing ulcers, cellulitis, subcutaneous nodules, ecchymoses, gummas, abscesses, and granulomata.[97] Diagnosis of SSTI due to *Cryptococcus* is made by skin biopsy, blood culture, or a positive serum cryptococcal antigen.[97] Given that cutaneous involvement by *Cryptococcus* could be a harbinger of disseminated disease including meningitis, cerebrospinal fluid analysis for cryptococcal antigen and fungal cultures is recommended.[98]

Treatment guidelines for cryptococcosis have been published.[98] Inasmuch as cryptococcal SSTIs generally represent disseminated disease in immunosuppressed persons, amphotericin B is the cornerstone of initial therapy.[98] Ideally, flucytosine, with therapy guided by levels, is also used, although bone marrow suppression can be a significant issue in patients with compromised bone marrow function.[99] Subsequently, consolidation therapy with high dose fluconazole (6 mg/kg/d) should be given for a minimum of 8 weeks followed by maintenance therapy with lower doses of fluconazole typically for at least 1 year. There are minimal data to guide therapy of primary cutaneous cryptococcosis, which seems to have less mortality compared with the disseminated form and may respond well to azole-based therapy.[98]

HERPES VIRUSES

Herpes simplex virus (HSV) and varicella zoster virus (VZV) are common causes of both primary and recurrent skin infections in patients with a variety of immunodeficiencies.[14,100] Although HSV and VZV incidence has been dramatically decreased with near universal acyclovir-based prophylaxis among profoundly immunosuppressed individuals, HSV and VZV infections remain challenging both diagnostically and therapeutically.

HSV disease primarily involves the mucocutaneous areas in and around the mouth (HSV-1) and genital areas (HSV-2). Typically, HSV disease begins as papules that rupture after a few days, resulting in ulcers that crust within 96 hours, although crusting can take much longer in immunocompromised patients.[14] Unusual manifestations of HSV disease can occur in immunocompromised patients such as the "knife-cut" sign involving intertriginous areas or disseminated infection.[101,102] Immunosuppressed populations, especially those with cancer and transplant recipients, are prone to having recurrent HSV infections and potentially antiviral resistance.[103] Newer cancer therapies, such as chimeric antigen receptor T-cell therapy, also pose risks for reactivation of HSV virus such that prophylaxis may be needed for such patients.[104] The diagnosis of HSV infection can often be made clinically based on characteristic skin lesions, although polymerase chain reaction-based testing of swabbed lesions can be helpful in atypical circumstances.[105] Polymerase chain reaction testing of the blood or of fluid or tissue of target organs is used in disseminated disease[105]

Therapy with acyclovir and acyclovir analogues is recommended for immunocompromised patients with HSV infection with intravenous therapy used in more severe mucocutaneous or disseminated disease.[105] When disease develops while taking acyclovir prophylaxis and/or does not respond to intravenous acyclovir, then resistance should be suspected, although in vitro confirmation can be problematic.[106] Foscarnet or cidofovir are used to treat acyclovir resistant HSV disease, but results are suboptimal and side effects are common.[103]

VZV skin infection, typically in form of reactivation, causes significant morbidity in the immunocompromised patient.[107,108] Reactivation VZV tends to manifest as a painful, dermatomal rash that turns into fluid-filled blisters that break open and subsequently scab in 7 to 10 days. However, zoster can be quite atypical in immunocompromised patients, including unusual morphologies and nondermatomal distributions. Moreover, complications such as disseminated disease and postherpetic neuralgia are more common in immunocompromised patients.[107] Therefore, a high index of suspicion for VZV should be maintained in immunocompromised patients. Diagnosis and treatment of VZV are quite similar to those outlined elsewhere in this article for HSV.[107] A major advancement for immunosuppressed patients has been the finding that recombinant VZV vaccine, currently marketed as Shingrix, is highly effective both in preventing VZV recurrence and VZV complications, even in patients with significant immunocompromise, such as those having undergone autologous stem cell transplantation.[109]

Leishmania spp.

Cutaneous leishmaniasis (CL) is a vector-born infection caused by a group of protozoans broadly distributed in South America, southern Europe, Africa, and eastern Asia. Immunosuppressed patients are more likely to develop CL and for the CL to be more severe and ulcerative compared with immunocompetent patients.[110] Use of anti–tumor necrosis factor-α monoclonal antibodies seem to be particularly associated with CL, whereas reports of CL in leukemia or stem cell transplantation are rare.[111,112] Treatment descriptions of CL in non-HIV immunosuppressive conditions are mostly case reports. Treatment is typically with amphotericin B–based medications with limited information indicating that treatment outcomes are improved relative to HIV-infected individuals but not equivalent to those in the immunocompetent population.[110]

NONINFECTIOUS DISEASE SKIN PATHOLOGIES

It is important to note that there are a range of noninfectious pathologies that can mimic skin infections in immunosuppressed hosts, from malignancy involvement to side effects of medications to autoimmune conditions.[72] The neutrophilic dermatoses, which include pyoderma gangrenosum and Sweet's syndrome, are critically important for clinicians to remember given that these disorders can progress to very severe inflammatory states including necrotizing fasciitis (**Fig. 7**).[113,114] Generally, these patients have hematological malignancies, autoimmune disorders, or are on proinflammatory medication (eg, granulocyte colony stimulating factor).[113]

Sweet's syndrome lesions are debilitating, well-defined red plaques or nodules, sometimes with pustules on the surface. They may occur anywhere on the body, including the face, and are associated with fever and neutrophilia. Lesions are frequently misdiagnosed as abscesses and incorrectly treated with antibiotics.[113] Diagnosis is made by merging the clinical picture with a skin biopsy showing a neutrophilic infiltrate, absence of leukocytoclastic vasculitis, and negative cultures for a micro-organism.

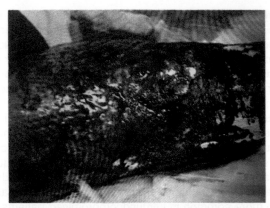

Fig. 7. Necrotic arm lesion in patient with acute myelogenous leukemia. Biopsy showed neutrophilic infiltrate with negative stains and cultures for microbes. The patient responded well to corticosteroids and was thus diagnosed with Sweet's syndrome.

Corticosteroids are the mainstay of treatment for neutrophilic dermatoses with improvement typically occurring in 2 or 3 days with the worst of the lesions disappearing within 1 to 4 weeks. However, recurrence are common upon corticosteroid tapering, particularly in patients with an underlying malignancy, and the optimal treatment approach in this setting is not established.[113]

SUMMARY

Owing to the diversity of pathogens, unusual presentations, and rising rates of antimicrobial resistance, SSTIs in the non-HIV immunocompromised patient are a major clinical challenge. Moreover, an SSTI in an immunocompromised patient may be the first clue to a potentially deadly, disseminated infection. Familiarity with the distinct pathogens causing SSTIs along with diagnostic and therapeutic strategies can assist medical practitioners in optimizing outcomes.

CLINICS CARE POINTS

- Outcomes of SSTIs in non-HIV immunocompromised patients are worse compared with immunocompetent persons.
- SSTIs in non-HIV immunocompromised patients are caused by a broader array of pathogens compared with immunocompetent persons.
- Antimicrobial resistance rates are higher in pathogens causing SSTIs in non-HIV immunocompromised patients compared with those causing disease in immunocompetent persons.

DISCLOSURE

The authors have nothing to disclose.

REFERENCES

1. Lopez FA, Sanders CV. Dermatologic infections in the immunocompromised (non-HIV) host. Infect Dis Clin North Am 2001;15(2):671–702, xi.

2. Ungaro R, Mikulska M. The skin and soft tissue infections in hematological patients. Curr Opin Infect Dis 2020;33(2):101–9.
3. Keung EZ, Liu X, Nuzhad A, et al. Immunocompromised status in patients with necrotizing soft-tissue infection. JAMA Surg 2013;148(5):419–26.
4. Linder KA, Alkhouli L, Ramesh M, et al. Effect of underlying immune compromise on the manifestations and outcomes of group a streptococcal bacteremia. J Infect 2017;74(5):450–5.
5. Vigil KJ, Johnson JR, Johnston BD, et al. Escherichia coli pyomyositis: an emerging infectious disease among patients with hematologic malignancies. Clin Infect Dis 2010;50(3):374–80.
6. Guarana M, Nucci M. Acute disseminated candidiasis with skin lesions: a systematic review. Clin Microbiol Infect 2018;24(3):246–50.
7. Bernardeschi C, Foulet F, Ingen-Housz-Oro S, et al. Cutaneous invasive aspergillosis: retrospective multicenter study of the French Invasive-Aspergillosis Registry and literature review. Medicine (Baltimore) 2015;94(26):e1018.
8. Burke VE, Lopez FA. Approach to skin and soft tissue infections in non-HIV immunocompromised hosts. Curr Opin Infect Dis 2017;30(4):354–63.
9. Gunaydin SD, Arikan-Akdagli S, Akova M. Fungal infections of the skin and soft tissue. Curr Opin Infect Dis 2020;33(2):130–6.
10. Pettit CJ, Mazurek K, Kaffenberger B. Cutaneous manifestations of infections in solid organ transplant recipients. Curr Infect Dis Rep 2018;20(7):16.
11. Nesher L, Rolston KV. The current spectrum of infection in cancer patients with chemotherapy related neutropenia. Infection 2014;42(1):5–13.
12. White L, Ybarra M. Neutropenic fever. Hematol Oncol Clin North Am 2017;31(6): 981–93.
13. Chamilos G, Lionakis MS, Kontoyiannis DP. Call for action: invasive fungal infections associated with ibrutinib and other small molecule kinase inhibitors targeting immune signaling pathways. Clin Infect Dis 2018;66(1):140–8.
14. Tan HH, Goh CL. Viral infections affecting the skin in organ transplant recipients: epidemiology and current management strategies. Am J Clin Dermatol 2006; 7(1):13–29.
15. Diaz MAA, Huff TN, Libertin CR. Nontuberculous mycobacterial infections of the lower extremities: a 15-year experience. J Clin Tuberc Other Mycobact Dis 2019; 15:100091.
16. Noguchi H, Matsumoto T, Kimura U, et al. Cutaneous cryptococcosis. Med Mycol J 2019;60(4):101–7.
17. Bodey GP. The changing face of febrile neutropenia-from monotherapy to moulds to mucositis. Fever and neutropenia: the early years. J Antimicrob Chemother 2009;63(Suppl 1):i3–13.
18. Kaya H, Yoshida T. A case of intravascular lymphoma complicated with Fournier's syndrome due to multidrug-resistant Pseudomonas aeruginosa. J Clin Exp Hematop 2011;51(2):115–8.
19. Emmett C, Kane G. Necrotising fasciitis caused by p aeruginosa in a male patient with chronic lymphocytic leukaemia. BMJ Case Rep 2013;2013. bcr2012008133.
20. Maravelas R, Melgar TA, Vos D, et al. Pyomyositis in the united states 2002-2014. J Infect 2020;80(5):497–503.
21. Vaiman M, Lazarovitch T, Heller L, et al. Ecthyma gangrenosum and ecthyma-like lesions: review article. Eur J Clin Microbiol Infect Dis 2015;34(4):633–9.
22. Hakki M, Humphries RM, Hemarajata P, et al. Fluoroquinolone prophylaxis selects for meropenem-nonsusceptible Pseudomonas aeruginosa in patients

with hematologic malignancies and hematopoietic cell transplant recipients. Clin Infect Dis 2019;68(12):2045–52.

23. Gudiol C, Albasanz-Puig A, Laporte-Amargos J, et al. Clinical predictive model of multidrug resistance in neutropenic cancer patients with bloodstream infection due to Pseudomonas aeruginosa. Antimicrobial Agents Chemother 2020; 64(4):e02494-19.

24. Bassetti M, Castaldo N, Cattelan A, et al. Ceftolozane/tazobactam for the treatment of serious Pseudomonas aeruginosa infections: a multicentre nationwide clinical experience. Int J Antimicrob Agents 2019;53(4):408–15.

25. McCarthy KL, Paterson DL. Increased risk of death with recurrent Pseudomonas aeruginosa bacteremia. Diagn Microbiol Infect Dis 2017;88(2):152–7.

26. Fabre V, Amoah J, Cosgrove SE, et al. Antibiotic therapy for Pseudomonas aeruginosa bloodstream infections: how long is long enough? Clin Infect Dis 2019; 69(11):2011–4.

27. Brooke JS. Stenotrophomonas maltophilia: an emerging global opportunistic pathogen. Clin Microbiol Rev 2012;25(1):2–41.

28. Jeon YD, Jeong WY, Kim MH, et al. Risk factors for mortality in patients with Stenotrophomonas maltophilia bacteremia. Medicine (Baltimore) 2016;95(31): e4375.

29. Bin Abdulhak AA, Zimmerman V, Al Beirouti BT, et al. Stenotrophomonas maltophilia infections of intact skin: a systematic review of the literature. Diagn Microbiol Infect Dis 2009;63(3):330–3.

30. Boktour M, Hanna H, Ansari S, et al. Central venous catheter and Stenotrophomonas maltophilia bacteremia in cancer patients. Cancer 2006;106(9):1967–73.

31. Son YM, Na SY, Lee HY, et al. Ecthyma gangrenosum: a rare cutaneous manifestation caused by Stenotrophomonas maltophilia in a leukemic patient. Ann Dermatol 2009;21(4):389–92.

32. Safdar A, Rolston KV. Stenotrophomonas maltophilia: changing spectrum of a serious bacterial pathogen in patients with cancer. Clin Infect Dis 2007; 45(12):1602–9.

33. Aitken SL, Sahasrabhojane PV, Kontoyiannis DP, et al. Alterations of the oral microbiome and cumulative carbapenem exposure are associated with Stenotrophomonas maltophilia infection in patients with acute myeloid leukemia receiving chemotherapy. Clin Infect Dis 2020. https://doi.org/10.1093/cid/ciaa778.

34. Biagi M, Tan X, Wu T, et al. Activity of potential alternative treatment agents for Stenotrophomonas maltophilia isolates nonsusceptible to levofloxacin and/or trimethoprim-sulfamethoxazole. J Clin Microbiol 2020;58(2):e01603-19.

35. Rolston KVI, Gerges B, Shelburne S, et al. Activity of cefiderocol and comparators against isolates from cancer patients. Antimicrobial Agents Chemother 2020;64(5):e01955-19.

36. Bao H, Qiao Y, Liu D, et al. The clinical impact of Stenotrophomonas maltophilia bacteremia on the 30-day mortality rate in patients with hematologic disorders: a single-institution experience. Infection 2020;48(2):205–12.

37. Klastersky J, Ameye L, Maertens J, et al. Bacteraemia in febrile neutropenic cancer patients. Int J Antimicrob Agents 2007;30(Suppl 1):S51–9.

38. Montassier E, Batard E, Gastinne T, et al. Recent changes in bacteremia in patients with cancer: a systematic review of epidemiology and antibiotic resistance. Eur J Clin Microbiol Infect Dis 2013;32(7):841–50.

39. Gudiol C, Bodro M, Simonetti A, et al. Changing aetiology, clinical features, antimicrobial resistance, and outcomes of bloodstream infection in neutropenic cancer patients. Clin Microbiol Infect 2013;19(5):474–9.
40. Ioannou P, Tsagkaraki E, Athanasaki A, et al. Gram-negative bacteria as emerging pathogens affecting mortality in skin and soft tissue infections. Hippokratia 2018;22(1):23–8.
41. Kuehl R, Tschudin-Sutter S, Siegemund M, et al. High mortality of non-Fournier necrotizing fasciitis with enterobacteriales: time to rethink classification? Clin Infect Dis 2019;69(1):147–50.
42. Baker TM, Satlin MJ. The growing threat of multidrug-resistant gram-negative infections in patients with hematologic malignancies. Leuk Lymphoma 2016; 57(10):2245–58.
43. Yahav D, Duskin-Bitan H, Eliakim-Raz N, et al. Monomicrobial necrotizing fasciitis in a single center: the emergence of gram-negative bacteria as a common pathogen. Int J Infect Dis 2014;28:13–6.
44. Rahim GR, Gupta N, Maheshwari P, et al. Monomicrobial Klebsiella pneumoniae necrotizing fasciitis: an emerging life-threatening entity. Clin Microbiol Infect 2019;25(3):316–23.
45. Albasanz-Puig A, Rodriguez-Pardo D, Pigrau C, et al. Necrotizing fasciitis in haematological patients: a different scenario. Ann Hematol 2020;99(8):1741–7.
46. CDC. Antibiotic resistant threats in the united states. 2019. Available at: https://www.cdc.gov/drugresistance/pdf/threats-report/2019-ar-threats-report-508.pdf. Accessed June 27, 2020.
47. Harris PNA, Tambyah PA, Lye DC, et al. Effect of piperacillin-tazobactam vs meropenem on 30-day mortality for patients with e coli or Klebsiella pneumoniae bloodstream infection and ceftriaxone resistance: a randomized clinical trial. JAMA 2018;320(10):984–94.
48. Tamma PD, Doi Y, Bonomo RA, et al. A primer on AmpC beta-lactamases: necessary knowledge for an increasingly multidrug-resistant world. Clin Infect Dis 2019;69(8):1446–55.
49. Alosaimy S, Jorgensen SCJ, Lagnf AM, et al. Real-world multicenter analysis of clinical outcomes and safety of meropenem-vaborbactam in patients treated for serious gram-negative bacterial infections. Open Forum Infect Dis 2020;7(3): ofaa051.
50. Alraddadi BM, Saeedi M, Qutub M, et al. Efficacy of ceftazidime-avibactam in the treatment of infections due to carbapenem-resistant enterobacteriaceae. BMC Infect Dis 2019;19(1):772.
51. Bhusal Y, Mihu CN, Tarrand JJ, et al. Incidence of fluoroquinolone-resistant and extended-spectrum beta-lactamase-producing Escherichia coli at a comprehensive cancer center in the united states. Chemotherapy 2011;57(4):335–8.
52. Rolston KVI, Jamal MA, Nesher L, et al. In vitro activity of ceftaroline and comparator agents against gram-positive and gram-negative clinical isolates from cancer patients. Int J Antimicrob Agents 2017;49(4):416–21.
53. Daley CL, Iaccarino JM, Lange C, et al. Treatment of nontuberculous mycobacterial pulmonary disease: an official ATS/ERS/ESCMID/IDSA clinical practice guideline. Eur Respir J 2020;56(1):2000535.
54. Wentworth AB, Drage LA, Wengenack NL, et al. Increased incidence of cutaneous nontuberculous mycobacterial infection, 1980 to 2009: a population-based study. Mayo Clin Proc 2013;88(1):38–45.
55. Franco-Paredes C, Marcos LA, Henao-Martinez AF, et al. Cutaneous mycobacterial infections. Clin Microbiol Rev 2018;32(1):e00069-18.

56. Al-Anazi KA, Al-Jasser AM, Al-Anazi WK. Infections caused by non-tuberculous mycobacteria in recipients of hematopoietic stem cell transplantation. Front Oncol 2014;4:311.

57. Prevots DR, Marras TK. Epidemiology of human pulmonary infection with nontuberculous mycobacteria: a review. Clin Chest Med 2015;36(1):13–34.

58. Sotello D, Garner HW, Heckman MG, et al. Nontuberculous mycobacterial infections of the upper extremity: 15-year experience at a tertiary care medical center. J Hand Surg Am 2018;43(4):387 e1–87 e8.

59. Jurairattanaporn N, Vachiramon V, Bruminhent J. Mycobacterium haemophilum skin and soft tissue infection in a kidney transplant recipient: a case report and summary of the literature. Transpl Infect Dis 2020;e13315. https://doi.org/10.1111/tid.13315.

60. Nookeu P, Angkasekwinai N, Foongladda S, et al. Clinical characteristics and treatment outcomes for patients infected with mycobacterium haemophilum. Emerg Infect Dis 2019;25(9):1648–52.

61. Li JJ, Beresford R, Fyfe J, et al. Clinical and histopathological features of cutaneous nontuberculous mycobacterial infection: a review of 13 cases. J Cutan Pathol 2017;44(5):433–43.

62. Daley CL, Iaccarino JM, Lange C, et al. Treatment of nontuberculous mycobacterial pulmonary disease: an official ATS/ERS/ESCMID/IDSA clinical practice guideline. Clin Infect Dis 2020;71(4):905–13.

63. El Helou G, Hachem R, Viola GM, et al. Management of rapidly growing mycobacterial bacteremia in cancer patients. Clin Infect Dis 2013;56(6):843–6.

64. Hemmersbach-Miller M, Catania J, Saullo JL. Updates on nocardia skin and soft tissue infections in solid organ transplantation. Curr Infect Dis Rep 2019; 21(8):27.

65. Coussement J, Lebeaux D, Rouzaud C, et al. Nocardia infections in solid organ and hematopoietic stem cell transplant recipients. Curr Opin Infect Dis 2017; 30(6):545–51.

66. Brown-Elliott BA, Brown JM, Conville PS, et al. Clinical and laboratory features of the nocardia spp. Based on current molecular taxonomy. Clin Microbiol Rev 2006;19(2):259–82.

67. De La Cruz O, Minces LR, Silveira FP. Experience with linezolid for the treatment of nocardiosis in organ transplant recipients. J Infect 2015;70(1):44–51.

68. Davidson N, Grigg MJ, McGuinness SL, et al. Safety and outcomes of linezolid use for nocardiosis. Open Forum Infect Dis 2020;7(4):ofaa090.

69. Kontoyiannis DP, Marr KA, Park BJ, et al. Prospective surveillance for invasive fungal infections in hematopoietic stem cell transplant recipients, 2001-2006: overview of the transplant-associated infection surveillance network (transnet) database. Clin Infect Dis 2010;50(8):1091–100.

70. Pappas PG, Alexander BD, Andes DR, et al. Invasive fungal infections among organ transplant recipients: results of the transplant-associated infection surveillance network (transnet). Clin Infect Dis 2010;50(8):1101–11.

71. Krishnan N, Patel B, Palfrey W, et al. Rapidly progressive necrotizing cellulitis secondary to candida tropicalis infection in an immunocompromised host. IDCases 2020;19:e00691.

72. Farmakiotis D, Ciurea AM, Cahuayme-Zuniga L, et al. The diagnostic yield of skin biopsy in patients with leukemia and suspected infection. J Infect 2013; 67(4):265–72.

73. Pappas PG, Kauffman CA, Andes DR, et al. Clinical practice guideline for the management of candidiasis: 2016 update by the Infectious Diseases Society of America. Clin Infect Dis 2016;62(4):e1–50.
74. Farmakiotis D, Tarrand JJ, Kontoyiannis DP. Drug-resistant candida glabrata infection in cancer patients. Emerg Infect Dis 2014;20(11):1833–40.
75. McCullers JA, Vargas SL, Flynn PM, et al. Candidal meningitis in children with cancer. Clin Infect Dis 2000;31(2):451–7.
76. Corsi-Vasquez G, Ostrosky-Zeichner L. Candida auris: what have we learned so far? Curr Opin Infect Dis 2019;32(6):559–64.
77. Maddy AJ, Sanchez N, Shukla BS, et al. Dermatological manifestations of fungal infection in patients with febrile neutropaenia: a review of the literature. Mycoses 2019;62(9):826–34.
78. Shields BE, Rosenbach M, Brown-Joel Z, et al. Angioinvasive fungal infections impacting the skin: background, epidemiology, and clinical presentation. J Am Acad Dermatol 2019;80(4):869–880 e5.
79. Nucci M, Anaissie E. Cutaneous infection by fusarium species in healthy and immunocompromised hosts: implications for diagnosis and management. Clin Infect Dis 2002;35(8):909–20.
80. Campo M, Lewis RE, Kontoyiannis DP. Invasive fusariosis in patients with hematologic malignancies at a cancer center: 1998-2009. J Infect 2010;60(5):331–7.
81. Berger AP, Ford BA, Brown-Joel Z, et al. Angioinvasive fungal infections impacting the skin: diagnosis, management, and complications. J Am Acad Dermatol 2019;80(4):883–898 e2.
82. Lionakis MS, Lewis RE, Kontoyiannis DP. Breakthrough invasive mold infections in the hematology patient: current concepts and future directions. Clin Infect Dis 2018;67(10):1621–30.
83. Patterson TF, Thompson GR 3rd, Denning DW, et al. Practice guidelines for the diagnosis and management of aspergillosis: 2016 update by the infectious diseases society of America. Clin Infect Dis 2016;63(4):e1–60.
84. Mellouli F, Ksouri H, Barbouche R, et al. Successful treatment of fusarium solani ecthyma gangrenosum in a patient affected by leukocyte adhesion deficiency type 1 with granulocytes transfusions. BMC Dermatol 2010;10:10.
85. Smith JA, Jt Riddell, Kauffman CA. Cutaneous manifestations of endemic mycoses. Curr Infect Dis Rep 2013;15(5):440–9.
86. Ashraf N, Kubat RC, Poplin V, et al. Re-drawing the maps for endemic mycoses. Mycopathologia 2020. https://doi.org/10.1007/s11046-020-00431-2.
87. Karimi K, Wheat LJ, Connolly P, et al. Differences in histoplasmosis in patients with acquired immunodeficiency syndrome in the united states and brazil. J Infect Dis 2002;186(11):1655–60.
88. Miller R, Assi M, ASTIDCo Practice. Endemic fungal infections in solid organ transplant recipients-guidelines from the American Society of Transplantation Infectious Diseases community of practice. Clin Transplant 2019;33(9):e13553.
89. Connolly PA, Durkin MM, Lemonte AM, et al. Detection of histoplasma antigen by a quantitative enzyme immunoassay. Clin Vaccine Immunol 2007;14(12):1587–91.
90. Castillo CG, Kauffman CA, Miceli MH. Blastomycosis. Infect Dis Clin North Am 2016;30(1):247–64.
91. Patel M, Lander JK. North American blastomycosis in an immunocompromised patient. Cutis 2019;104(6):E18–21.

92. Connolly P, Hage CA, Bariola JR, et al. Blastomyces dermatitidis antigen detection by quantitative enzyme immunoassay. Clin Vaccine Immunol 2012; 19(1):53–6.

93. Garcia Garcia SC, Salas Alanis JC, Flores MG, et al. Coccidioidomycosis and the skin: a comprehensive review. An Bras Dermatol 2015;90(5):610–9.

94. Wheat LJ, Freifeld AG, Kleiman MB, et al. Clinical practice guidelines for the management of patients with histoplasmosis: 2007 update by the infectious diseases society of America. Clin Infect Dis 2007;45(7):807–25.

95. Chapman SW, Dismukes WE, Proia LA, et al. Clinical practice guidelines for the management of blastomycosis: 2008 update by the infectious diseases society of America. Clin Infect Dis 2008;46(12):1801–12.

96. Galgiani JN, Ampel NM, Blair JE, et al. 2016 Infectious Diseases Society of America (IDSA) clinical practice guideline for the treatment of coccidioidomycosis. Clin Infect Dis 2016;63(6):e112–46.

97. Ilyas M, Sharma A. Cutaneous fungal infections in solid organ transplant recipients. Transplant Rev (Orlando) 2017;31(3):158–65.

98. Perfect JR, Dismukes WE, Dromer F, et al. Clinical practice guidelines for the management of crantyptococcal disease: 2010 update by the infectious diseases society of America. Clin Infect Dis 2010;50(3):291–322.

99. Baddley JW, Forrest GN, ASTIDCo Practice. Cryptococcosis in solid organ transplantation-guidelines from the American Society of Transplantation Infectious Diseases community of practice. Clin Transplant 2019;33(9):e13543.

100. Ilyas M, Maganty N, Sharma A. Cutaneous infections from viral sources in solid organ transplant recipients. J Clin Virol 2017;97:33–7.

101. Cohen PR. The "knife-cut sign" revisited: a distinctive presentation of linear erosive herpes simplex virus infection in immunocompromised patients. J Clin Aesthet Dermatol 2015;8(10):38–42.

102. Fernandez-Nieto D, Jimenez-Cauhe J, Ortega-Quijano D, et al. A case of atypical disseminated herpes simplex virus 1 with hepatitis in a liver transplant recipient: the need for dermatologic evaluation. Dermatol Online J 2020;26(2). 13030/qt3k90n5s9.

103. Anton-Vazquez V, Mehra V, Mbisa JL, et al. Challenges of aciclovir-resistant HSV infection in allogeneic bone marrow transplant recipients. J Clin Virol 2020;128:104421.

104. Vora SB, Waghmare A, Englund JA, et al. Infectious complications following cd19 chimeric antigen receptor t-cell therapy for children, adolescents, and young adults. Open Forum Infect Dis 2020;7(5):ofaa121.

105. Lee DH, Zuckerman RA, ASTIDCo Practice. Herpes simplex virus infections in solid organ transplantation: guidelines from the American Society of Transplantation Infectious Diseases community of practice. Clin Transplant 2019;33(9):e13526.

106. Piret J, Boivin G. Antiviral resistance in herpes simplex virus and varicella-zoster virus infections: diagnosis and management. Curr Opin Infect Dis 2016;29(6):654–62.

107. Pergam SA, Limaye AP, ASTIDCo Practice. Varicella zoster virus in solid organ transplantation: guidelines from the American Society of Transplantation Infectious Diseases community of practice. Clin Transplant 2019;33(9):e13622.

108. Xue E, Xie H, Leisenring WM, et al. High incidence of herpes zoster after cord blood hematopoietic cell transplant despite longer duration of antiviral prophylaxis. Clin Infect Dis 2020. https://doi.org/10.1093/cid/ciaa222.

109. Bastidas A, de la Serna J, El Idrissi M, et al. Effect of recombinant zoster vaccine on incidence of herpes zoster after autologous stem cell transplantation: a randomized clinical trial. JAMA 2019;322(2):123-33.
110. van Griensven J, Carrillo E, Lopez-Velez R, et al. Leishmaniasis in immunosuppressed individuals. Clin Microbiol Infect 2014;20(4):286-99.
111. Marcoval J, Penin RM, Sabe N, et al. Cutaneous leishmaniasis associated with anti-tumour necrosis factor-alpha drugs: an emerging disease. Clin Exp Dermatol 2017;42(3):331-4.
112. Gajurel K, Dhakal R, Deresinski S. Leishmaniasis in solid organ and hematopoietic stem cell transplant recipients. Clin Transplant 2017;31(1). https://doi.org/10.1111/ctr.12867.
113. Cohen PR. Neutrophilic dermatoses: a review of current treatment options. Am J Clin Dermatol 2009;10(5):301-12.
114. Kroshinsky D, Alloo A, Rothschild B, et al. Necrotizing sweet syndrome: a new variant of neutrophilic dermatosis mimicking necrotizing fasciitis. J Am Acad Dermatol 2012;67(5):945-54.

Infectious Complications of Bite Injuries

Sarah E. Greene, MD, PhD, Stephanie A. Fritz, MD, MSCI*

KEYWORDS

- Bite • Mammal • Dog • Cat • Human • Skin infection • *Pasteurella* • *Eikenella*

KEY POINTS

- Skin and soft tissue infection is the most frequent complication following a bite injury; these infections often are polymicrobial and are caused by aerobic and anaerobic microorganisms comprising the oral flora of the perpetrator as well as the skin flora of the victim.
- The risk for infection is influenced by the type, location, and extent of the injury; patient comorbidities; and time elapsed from the bite injury to presentation to medical attention.
- Cat bites commonly inflict puncture wounds and frequently are contaminated by *Pasteurella* species, posing high risk for subsequent infection.
- Irrigation and debridement are the mainstays of bite injury management. Administration of preemptive antibiotic therapy is controversial and generally is recommended for high-risk injuries or injuries occurring in patients at high risk for infection.
- The risk for tetanus and rabies transmission and the need for prophylaxis should be considered in patients sustaining an animal bite.

INTRODUCTION

Bites are a common cause of injury and medical visits in children and adults. It is estimated that 50% of Americans will experience a mammalian bite injury throughout their lifetime.[1] Although lack of national reporting precludes defining the exact incidence of bite injuries, studies have demonstrated that a majority of bite injuries inflicted by mammals result from dog bites and less frequently from cat and human bites. Other mammals, including rodents, horses, and nonhuman primates, account for a very small proportion of these injuries. In more than half of cases, the animal or other human inflicting the bite injury is known to the victim.[2–4] Depending on the type and location of bite, a substantial proportion of these injuries subsequently progresses to symptomatic infection.

Department of Pediatrics, Washington University School of Medicine, 660 South Euclid Avenue, Campus Box 8116, St Louis, MO 63110, USA
* Corresponding author.
E-mail address: fritz.s@wustl.edu

Infect Dis Clin N Am 35 (2021) 219–236
https://doi.org/10.1016/j.idc.2020.10.005
0891-5520/21/© 2020 Elsevier Inc. All rights reserved.

id.theclinics.com

EPIDEMIOLOGY AND MECHANISMS OF INJURY
Dog Bites

An estimated 4.5 million dog bites occur in the United States annually, at a cost of $165 million.[5,6] Of these, 750,000 dog bite injuries require emergency department (ED) attention, representing approximately 1% of ED visits overall.[6,7] Approximately 1% to 2.5% of ED visits for dog bite injuries result in hospitalization.[7,8] According to the Healthcare Cost and Utilization Project, nearly 60% of patients hospitalized for dog bite injuries require a surgical procedure, most frequently debridement, and 43% of hospitalizations are due to infectious complications of the bite.[8] Compared with hospitalizations for other types of injury, dog bites result in longer and more expensive hospitalizations.[8]

Men more often are victims of dog bites than women. Children less than 19 years of age account for 50% of dog bites, with the highest incidence occurring in children aged 5 years to 9 years.[3,7,9] Younger children are more likely to be bitten on their head and neck, likely given the proximity to the dog's jaw, compared with children greater than 10 years, who more often are bitten on the arm or hand.[3,4,10,11] The incidence of dog bites requiring ED utilization varies by region, but there are 4 times as many ED visits for dog bite injuries in rural areas than in urban settings.[8] ED visits for dog bite injuries are more common in the summer months and on weekends.[7,9]

Injuries resulting from dog bites range from abrasions to puncture wounds to lacerations (many with tissue avulsion). Larger dogs can cause crush injury with extensive tissue damage.[12–14] Approximately 20 people die from dog bite injuries in the United States each year, and 55% of deaths are in children.[15] These fatalities typically result from exsanguination or asphyxia or less commonly from sepsis or craniocerebral trauma.[12,16–20]

Cat Bites

Cats are estimated to cause 5% to 15% of bite injuries, with the caveat that minor cat bites likely are under-reported. Cat bites occur more commonly in women.[2,21,22] These injuries most commonly are sustained on the hand and arm.[21] In 1 study using animal control surveillance data, although 45% of people injured by dog bites reported that the incident was provoked, 89% of cat bites occurred via a provoked incident.[23] Given their small sharp teeth, cats most commonly inflict puncture wounds.

Human Bites

Human bites represent a small fraction of bite injuries overall. Human bites are most frequent in small children, who commonly are bit by other small children in day care or preschool settings. These injuries most often are occlusion bites, in which the upper and lower teeth meet and damage tissue between them, resulting in contusions or lacerations.[24,25] Human bites also occur in adolescents and adults, typically on the dominant hand resulting from a fist-to-tooth encounter (ie, a fight bite), which occurs when a closed fist contacts an opponent's teeth. These injuries can result in serious damage to the structures of the hand, especially metacarpophalangeal joints and tendons. An estimated 50% of fight bites cause metacarpophalangeal joint damage.[25]

INFECTIONS RESULTING FROM BITE INJURIES

Infections resulting from animal and human bites most commonly manifest as skin and soft tissue infections. The risk for infection is influenced by the type, location, and extent of the injury; patient comorbidities; and time elapsed from the bite injury to seeking medical attention.[26,27] For example, bite injuries greater than 3 cm, as well as bites to the hand, pose increased risk for infection.[2,11] The incidence of infection after a dog bite injury is estimated to range from 2% to 25%.[2,27,28] Although the incidence of cat bite injuries reportedly is less than that of dog bite injuries, given the mechanism of small-bore deep puncture wounds that are difficult to irrigate, as well as the virulent feline oral flora (discussed later), the incidence of infection from cat bites is considerably higher, ranging from 30% to 50%.[2,27–29] The first signs of infection appear earlier after cat bites than dog bites, developing within a median of 12 hours and 24 hours, respectively.[22] In 1 study of patients presenting with cat bite injuries, clinical signs of infection developed within 3 hours from the time of the bite injury in more than 50% of cases.[21] In 1 study of patients presenting to the ED with skin infection resulting from dog and cat bites, one-third of patients required hospitalization and intravenous antibiotic administration.[22] The estimated incidence of human bite wound infection is 2% to 25%.[2,25,27,28]

Local Infections at the Site of the Bite Injury

Presenting symptoms of infection at the site of the bite injury most frequently include severe pain, edema, and erythema.[21] Bacteria from the inoculation of skin and oral flora result in local purulent and nonpurulent cellulitis, skin and subcutaneous abscess, lymphangitis, fasciitis, or myositis, depending on the depth of the bite or the degree of spread of the infection. Bites that breach a joint capsule also can cause tendonitis or septic arthritis, whereas those that penetrate bone can cause osteomyelitis.[24]

Pathogens Associated with Local Bite Injury Infections

Infections resulting from animal bites are caused by the bacteria from the oral flora of a perpetrator's mouth as well as from human skin flora of the victim. Due to the abundant bacteria in the oral cavity, infections from animal bites often are polymicrobial, with a median of 5 distinct species per wound culture.[22] Animal oral flora is composed of a variety of aerobic bacteria, including *Staphylococcus*, *Streptococcus*, *Pasteurella*, *Moraxella*, *Corynebacterium*, and *Neisseria* spp. This is true for most mammals with some microbial species variation by animal. Human oral flora includes these bacteria as well as *Eikenella* and *Haemophilus* spp. Infections resulting from human bites also are polymicrobial, with a median of 4 species recovered per wound culture.[24] *Candida* spp also have been recovered from human bite injury infections.[24] Anaerobic bacteria are abundant in animal and human oral flora as well, including species from the genera *Bacteroides*, *Fusobacteria*, *Porphyromonas*, *Peptostreptococcus*, and *Prevotella*.[22,30]

Infections resulting from dog bites are more often caused by human skin flora, whereas those resulting from cat bites are more likely to be due to organisms comprising a cat's oral flora. For example, 1 study isolated *Staphylococcus aureus* from 20% of dog bites and 4% of cat bites, and *Streptococcus pyogenes* from 12% of dog bites and no cat bites.[22] Because there is overlap in the microbiota of these 2 body sites, determining whether the contamination originated from patient's skin or animal oral flora can be challenging.

Pasteurella spp often are present in the oral flora of animals, recovered from the mouths of 70% to 90% of cats and 20% to 50% of dogs and thus are the organisms isolated most commonly from bite wound cultures.[22,31] *Pasteurella* spp are isolated from 50% of infected dog bites (most commonly *P canis*) and 75% of infected cat bites (most often *P multocida*, subspecies *multocida* and *septica*).[22,28] *P multocida* subspecies *septica* is associated with developing systemic infection, especially central nervous system infection, although the pathogenesis of this increased virulence is unknown.[11,28,32] When *P multocida* species do cause systemic infection, often it is due to bacteremia extending from a localized infection and often in immunocompromised hosts.[31]

Capnocytophaga is an anaerobic bacterium that can cause both local and systemic infection. Although this microbe classically is identified with dog bites, it is present in the oral flora of both dogs and cats and causes infections after bites from both as well. These infections can be particularly severe in people with functional or anatomic asplenia or other immunocompromising conditions.[11,22,28,33–35]

Cat bite infections also have been reported to be caused by *Erysipelothrix rhusiopathiae*.[22] This gram-positive organism is carried by a wide range of farm and marine animals as well as cats and dogs. Although cellulitis from this organism most commonly occurs in fisherman, it can be spread by animal bites as well. *E rhusiopathiae* rarely causes systemic infection and endocarditis. Cat bites also can transmit *Sporothrix schenckii*.[28] This dimorphic fungus causes cutaneous lesions that spread proximally along the lymphatic system (sporotrichoid spread).

Systemic Infections

Animal bites can result in rabies infection, which almost universally is fatal. Rabies is spread via contact with the saliva of an infected animal, usually through a bite. This virus also can be spread by contact with the central nervous system or peripheral nervous system tissue of an infected animal or by organ transplantation, although these modes of transmission are rare.[36] Globally, dogs are the primary cause of rabies transmission, and rabies infections from dog bites cause 59,000 deaths annually.[37] In the United States, there are 5000 cases of rabies in animals annually, 90% of which are reported in wild animals, primarily bats, raccoons, skunks, and foxes.[38] Although all mammals can become infected with rabies, rabbits and rodents rarely transmit rabies.[39] Animal vaccination and pest control have reduced rabies carriage by domestic and wild animals in the United States, and there are now only 1 to 2 deaths from rabies annually, mostly from international dog bite exposure or local bat exposure.[38]

Although implementation of human vaccination programs has resulted in a low incidence of tetanus in the United States, animal bites can result in transmission of *Clostridium tetani,* leading to the development of tetanus. This is seen with deep penetrating wounds, those with soil contamination, and crush injury that leads to devascularized tissue, thus supporting the growth of anaerobic bacteria.[30,40–42]

Although usually spread by animal urine or contact with infected water, animal bites can transmit *Leptospira*, leading to leptospirosis. This has been reported mostly from bites by rats, mice, or dogs.[43] *Leptospira* spirochetes usually are not found in saliva, and thus it is unclear whether infections that result from bites are transmitted by saliva or from transfer of blood or urine around an animal's mouth via the bite. Leptospirosis manifests as a febrile illness that can be severe and result in damage to the liver, kidneys, and brain; in pregnant women, the organism is able to cross the placenta and infect the fetus. Tularemia is a severe systemic illness caused by *Francisella tularensis*. Although most commonly transmitted by tick bites, *F tularensis* also can be carried by cats, dogs, rabbits, and rodents and can be spread to humans by the bites of these animals.[28,44]

Dog Bites

Although uncommon, dog bites can transmit *Blastomyces dermatitidis*.[28] This dimorphic fungus causes blastomycosis, which can present with cutaneous lesions and can disseminate, predominantly to bone, lung, and brain.

Cat Bites

Cat bites can transmit *Bartonella henselae*, which causes cat-scratch disease.[28,45–47] This entity can present with a wide range of manifestations, including prolonged fever, lymphadenopathy, Parinaud oculoglandular syndrome, and culture-negative endocarditis.[48] Cat fleas transmit *B henselae* to cats, who in turn transmit it to humans via scratch or bite. Most patients diagnosed with cat-scratch disease report having cat exposure.

Human Bites

Given the potential for mixing of bodily fluids via a bite injury, specifically blood and saliva, there is the potential for transmission of any systemic viral illness during a bite encounter. Human immunodeficiency virus (HIV) is present in the blood of people with untreated HIV, but HIV is not transmitted by saliva. The risk of HIV transmission from a needlestick is 0.3%, and the risk of transmission via blood onto nonintact skin is less than 0.1%.[49] Thus, the risk of HIV transmission via bite injury is extremely low, although there are a handful of case reports citing transmission of HIV through a bite injury.[50,51] Most of these cases involve serious bites from an HIV-positive biter to HIV-negative bite recipients, often when the biter has blood in his or her mouth. There is likely some selection bias because biters usually do not present for medical care, whereas bite recipients seek care and medical follow-up. Although assessed case by case, postexposure prophylaxis (PEP) to prevent HIV transmission is not recommended routinely after a bite.[50]

Hepatitis B and hepatitis C viruses are present in blood and can be transmitted via bite; however, this also is rare.[52,53] The rate of transmission after a needlestick is estimated to be 6% to 30% for hepatitis B and 1.8% for hepatitis C[49]; the risk of transmission from a bite is substantially lower because there often is not significant blood exchange. The vaccination status of the bite victim is critical in assessing risk of hepatitis B transmission. Following a bite injury, PEP with a hepatitis B vaccination series, and in some cases the addition of hepatitis B immunoglobulin (HBIG) warrants consideration depending on the biter's hepatitis B infection status and victim's vaccination status.[54] If the biter is known to have acute hepatitis B (hepatitis B surface antigen positive), unvaccinated bite victims should receive the hepatitis B vaccine series and HBIG, wherease a previously vaccinated victim should receive 1 dose of the hepatitis B vaccine. If the hepatitis B status of the biter is unknown, an unvaccinated bite victim should receive the hepatitis B series, whereas vaccinated victims require no further intervention. Bites with this type of exposure also can prompt consideration of testing for seroconversion for hepatitis C, although this is not performed commonly.

Rodent Bites

Rodent bites are uncommon, although the exact incidence is not tracked nationally. Rodent oral flora is similar to that of other mammals, as described previously, and thus rodent bites can cause infections similar to those resulting from dog or cat bites. Additionally, 50% of wild rats carry the causative agents of rat-bite fever: *Streptobacillus moniliformis* in North America or *Spirillum minus* in Asia.[55] This systemic illness causes fever, arthralgias, headache, and rash and can be severe, with a 13% mortality rate if untreated.[55] These organisms are challenging to isolate in the clinical microbiology laboratory, complicating the ability to diagnose this infection. Approximately 50% of cases of rat-bite fever occur in children, although laboratory workers and pet shop owners also contract this infection.[55]

Nonhuman Primate Bites

The oral flora of nonhuman primates is similar to that of humans and thus bite injuries can cause similar types of infections to those of humans. Of important consideration are macaques, classified as Old World monkeys, although they have a broad geographic distribution. Macaques can carry herpesvirus B virus (B virus). Like other herpes viruses, B virus establishes a latent infection, and thus can be spread by blood and mucosal secretions of asymptomatic macaques. More frequently, however, B virus is spread by fluid from cutaneous vesicles or bodily fluids of sick animals. B virus can be transmitted to humans by bite or exposure to animal secretions, and most cases occur in people working with macaques in animal facilities. There also has been 1 case reported of human-to-human transmission via transmission of viral material from a skin lesion.[56] B virus infection causes flulike illness, rash, and a variety of central nervous system manifestations. Importantly, B virus poses a 40% to 80% mortality rate. Thus, prophylaxis with acyclovir or valacyclovir is recommended after certain exposures with macaques, and treatment with acyclovir or ganciclovir is recommended for documented disease.[57]

Insect Bites

There are a variety of systemic infections that can be spread by insects. Some of these cause local infections that then spread systemically, although most transmit bacteria, viruses, or parasites that cause systemic disease (**Table 1**). All can be prevented with methods that reduce the occurrence of bites, such as bed netting or insect repellent to reduce the number of bites and vector elimination with reduction of standing water or pesticides targeting the insect vector. Additionally, some of these diseases can be prevented with vaccines or prophylactic medication (see **Table 1**).

BITE WOUND MANAGEMENT
Evaluation, Irrigation, and Debridement

The initial evaluation of a patient who has sustained a bite injury includes a thorough history to document the species of animal, whether the animal was known to the victim or foreign (and for a foreign animal, whether it was domestic or wild), whether the immunization status of the animal is known, whether the incident was provoked, and the patient's comorbidities, immunization status, and history of medication allergies.

During the physical examination, bite injuries should be assessed carefully, noting the size and depth of the injury. For bites to the hand or over a joint, assessment of range of motion and examination for injury to the joint capsule, bone, or any nearby neurovascular structures or tendons should be completed. The objective of this evaluation is to assess the risk of septic arthritis, osteomyelitis, or tendonitis as well as need for surgical exploration, debridement, and repair of these structures. Diagnostic imaging should be considered for penetrating injuries, particularly to evaluate for joint or bone penetration or fracture or presence of foreign material. Microbiologic cultures generally should not be obtained from the site of an acute bite injury unless signs of infection are present on presentation.[4,25,58]

The surface of the bite injury should be cleansed, followed by copious irrigation with sterile saline. Puncture wounds should be irrigated gently, avoiding high-pressure irrigation.[27] In addition to cleansing the wound and decreasing the microbial burden, irrigation also allows for the removal of foreign material, which can include teeth fragments resulting from bites by older animals with poor dentition. Superficial devitalized tissue should also be debrided.[11]

Table 1
Infectious entities spread by insects

Insect Vector	Disease	Organism	Geographic Distribution	Prevention and Therapy
Mosquito - Anopheles	Malaria[68]	*Plasmodium falciparum* *Plasmodium vivax* *Plasmodium ovale* *Plasmodium malariae*	South and central America, sub-Saharan Africa, Middle east, Asia	Treatment: • Artemether-lumefantrine[a,b] • Atovaquone-proguanil • Mefloquine
Mosquito - Anopheles	Lymphatic filariasis[69]	*Wuchereria bancrofti* *Brugia spp*	South America, Caribbean, Africa, Asia	Varies by location/ co-infections • Diethylcarbamazine (DEC) • Vermectin • Albendazole
Mosquitos–Aedes	Zika	Zika virus (*Flavivirus*)	Africa, South America, Asia	Supportive care
Mosquitos -Aedes	Dengue	Dengue virus (*Flavivirus*)	Worldwide in tropics	Prevention: vaccine for people >9 months old • Supportive care • Avoid aspirin and non-steroidal anti-inflammatory drugs
Mosquitos -Aedes	Yellow fever	Yellow fever virus (*Flavivirus*)	South America, Africa	• Supportive care • Avoid aspirin and non-steroidal anti-inflammatory drugs
Mosquitos -Aedes	Chikungunya	Chickungunya virus (*Alphavirus*)	South America, Africa, Asia	• Supportive care
Mosquitos -Aedes	La Crosse (California encephalitis group)	La Crosse virus (*Bunyavirus*)	North America	• Supportive care
Mosquito-Culex	Eastern and Western equine encephalitis	Eastern and Western equine encephalitis virus (*Alphavirus*)	North America	• Supportive care
Mosquito-Culex	West Nile virus;	West Nile virus (*Flavivirus*);	Americas, Africa, Europe, Middle East, Asia	Supportive care
Tsetse fly	African sleeping sickness[70]	*Trypanosoma brucei* (*T. b. gambiense* *T. b. rhodesiense*)	Equatorial Africa	• Pentamidine[a] • Other medications available internationally or from Center for Disease Control and Prevention

(continued on next page)

Table 1
(continued)

Insect Vector	Disease	Organism	Geographic Distribution	Prevention and Therapy
Black fly	Onchocerciasis (river blindness)[71]	*Onchocerca volvulus*	South America, Middle East, Africa	• Ivermectin • Doxycycline
Sand fly	Leishmaniasis[72]	*Leishmania* spp	South and Central America, Middle East, Asia, Africa,	• Amphotericin[a] • Miltefosine • Paromomycin • Pentamidine • Azoles • Pentavalent antimony
Deerfly	Loiasis[73]	*Loa loa*	Central and West Africa	• diethylcarbamazine (DEC) - unless patient has a high microfilaria burden
Riduviid (kissing bug)	Chagas disease[74]	*Trypanosoma cruzi*	South and Central America, Southern USA	• Benznidazole • Nifurtimox
Tick–Ixodes	Babesiosis[75]	*Babesia microti*	North America	• Azithromycin-Atovaquone • Clindamycin-Quinine

Table 1
(continued)

Insect Vector	Disease	Organism	Geographic Distribution	Prevention and Therapy
Tick– *Ixodes*	Lyme disease	*Borrelia burgdorferi*	North America, Europe, Asia	• Amoxicillin • Cefuroxime • Doxycycline
Tick– *Ixodes*	Anaplasmosis	*Anaplasma phagocytophilum*	North America	• Doxycycline
Tick– *Ixodes*	Crimean-Congo hemorrhagic fever	Crimean-Congo hemorrhagic fever virus (*Nairovirus*)	Europe, Asia, Middle East, Africa	• Prevention: vaccine (not available in USA) • Supportive care
Tick– *Ixodes*	Powassan	Powassan virus (*Flavivirus*)	North America	• Supportive care
Tick– *Ixodes*	Kyasanur forest disease	Kyasanur forest disease virus (*Flavivirus*)	India	• Supportive care
Tick– *Ixodes*	Omsk hemorrhagic fever	Omsk hemorrhagic fever virus (*Flavivirus*)	Russia	• Supportive care
Tick– *Ixodes*	Tick-borne encephalitis	Tick-borne encephalitis virus (*Flavivirus*)	Europe	• Supportive care
Tick–*Amblyomma*	Ehrlichiosis	*Ehrlichia chaffeensis, ewingii, muris*	North America	• Doxycycline
Tick– *Amblyomma*	Southern tick–associated rash illness	Unknown	North America	• Doxycycline • (Amoxicillin)
Tick–*Dermacentor*	Rocky Mountain spotted fever	*Rickettsia rickettsii*	North America	• Doxycycline
Tick– *Dermacentor*	Colorado tick fever	Colorado tick fever virus (*Coltivirus*)	North America	• Supportive care
Tick–*Ornithodoros*	Tick-borne relapsing fever	*Borrelia* spp	North America	• Tetracyclines • Ceftriaxone • (Fluoroquinolones)
Tick		Bourbon virus (*Thogotovirus*)	USA (Midwest and South)	• Supportive care

(continued on next page)

Table 1
(continued)

Insect Vector	Disease	Organism	Geographic Distribution	Prevention and Therapy
Tick		Heartland virus (*Phlebovirus*)	USA (Midwest and South)	• Supportive care
Tick	African tick-bite fever	*Rickettsia africae*	Sub-Saharan Africa, Caribbean	• Doxycycline
Tick	Mediterranean spotted fever	*Rickettsia conorii*	Europe, Middle east, India, Africa	• Doxycycline
Tick	Queensland tick typhus	*Rickettsia australis*	Australia	• Doxycycline
Louse	Japanese spotted fever	*Rickettsia japonica*	Japan, Korea	• Doxycycline
Tick and deer fly	Tularemia	*F tularensis*	North America, Europe, Asia	• Aminoglycosides • Tetracyclines • (Fluoroquinolones)
Louse	Trench fever	*Bartonella quintana*	Areas with overcrowding	• Doxycycline and gentamicin
Louse	Louse-borne relapsing fever	*Borrelia recurrentis*	Northern Africa	• Doxycycline
Louse	Typhus	*Rickettsia prowazekii*	Areas with overcrowding	• Doxycycline • Tetracycline • Chloramphenicol
Flea	Murine typhus	*Rickettsia typhi*	Worldwide tropical/subtropical climates	• Doxycycline
Chigger	Scrub typhus	*Orientia tsutsugamushi*	Southeast Asia	• Doxycycline

Color coded by type of infection: pink for virus, purple for bacteria, blue for parasite.

[a] Approach depends on specific species and form/stage of disease.

[b] Approach varies by location infection acquired and local resistance pattern.

Information from Center for Disease Control and Prevention.[76]

Primary Wound Closure

There is limited evidence to guide the practice of bite wound closure after irrigation and debridement, and there is concern for increased risk of infection with primary closure. Bite injuries that occurred more than 24 hours prior to seeking medical attention and those that demonstrate signs of infection should not be closed. Additionally, due to the high risk for infection, puncture wounds and bites to the hand should not be closed. For the purposes of cosmesis, and, given the lower risk of infection, primary wound closure often is performed for bite injuries to the face.[4,30,59]

Considerations for Tetanus and Rabies Prophylaxis Following Animal Bites

Because tetanus potentially can be transmitted by cat and dog bites, the Advisory Committee on Immunization Practices recommends administering a tetanus toxoid–containing vaccine to patients sustaining an animal bite injury who have received less than 3 doses of a tetanus toxoid–containing vaccine. For patients who have received 3 or more prior doses of a tetanus toxoid–containing vaccine but have not been immunized against tetanus in the prior 5 years, a booster dose also is recommended. Tetanus immune globulin also should be administered to patients who have received less than 3 doses of a tetanus toxoid–containing vaccine and those with HIV infection or another severe immunocompromising condition (regardless of tetanus immunization history).[40,60]

After a bite from a rabid animal, cleansing the wound and administering PEP with rabies immunoglobulin and rabies vaccination can prevent rabies transmission. Considerations for rabies prophylaxis after an animal bite include whether the immunization status of the animal is known, whether the animal is available to be observed, and the local epidemiology. If the bite is from a domestic dog, cat, or ferret, the animal can be quarantined for 10 days and monitored for symptoms of rabies. If the animal remains well for the 10 days following the bite, there is no need for rabies PEP for the patient who was bitten.[61] For bites or exposures to other animals, the type of exposure and local rabies carriage among that species inform the need for rabies PEP, which should be made through consultation with local health officials.[61] Given the high risk for rabies carriage and transmission, rabies prophylaxis is indicated for patients who sustain bites from bats, foxes, raccoons, and skunks.[38]

Preemptive Antibiotic Therapy

Preemptive early antimicrobial therapy aims to decrease the bacterial burden and prevent contaminated bite wounds from progressing to symptomatic infection. Despite the frequency with which bites need medical attention, there is a paucity of data to inform evidence-based practice regarding preemptive antibiotic therapy; many published trials included small numbers of patients and did not employ antibiotic regimens that currently are considered standard of care.[62] Studies have demonstrated a lower incidence of infection when preemptive antibiotics were administered for high risk bites, although little benefit for lower-risk wounds. For example, in a randomized trial of patients sustaining human hand bite injuries, infection developed in 7 of 15 patients (46%) who received placebo, whereas none of the 33 patients who received oral or intravenous antibiotics developed infection.[63] In a placebo-controlled trial evaluating the effectiveness of amoxicillin-clavulanate after mammalian bites, among the subgroup of adults, subsequent infection occurred in 60% of patients receiving placebo and 33% of patients receiving amoxicillin-clavulanate; there was no statistically significant difference between treatment arms among children.[64] In this study, the benefit of preemptive antibiotic therapy was greatest for injuries presenting 9 hours to 24 hours after the bite compared with those presenting within the first 9 hours. In another small study, preemptive oxacillin administered to patients with uncomplicated cat bites resulted in a lower incidence of infection compared with placebo; 4 of 6 (66%) patients receiving placebo, but none of 5 patients treated with preemptive oxacillin, developed infection.[65] In another study, however, treatment with preemptive oxacillin administered to patients with uncomplicated dog bite injuries did not reduce the infection incidence compared with placebo.[66] Similarly, in another study of patients with uncomplicated human bites, preemptive antibiotics, compared with placebo, did not reduce the incidence of infection.[67]

Considerations for preemptive early antibiotic therapy following a bite injury include the type and extent of the injury, the location of the bite, and comorbidities of the patient (**Box 1**). High-risk bites include those with extensive edema or crush injury, because decreased blood flow can increase risk of infection. Wounds that have been closed surgically (commonly those on the face or genitals) also warrant prophylactic antibiotics because closure can increase risk of infection. In a prospective study of 87 pediatric patients with facial dog bite injuries, all patients underwent primary repair of the injury at the time of presentation and received concomitant antibiotics; none of these patients developed subsequent wound infections.[59] Bites sustained by asplenic or immunocompromised patients, as well as those with advanced liver disease, also should receive preemptive antibiotics to prevent infection. Lastly, puncture wounds (eg, from cat bites) and those on the hand or feet have higher risk of infection and complications; thus, prophylactic antibiotics are indicated.[2,30] Patients should be re-evaluated 48 hours after initial presentation to assess for worsening injury or developing infection.

Choice and Duration of Preemptive Antibiotic Therapy

A wide range of bacteria cause infections in bite wounds, as discussed previously, and these infections often are polymicrobial. Therefore, if preemptive antibiotics are warranted, therapy should target the most likely infecting organisms and include activity against both aerobes and anaerobes. Typically, a β-lactam/β-lactamase inhibitor combination, such as amoxicillin-clavulanate (or ampicillin-sulbactam, if intravenous therapy is indicated), is the first-line agent (**Box 2**). This provides broad activity against most streptococcal spp and staphylococcal spp (albeit not against methicillin-resistant S aureus). The β-lactamase inhibitor also provides broader gram-negative

---

Box 1
Scenarios for which antibiotics are indicated following a bite injury

- Bites resulting in moderate to severe injury, including crush injury
- Preexisting or resultant edema of the affected area
- Puncture wounds
- Bites to the face, hand, foot, or genitals
- Bites that may have penetrated the joint capsule, tendons, or bone
- Patients who are at increased risk of infection, including patients with:
  - Asplenia (anatomic or functional)
  - Immunocompromising conditions
  - Advanced liver disease
  - Implants (eg, artificial heart valves)
- Signs and symptoms of infection

Box 2
Suggested antibiotic therapy following animal and human bites

Animal bites
  Oral therapy
    Amoxicillin-clavulanate
    Trimethoprim-sulfamethoxazole plus clindamycin
    Doxycycline
    Ciprofloxacin or levofloxacin plus clindamycin or metronidazole
    Moxifloxacin
    Cefuroxime plus clindamycin or metronidazole
  Intravenous therapy
    Ampicillin-sulbactam
    Piperacillin-tazobactam
    Ertapenem
    Ceftriaxone plus clindamycin or metronidazole

Human bites
  Oral therapy
    Amoxicillin-clavulanate
    Doxycycline
    Ciprofloxacin or levofloxacin plus clindamycin or metronidazole
    Moxifloxacin
  Intravenous therapy
    Ampicillin-sulbactam
    Ertapenem

Data from Refs.[22,24,30]

---

and anaerobic coverage, which is important in the setting of polymicrobial contamination and possible infection. If the patient reports a β-lactam allergy, a combination of clindamycin and trimethoprim-sulfamethoxazole is the second-line therapy. This combination provides similar anti-streptococcal, anti-staphylococcal, and anti-anaerobic activity but less gram-negative activity. Both of the aforementioned regimens provide coverage for *P multocida*, which is of particular concern after animal bites. Importantly, first-generation cephalosporins and macrolides do not provide adequate activity against *Eikenella corrodens* and *P multocida* and thus should not be prescribed.[30]

There also is a paucity of data to inform duration of preemptive antibiotic treatment. The studies, discussed previously, evaluating the effectiveness of preemptive antibiotics to prevent symptomatic infection after a bite injury typically prescribed 5 days of therapy.[63,65,66] There recently has been a desire, however, to shorten antibiotic duration in an effort to reduce side effects, the risk of *C difficile* infection, development of antimicrobial resistance, impact on gut microbiota, and cost. In general, although there is some practice variation, 3 days to 5 days of therapy typically are recommended when preemptive antibiotic therapy is indicated.[30]

Treatment of Infections Resulting from Bite Wounds

If an infection does develop at the site of a bite injury, aerobic and anaerobic cultures should be obtained to identify the causative agent(s) and discern antibiotic susceptibilities. Empiric therapy should target the most common organisms causing bite wound infections, as described previously. Duration of therapy is dictated by the location and severity of infection. For localized infection (eg, cellulitis or skin abscess), 10 days to 14 days of therapy is recommended, whereas more extended courses are recommended for invasive infections. Specifically, patients with septic arthritis typically are treated with antibiotic therapy for 3 weeks, and those with osteomyelitis for 4 weeks to 6 weeks, depending on their clinical course and inflammatory markers.

SUMMARY

Prevention of injuries resulting from animal and human bites is a public health priority. Although skin and soft tissue infections are the most common entities, potential for systemic infection also should be considered, particularly in high-risk hosts with immunocompromising conditions who have sustained a bite injury. Although irrigation and debridement are the mainstay of therapy upon acute presentation, patients sustaining bite wounds posing high risk for subsequent infection generally should be prescribed preemptive antibiotic therapy with broad activity against aerobic and anaerobic bacteria. Well-designed and well-executed trials are needed to inform the clinical practice of preemptive antibiotic therapy and illuminate the optimal type of injury and patient populations for whom this practice should be employed.

CLINICS CARE POINTS

- Cat bites commonly result in puncture wounds and pose a high risk for subsequent infection.
- Irrigation and debridement are the mainstays of management for patients presenting with bite injuries.
- There is a paucity of data to inform the type of injury and patient for whom preemptive antibiotic therapy is most beneficial. Preemptive antibiotics are recommended for patients with immunocompromising comorbidities and those sustaining bites resulting in moderate to severe injury; puncture wounds; bites to the face, hand, foot, or genitals; or bites that may have penetrated the joint capsule, tendons, or bone.

DISCLOSURE

This work was supported in part by a grant from the Agency for Healthcare Research and Quality (R01-HS024269). The content is solely the responsibility of the authors and does not necessarily represent the official views of the Agency for Healthcare Research and Quality. The authors have nothing to disclose.

REFERENCES

1. Goldstein EJ. Bite wounds and infection. Clin Infect Dis 1992;14(3):633–40.
2. Jaindl M, Grunauer J, Platzer P, et al. The management of bite wounds in children–a retrospective analysis at a level I trauma centre. Injury 2012;43(12):2117–21.
3. Weiss HB, Friedman DI, Coben JH. Incidence of dog bite injuries treated in emergency departments. JAMA 1998;279(1):51–3.
4. Gurunluoglu R, Glasgow M, Arton J, et al. Retrospective analysis of facial dog bite injuries at a Level I trauma center in the Denver metro area. J Trauma Acute Care Surg 2014;76(5):1294–300.
5. Quinlan KP, Sacks JJ. Hospitalizations for dog bite injuries. JAMA 1999;281(3):232–3.
6. Sacks JJ, Kresnow M, Houston B. Dog bites: how big a problem? Inj Prev 1996;2(1):52–4.
7. Loder RT. The demographics of dog bites in the United States. Heliyon 2019;5(3):e01360.

8. Holmquist L, Elixhauser A. Emergency department visits and inpatient stays involving dog bites, 2008: statistical brief #101. healthcare cost and utilization project (HCUP) statistical briefs. Rockville (MD): 2006. Available at https://hcup-us.ahrq.gov/reports/statbriefs/sb101.pdf.

9. Holzer KJ, Vaughn MG, Murugan V. Dog bite injuries in the USA: prevalence, correlates and recent trends. Inj Prev 2019;25(3):187–90.

10. Centers for Disease C, Prevention. Nonfatal dog bite-related injuries treated in hospital emergency departments–United States, 2001. MMWR Morb Mortal Wkly Rep 2003;52(26):605–10.

11. Oehler RL, Velez AP, Mizrachi M, et al. Bite-related and septic syndromes caused by cats and dogs. Lancet Infect Dis 2009;9(7):439–47.

12. Tsokos M, Byard RW, Puschel K. Extensive and mutilating craniofacial trauma involving defleshing and decapitation: unusual features of fatal dog attacks in the young. Am J Forensic Med Pathol 2007;28(2):131–6.

13. Bini JK, Cohn SM, Acosta SM, et al. Mortality, mauling, and maiming by vicious dogs. Ann Surg 2011;253(4):791–7.

14. Sacks JJ, Sinclair L, Gilchrist J, et al. Breeds of dogs involved in fatal human attacks in the United States between 1979 and 1998. J Am Vet Med Assoc 2000; 217(6):836–40.

15. Langley RL. Human fatalities resulting from dog attacks in the United States, 1979-2005. Wilderness Environ Med 2009;20(1):19–25.

16. Santoro V, Smaldone G, Lozito P, et al. A forensic approach to fatal dog attacks. A case study and review of the literature. Forensic Sci Int 2011;206(1–3):e37–42.

17. Fonseca G, Mora E, Lucena J, et al. Forensic studies of dog attacks on humans: a focus on bite mark analysis. Res Rep Forensic Med Sci 2015;5:39–51.

18. Calkins CM, Bensard DD, Partrick DA, et al. Life-threatening dog attacks: a devastating combination of penetrating and blunt injuries. J Pediatr Surg 2001; 36(8):1115–7.

19. Sacks JJ, Lockwood R, Hornreich J, et al. Fatal dog attacks, 1989-1994. Pediatrics 1996;97(6 Pt 1):891–5.

20. Centers for Disease C, Prevention. Dog-bite-related fatalities–United States, 1995-1996. MMWR Morb Mortal Wkly Rep 1997;46(21):463–7.

21. Westling K, Farra A, Cars B, et al. Cat bite wound infections: a prospective clinical and microbiological study at three emergency wards in Stockholm, Sweden. J Infect 2006;53(6):403–7.

22. Talan DA, Citron DM, Abrahamian FM, et al. Bacteriologic analysis of infected dog and cat bites. Emergency medicine animal bite infection study group. N Engl J Med 1999;340(2):85–92.

23. Patrick GR, O'Rourke KM. Dog and cat bites: epidemiologic analyses suggest different prevention strategies. Public Health Rep 1998;113(3):252–7.

24. Talan DA, Abrahamian FM, Moran GJ, et al. Clinical presentation and bacteriologic analysis of infected human bites in patients presenting to emergency departments. Clin Infect Dis 2003;37(11):1481–9.

25. Patil PD, Panchabhai TS, Galwankar SC. Managing human bites. J Emerg Trauma Shock 2009;2(3):186–90.

26. Esposito S, Picciolli I, Semino M, et al. Dog and cat bite-associated infections in children. Eur J Clin Microbiol Infect Dis 2013;32(8):971–6.

27. Sartelli M, Guirao X, Hardcastle TC, et al. 2018 WSES/SIS-E consensus conference: recommendations for the management of skin and soft-tissue infections. World J Emerg Surg 2018;13:58.

28. Abrahamian FM, Goldstein EJ. Microbiology of animal bite wound infections. Clin Microbiol Rev 2011;24(2):231–46.
29. Dire DJ. Cat bite wounds: risk factors for infection. Ann Emerg Med 1991;20(9): 973–9.
30. Stevens DL, Bisno AL, Chambers HF, et al. Practice guidelines for the diagnosis and management of skin and soft tissue infections: 2014 update by the infectious diseases society of America. Clin Infect Dis 2014;59(2):147–59.
31. Giordano A, Dincman T, Clyburn BE, et al. Clinical features and outcomes of pasteurella multocida infection. Medicine 2015;94(36):e1285.
32. Weber DJ, Wolfson JS, Swartz MN, et al. Pasteurella multocida infections. Report of 34 cases and review of the literature. Medicine 1984;63(3):133–54.
33. Zajkowska J, Krol M, Falkowski D, et al. Capnocytophaga canimorsus - an underestimated danger after dog or cat bite - review of literature. Przegl Epidemiol 2016;70(2):289–95.
34. Lion C, Escande F, Burdin JC. Capnocytophaga canimorsus infections in human: review of the literature and cases report. Eur J Epidemiol 1996;12(5):521–33.
35. Pers C, Gahrn-Hansen B, Frederiksen W. Capnocytophaga canimorsus septicemia in Denmark, 1982-1995: review of 39 cases. Clin Infect Dis 1996; 23(1):71–5.
36. Centers for Disease Control and Prevention NCfEaZID. Questions and answers - human rabies due to organ transplantation 2013. Available at: https://www.cdc.gov/rabies/resources/news/2013-03-15.html. Accessed July 2020.
37. WHO. Rabies: epidemiology and burden of disease 2018. Available at: http://www.who.int/rabies/epidemiology/en/. Accessed July 2020.
38. Centers for Disease Control and Prevention NCfEaZID. Rabies in the U.S.: public health importance of rabies 2018. Available at: https://www.cdc.gov/rabies/location/usa/index.html. Accessed July 2020.
39. Centers for Disease Control and Prevention NCfEaZID. Other wild animals 2019. Available at: https://www.cdc.gov/rabies/exposure/animals/other.html. Accessed July 2020.
40. Liang JL, Tiwari T, Moro P, et al. Prevention of pertussis, tetanus, and diphtheria with vaccines in the United States: recommendations of the advisory committee on immunization practices (ACIP). MMWR Recomm Rep 2018;67(2):1–44.
41. Moynan D, O'Riordan R, O'Connor R, et al. Tetanus - a rare but real threat. IDCases 2018;12:16–7.
42. Radjou A, Hanifah M, Govindaraj V. Tetanus following dog bite. Indian J Community Med 2012;37(3):200–1.
43. Bedard BA, Kennedy BS, Weimer AC, et al. Leptospirosis and an animal bite. Ann Trop Med Public Health 2014;7(3):182–4.
44. Petersson E, Athlin S. Cat-bite-induced Francisella tularensis infection with a false-positive serological reaction for Bartonella quintana. JMM Case Rep 2017;4(2):e005071.
45. Westling K, Farra A, Jorup C, et al. Bartonella henselae antibodies after cat bite. Emerg Infect Dis 2008;14(12):1943–4.
46. Jacomo V, Kelly PJ, Raoult D. Natural history of Bartonella infections (an exception to Koch's postulate). Clin Diagn Lab Immunol 2002;9(1):8–18.
47. Nelson CA, Saha S, Mead PS. Cat-scratch disease in the United States, 2005-2013. Emerg Infect Dis 2016;22(10):1741–6.
48. Okaro U, Addisu A, Casanas B, et al. Bartonella species, an emerging cause of blood-culture-negative endocarditis. Clin Microbiol Rev 2017;30(3):709–46.

49. Centers for Disease Control and Prevention NCfID. Exposure to blood: what healthcare personnel need to know 2003. Available at: https://www.cdc.gov/hai/pdfs/bbp/exp_to_blood.pdf. Accessed July 2020.
50. Cresswell FV, Ellis J, Hartley J, et al. A systematic review of risk of HIV transmission through biting or spitting: implications for policy. HIV Med 2018;19(8): 532–40.
51. Bartholomew CF, Jones AM. Human bites: a rare risk factor for HIV transmission. AIDS 2006;20(4):631–2.
52. Dusheiko GM, Smith M, Scheuer PJ. Hepatitis C virus transmitted by human bite. Lancet 1990;336(8713):503–4.
53. MacQuarrie MB, Forghani B, Wolochow DA. Hepatitis B transmitted by a human bite. JAMA 1974;230(5):723–4.
54. Schillie S, Vellozzi C, Reingold A, et al. Prevention of hepatitis B virus infection in the United States: recommendations of the advisory committee on immunization practices. MMWR Recomm Rep 2018;67(1):1–31.
55. Elliott SP. Rat bite fever and Streptobacillus moniliformis. Clin Microbiol Rev 2007; 20(1):13–22.
56. Hilliard J. Monkey B virus. In: Arvin A, Campadelli-Fiume G, Mocarski E, et al, editors. Human herpesviruses: biology, therapy, and immunoprophylaxis. Cambridge (United Kingdom): 2007.
57. Cohen JI, Davenport DS, Stewart JA, et al. Recommendations for prevention of and therapy for exposure to B virus (cercopithecine herpesvirus 1). Clin Infect Dis 2002;35(10):1191–203.
58. Kennedy SA, Stoll LE, Lauder AS. Human and other mammalian bite injuries of the hand: evaluation and management. J Am Acad Orthop Surg 2015;23(1): 47–57.
59. Wu PS, Beres A, Tashjian DB, et al. Primary repair of facial dog bite injuries in children. Pediatr Emerg Care 2011;27(9):801–3.
60. Centers for Disease Control and Prevention NCfIaRD. Tetanus: for clinicians 2020. Available at: https://www.cdc.gov/tetanus/clinicians.html. Accessed July 2020.
61. Manning SE, Rupprecht CE, Fishbein D, et al. Human rabies prevention–United States, 2008: recommendations of the advisory committee on immunization practices. MMWR Recomm Rep 2008;57(RR-3):1–28.
62. Medeiros I, Saconato H. Antibiotic prophylaxis for mammalian bites. Cochrane Database Syst Rev 2001;(2):CD001738.
63. Zubowicz VN, Gravier M. Management of early human bites of the hand: a prospective randomized study. Plast Reconstr Surg 1991;88(1):111–4.
64. Brakenbury PH, Muwanga C. A comparative double blind study of amoxycillin/clavulanate vs placebo in the prevention of infection after animal bites. Arch Emerg Med 1989;6(4):251–6.
65. Elenbaas RM, McNabney WK, Robinson WA. Evaluation of prophylactic oxacillin in cat bite wounds. Ann Emerg Med 1984;13(3):155–7.
66. Elenbaas RM, McNabney WK, Robinson WA. Prophylactic oxacillin in dog bite wounds. Ann Emerg Med 1982;11(5):248–51.
67. Broder J, Jerrard D, Olshaker J, et al. Low risk of infection in selected human bites treated without antibiotics. Am J Emerg Med 2004;22(1):10–3.
68. Centers for Disease Control and Prevention GH. Treatment of malaria: guidelines for clinicians (United States) 2020. Available at: https://www.cdc.gov/malaria/resources/pdf/Malaria_Treatment_Guidelines.pdf. Accessed July 2020.

69. Centers for Disease Control and Prevention GH. Parasites - lymphatic filariasis: treatment 2018. Available at: https://www.cdc.gov/parasites/lymphaticfilariasis/treatment.html. Accessed July 2020.

70. Centers for Disease Control and Prevention GH. Parasites - African trypanosomiasis (also known as sleeping sickness): treatment 2020. Available at: https://www.cdc.gov/parasites/sleepingsickness/treatment.html. Accessed July 2020.

71. Prevention CfDCa. Parasites - onchocerciasis (also known as river blindness): treatment 2019. Available at: https://www.cdc.gov/parasites/onchocerciasis/treatment.html. Accessed July 2020.

72. Centers for Disease Control and Prevention GH. Parasites - leishmaniasis: treatment 2020. Available at: https://www.cdc.gov/parasites/leishmaniasis/treatment.html. Accessed July 2020.

73. Centers for Disease Control and Prevention GH. Parasites - loiasis: treatment 2015. Available at: https://www.cdc.gov/parasites/loiasis/treatment.html.

74. Centers for Disease Control and Prevention GH. Parasites - American trypanosomiasis (also known as chagas disease): treatment 2019. Available at: https://www.cdc.gov/parasites/chagas/treatment.html. Accessed July 2020.

75. Centers for Disease Control and Prevention GH. Parasites - babesiosis: treatment 2019. Available at: https://www.cdc.gov/parasites/babesiosis/treatment.html. Accessed July 2020.

76. Nabarro L, Morris-Jones S, Moore DAJ. Peters' Atlas of tropical medicine and parasitology. 7th edition. Elsevier; 2019.

Moving?

Make sure your subscription moves with you!

To notify us of your new address, find your **Clinics Account Number** (located on your mailing label above your name), and contact customer service at:

Email: journalscustomerservice-usa@elsevier.com

800-654-2452 (subscribers in the U.S. & Canada)
314-447-8871 (subscribers outside of the U.S. & Canada)

Fax number: 314-447-8029

Elsevier Health Sciences Division
Subscription Customer Service
3251 Riverport Lane
Maryland Heights, MO 63043

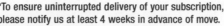

*To ensure uninterrupted delivery of your subscription, please notify us at least 4 weeks in advance of move.